KU-659-169

A CONSUMER'S GUIDE TO PRESCRIPTION MEDICINES

Dr Barrington Cooper and Dr Laurence Gerlis

With a Foreword by
T P Astill LLB, BPharmS, FRPharmS, FBIM
Director, National Pharmaceutical Association

● All commonly used medicines included ●
● All known side effects listed ●
● Key medical terms explained ●
● Easy-to-follow table of drug interactions ●

GUILD PUBLISHING
LONDON ▪ NEW YORK ▪ SYDNEY ▪ TORONTO

This edition published
1990 by Guild Publishing
by arrangement with
Hamlyn Publishing Group Limited,
Michelin House, 81 Fulham Road,
London SW3 6RB

© Charles Fowkes Ltd 1990

Edited, designed, and produced by Curtis Garratt Limited,
The Old Vicarage, Horton cum Studley, Oxford OX9 1BT

CN 8285

Preface

We have always felt that patient education is a vital part of the healing process in preventive and therapeutic medicine. Those patients who are best informed are also those for whom treatment is most likely to be successful.

The main purpose of this book is only to reinforce advice which a prescribing doctor has given already to a patient receiving that prescription. It confirms information about drug names and type, as well as the condition which is being treated.

As prescribing physicians, we have made conscious effort to provide information without, in any way, undermining the vitally important doctor-patient relationship. Thus, we have excluded injectable preparations and a small number of other sensitive areas of information. Our decision to use brand and generic names is not a statement of medical politics, but it is designed to help people who may have medication prescribed in either way. New European laws on product liability require a physician to explain possible side effects to patients, and this book will, to some extent, fulfil this role. Thus, *A Consumer's Guide to Prescription Medicines* should also be a valuable aid to doctors who are prescribing the medications listed.

Dr Barrington Cooper
Dr Laurence Gerlis
21 Devonshire Place
London W1

1989

In the introductory sections of this book, it has been emphasized that *A Consumer's Guide to Prescription Medicines* must **not** be used for self-prescription. Nor is it intended to be a substitute for the advice of a prescribing physician or the instructions on the medicine's package.

Every effort has been made to ensure that the information contained in the book is as accurate and up-to-date as possible at the time of going to press but medical and pharmaceutical knowledge continue to progress, and the use of a particular medicine may be different for every patient. **Always** consult your medical practitioner or other qualified medical specialist for advice.

The authors, editors, consultants, and publishers of this book can not be held liable for any errors or omissions, nor for any consequences of using it.

Foreword

It is no exaggeration to say that the last fifty years have seen a revolution in pharmacy and medicine. In the 'good old days', the family doctor would write a prescription which was usually in the form of a recipe and, quite deliberately, in semi-legible handwriting so that the patient could not read it — just in case the patient was able to decipher the writing, the names of the ingredients were in abbreviated Latin! The pharmacist would look at the prescription, nod sagely, and disappear out of sight behind his dispensary screen to make the pills or to mix the ingredients of the ointment or medicine. The name of the product never appeared on the label because everyone, including most patients, felt that it was undesirable for ordinary people to know what had been prescribed. It can now be revealed that what was in the bottle was probably innocuous and pharmacologically ineffective. The curative power of medicine in those days derived in large measure from the mystery and mystique which surrounded its preparation, coupled always with the doctor's bedside manner and confident reassurance.

Since then, there has been an enormous increase in scientific knowledge, especially of the way in which chemical substances affect the organs of the human body and of the way in which the body itself works. Antibiotics and other anti-infective agents have also been discovered, with the result that many hitherto fatal diseases have either disappeared altogether or can now be cured easily. Those who criticize the pharmaceutical industry forget too readily the former ravages of tuberculosis, polio, meningitis, septicaemia, typhoid fever, endocarditis, and other killing and crippling diseases. Many people suffering from asthma, epilepsy, hormone deficiency, or allergy can now lead a normal life whereas they would previously have been severely handicapped, confined to a wheelchair, or dead at an early age. Modern advances in surgery, such as organ transplants, have also been made possible by the drugs which control the body's natural tendency to reject 'invaders'.

Alongside this pharmaceutical revolution, there has also been a consumer revolution. Nowadays, you want to **know** what kind of drugs you are taking, and rightly so. While some people may regret the passing of the age of medicinal mystique, most of us prefer to be told precisely what is wrong with us and what is being provided to put us right. We want to know what effect the medicine is likely to have, what side effects might occur, and what precautions we need to take to ensure that the medicine behaves as it should. The modern medicine is certainly a powerful weapon for good, but its is also often complex in its chemistry and formulation. It is important, therefore, that patients are properly informed about their medicines, not only for their own peace of mind, but also so that the product gives them the maximum possible benefit with the minimum risk of harm.

For these reasons, I welcome warmly this new book by Dr Cooper and Dr Gerlis. In simple language it tells us what we need to know about our prescribed medicines. It reinforces and supplements what we have been told by our doctor and pharmacist; it will help us to understand why a particular medicine has been selected; and it tells us how it should be used. As the authors emphasize in their introduction, the book is **not** intended to be a substitute for professional advice. You should not hesitate to talk to your doctor or pharmacist if you are in serious doubt about any aspect of your treatment. But this book is a very usable source of reference and will fill reassuringly many gaps in our knowledge. It will help to remove those little apprehensions which many of us feel when we leave the surgery with the prescription and the pharmacy with our medicine.

T P Astill LLB, BPharmS, FRPharmS, FBIM
Director, National Pharmaceutical Association

How the book works

Apart from injectables and a small number of other medicines and appliances, all medicines which may be commonly prescribed through the National Health Service or private practice in the United Kingdom should be found in this book. They are arranged in strict alphabetical order throughout, with brand names, generic names, and any commonly used medical terms contained within the same sequence. There is also a chart to be found on page 719 which explains the way in which various drugs may interact with one another or with other substances such as alcohol. Some drugs are required to be prescribed by its generic, or scientific, name only and it is then up to the dispensing pharmacist to select a particular manufacturer's product. Other drugs are prescribed by a brand name. In this book, the main descriptions of any preparation are to be found under its commonly used brand name while the generic name will then cross refer to the main entry. In a small number of cases, where only a generic name exists, the main description will fall under that name.

Similarly, one particular medicine may be manufactured by more than one drug company under a variety of brand names. In such cases the authors have selected one preparation to be given the complete description, and then other preparations are, once again, cross-referred to the main entry. And, of course, the main entry also refers in its 'Other preparations' to any other manufacturers' version of the medicine. Thus, no matter what name has been used on the container of a medicine dispensed to a patient, it is a simple matter quickly to find a full description of the preparation.

The name of the medicine is given in bold type at the beginning of each entry, with the name of the manufacturing company in brackets on the next line. A short paragraph then follows describing the medicine in terms of its appearance, strength where this is relevant, what kind of drug it is — eg antacid, and what it is used to treat — eg dyspepsia. The usual dose or dose range is given for the particular uses of the medicine, including any variations that may be required to treat children, the elderly, or in any other special circumstances. The next section indicates whether the drug is available through the NHS, by private prescription, or over the counter without any prescription being needed. Any possible side effects that the medicine might produce are explained as well as any cautionary advice in its use. It is clearly stated if a medicine is not to be used for particular groups of patients, such as pregnant women, or to treat certain conditions or states. And any known interactions with other medicines or substances such as alcohol are also indicated. The components of the preparation are given in terms of their scientific names, and any other preparations of these components are also included at the end of the entry.

How to use this book (including how *not* to use it)

When a doctor prescribes a medicine for a patient, then he or she will always explain carefully to the patient how it is to be used. Similarly, the pharmacist will always write instructions for the drug's dose on the container, and the name of the drug will also be clearly visible. If you look up the name in *The Consumer's Guide to Prescription Medicines*, you will be able to confirm that you have understood the doctor's instructions fully so that you can be confident you are making the best possible use of the medicine. It will also help you to anticipate and prepare for any possible side effects, and ensure that you are not taking anything else which perhaps the doctor was not made aware of and which might interact with the prescription More importantly perhaps, the book will enable you to become better informed generally about the medicine(s) which has been prescribed to treat or prevent a particular condition.

A Consumer's Guide to Prescription Medicines is **not** a guide to self-prescription. Nor is it a 'home doctor'. The authors recognize clearly that it is the advice of the prescribing doctor, given after a careful investigation of the patient and his or her symptoms, which should always be followed by patients.If the information given in this book differs in any particular from the doctor's recommendations about a medicine, this must only be a basis for discussing such differences with the prescribing doctor or perhaps with the dispensing pharmacist.

The information contained in this book should not be followed in preference to the recommendations of the prescription even though it has been compiled by highly qualified physicians using the most up-to-date sources. There are few doctors or pharmacists who do not welcome well-informed questioning by their patients, and it is the purpose of this book to add to the information already given by the prescribing physician in the surgery and on the product's labelling. On the other hand, the authors have chosen not to include the names and addresses of the manufacturers of the drugs described because it is the policy of most drug companies not to respond directly to enquiries concerning their medicines from individual patients; generally, they will refer such enquiries back to the general practitioner.

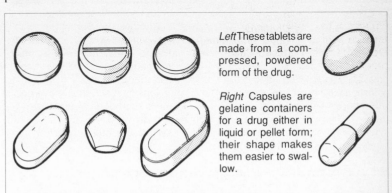

Left These tablets are made from a compressed, powdered form of the drug.

Right Capsules are gelatine containers for a drug either in liquid or pellet form; their shape makes them easier to swallow.

A selection of shapes and forms in which tablets, pills, and capsules may be supplied to help in their identification.

An annotated guide to understanding the entries

manufacturer's brand name or scientific name

manufacturer

general description including physical appearance, strength where appropriate, the type of drug, and the conditions it is used to treat

dose range, including any variations for children or the elderly (note: this is for guidance only and you should always follow the physician's advice)

Depixol
(Lundbeck)

A yellow tablet supplied at a strength of 3 mg and used as a sedative to treat schizophrenia and other mental disorders, especially withdrawal or apathy.

Dose: usually 1-3 tablets a day, up to a maximum of 6 tablets a day.

Availability: NHS and private prescription.

Side effects: muscle spasms, restlessness, hands shaking, dry mouth, urine retention, palpitations, low blood pressure, weight gain, changes in libido, low body temperature, breast swelling, menstrual changes, jaundice, blood and skin changes, drowsiness, rarely fits.

Caution: in pregnant women.

Not to be used for: children or for patients suffering from Parkinson's disease, severe hardening of the arteries, senility, advanced kidney, liver, or heart disease, or for very excitable or overactive patients, or for anyone who is intolerant of these drugs taken by mouth.

Not to be used with: alcohol, tranquillizers, pain killers, anti-hypertensives, anti-depressants, anti-convulsants, anti-diabetic drugs, LEVODOPA.

Contains: FLUPENTHIXOL DIHYDROCHLORIDE.

Other preparations: Depixol Injection, Depixol-Conc.

not all medicines are available through the National Health Service, while some are available over the counter without prescription

these are the most commonly noted side effects. In many cases, however, no side effects or only some will be experienced

circumstances where care should be exercised by certain groups of patients or those taking other medicines

any groups of patients who should **not** take this medicine

the active ingredients of the medicine

these are substances, such as alcohol or foods, or other drugs, with which this medicine should not be taken

this lists other forms of the same medicine, or equivalent drugs from a different manufacturer.

(note: CAPITALS indicate a separate entry in the book)

AAA Spray
(Rorer)

An aerosol used as an antibacterial and local anaesthetic to treat sore throat, minor infections of the nose and throat.

Dose: 2 sprays every 2-3 hours up to a maximum of 16 sprays in 24 hours; children over 6 years half adult dose.
Availability: NHS, private prescription, over the counter.
Side effects:
Caution:
Not to be used for: children under 6 years.
Not to be used with:
Contains: BENZOCAINE, CETALKONIUM CHLORIDE.
Other preparations:

Abidec
(Warner-Lambert)

Drops used as a multivitamin preparation to treat vitamin deficiencies.

Dose: adults and children over 1 year 0.6 ml a day; infants under 1 year half adult dose.
Availability: NHS, private prescription, over the counter.
Side effects:
Caution:
Not to be used for:
Not to be used with: LEVODOPA.
Contains: CALCIFEROL, THIAMINE HYDROCHLORIDE, RIBOFLAVINE, PYRIDOXINE HYDROCHLORIDE, NICOTINAMIDE, ASCORBIC ACID.
Other preparations: Abidec Capsules (not available on NHS).

ACE inhibitor (angiotension converting enzyme inhibitor)

a drug which blocks the production of water-retaining hormones and thus functions as a DIURETIC. Example captopril *see* CAPOTEN.

---

acebutolol *see* Secadrex, Sectral

Acepril *see* **Capoten**
(Duncan, Flockhart)

---

acetazolamide see Diamox, Diamox Sustets

---

acetic acid *see* **Aci-Jel, Phytex**

---

acetohexamide *see* **Dimelor**

---

acetomenaphthone *see* **Ketovite**

Acetoxyl
(Stiefel)

A gel used as an anti-bacterial and skin softener to treat acne.

Dose: wash and dry the affected area and apply the gel once a day.
Availability: NHS, private prescription, over the counter.
Side effects: irritation, peeling.
Caution: keep out of the eyes, nose, and mouth; children should use the weaker gel.
Not to be used for:
Not to be used with:
Contains: BENZOYL PEROXIDE.
Other preparations:

---

acetylcysteine *see* **Fabrol, Ilube, Parvolex**

Acezide *see* **Capozide**
(Duncan, Flockhart)

Achromycin
(Lederle)

An ointment, tablets, and syrup used as an antibiotic to treat outer ear, eye, or skin infections.

Dose: apply every 2 hours, or once a day or as needed for skin infections. Achromycin tablets for general infections 250-500 mg 4 times a day.
Availability: NHS and private prescription.
Side effects: additional infection.
Caution: in patients suffering from liver or kidney failure, perforated ear drum.
Not to be used for: children or pregnant women.
Not to be used with: milk, antacids, minerals, contraceptive pill.
Contains: TETRACYCLINE hydrochloride.
Other preparations: Achromycin Ophthalmic Oil Suspension.

Aci-Jel
(Cilag)

A jelly with applicator used as an antiseptic to treat non-specific vaginal infection.

Dose: 1 application into the vagina twice a day.
Availability: NHS and over the counter.
Side effects: irritation and inflammation.
Caution:
Not to be used for: children.
Not to be used with:
Contains: ACETIC ACID.
Other preparations:

---

acipimox *see* Olbetam

Acnegel
(Stiefel)

A gel used as an anti-bacterial and skin softener to treat acne.

Dose: wash and dry the affected area and apply the gel once a day.
Availability: NHS, private prescription, over the counter.
Side effects: irritation, peeling.
Caution: keep out of the eyes, nose, mouth.
Not to be used for:
Not to be used with:
Contains: BENZOYL PEROXIDE.
Other preparations: Acnegel Forte.

Acnidazil
(Janssen)

A cream used as an anti-bacterial and skin softener to treat acne.

Dose: wash and dry the affected area, and apply the cream once a day
for the first week, then twice a day for the next 4-8 weeks.
Availability: NHS, private prescription, over the counter.
Side effects: irritation, peeling.
Caution: keep out of the eyes, nose, mouth.
Not to be used for:
Not to be used with:
Contains: MICONAZOLE NITRATE, BENZOYL PEROXIDE.
Other preparations:

---

acrivastine *see* Semprex

---

acrosoxacin *see* Eradacin

Actal
(Winthrop)

A white tablet supplied at a strength of 360 mg and used as an antacid
to treat indigestion, dyspepsia.

Dose: 1-2 tablets when needed.
Availability: NHS (generic only), private prescription, and over the
counter.

Side effects: few; sodium overload is possible.
Caution:
Not to be used for: children.
Not to be used with: TETRACYCLINE antibiotics.
Contains: ALEXITOL SODIUM.
Other preparations: Actal Suspension.

Actidil
(Wellcome)

A white, scored tablet supplied a strength of 2.5 mg and used as an antihistamine to treat allergies.

Dose: adults 1-2 tablets 3 times a day; children use elixir.
Availability: NHS, private prescription, over the counter.
Side effects: drowsiness, reduced reactions, rarely skin eruptions.
Caution: in patients suffering from liver or kidney disease.
Not to be used for:
Not to be used with: alcohol, sedatives, some anti-depressants (MAOIS).
Contains: TRIPROLIDINE hydrochloride.
Other preparations: Actidil Elixir.

Actifed Compound
(Wellcome)

A linctus used as an antihistamine to treat cough, congestion.

Dose: adults 2 5 ml teaspoonsful 3 times a day; children 2-5 years $^1/_2$ teaspoonful 3 times a day, 6-12 years 1 teaspoonful 3 times a day.
Availability: private prescription and over the counter.
Side effects: drowsiness, reduced reactions.
Caution: in patients suffering from liver or kidney disease.
Not to be used for: children under 2 years.
Not to be used with: alcohol, sedatives, some anti-depressants (MAOIS).
Contains: TRIPROLIDINE hydrochloride, PSEUDOEPHEDRINE hydrochloride, DEXTROMETHORPHAN hydrobromide.
Other preparations: Actifed Expectorant, Actifed Tablets, Actifed Syrup.

Actinac
(Roussel)

A lotion used as an anti-bacterial, corticosteroid, and skin softener to treat acne and associated disorders.

Dose: apply to the affected area night and morning for 4 days, then at night only for 3 weeks after the spots have gone.
Availability: NHS and private prescription.
Side effects: severe reddening of the skin.
Caution: in pregnant women.
Not to be used for:
Not to be used with:
Contains: CHLORAMPHENICOL, HYDROCORTISONE acetate, BUTOXYETHYL NICOTINATE, ALLANTOIN, precipitated SULPHUR.
Other preparations:

Actonorm
(Wallace)

A white liquid supplied in 200 ml bottles and used as an antacid to treat indigestion, wind.

Dose: adults 5-20 ml after meals.
Availability: over the counter and private presecription.
Side effects: few; occasionally constipation or diarrhoea.
Caution:
Not to be used for: children.
Not to be used with: TETRACYCLINE antibiotics.
Contains: ALUMINIUM HYDROXIDE, MAGNESIUM HYDROXIDE, activated DIMETH-ICONE.
Other preparations:

Acupan
(3M Riker)

A white tablet supplied at a strength of 30 mg and used as an analgesic to relieve pain.

Dose: 1-3 tablets 3 times a day.
Availability: NHS and private prescription.

Side effects: nausea, nervousness, dry mouth, dizziness.
Caution: in patients suffering from kidney or liver disease.
Not to be used for: patients with a history of convulsions or patients suffering from heart attack.
Not to be used with: MAOIS, ANTI-CHOLINERGICS, SYMPATHOMIMETICS, TRI-CYCLICS.
Contains: NEFOPAM hydrochloride.
Other preparations: Acupan Injection.

---

acyclovir *see* Zovirax, Zovirax Ointment

Adalat
(Bayer)

An orange, liquid-filled capsule supplied at strengths of 5 mg, 10 mg and used as an anti-anginal treatment for angina, Raynaud's phenomenon.

Dose: 10 mg twice a day at first, then according to response up to 60 mg a day with or after food. For Raynaud's phenomenon 10 mg 3 times a day with food or after meals.
Availability: NHS and private prescription.
Side effects: headache, flushes, fluid retention, dizziness, chest pain, rarely jaundice, gum swelling.
Caution: in patients with weak hearts, liver disease, or low blood pressure.
Not to be used for: children, pregnant women, or patients suffering from severe low blood pressure.
Not to be used with: anti-hypertensives, CIMETIDINE, QUINIDINE.
Contains: NIFEDIPINE.
Other preparations: ADALAT RETARD (Bayer), BETA ADALAT (Bayer).

Adalat Retard
(Bayer)

A pink/grey tablet supplied at strengths of 10 mg, 20 mg and used as an anti-hypertensive to treat high blood pressure.

Dose: 20 mg twice a day at first, adjust to 10-40 mg twice a day according to response.
Availability: NHS and private prescription.
Side effects: headache, flushes, fluid retention, dizziness,chest pain,gum swelling, rarely jaundice.
Caution: in patients with weak heart or liver disease.
Not to be used for: children, pregnant women, or for patients suffering from severe low blood pressure.
Not to be used with: other anti-hypertensives, CIMETIDINE, QUINIDINE.
Contains: NIFEDIPINE.
Other preparations: ADALAT (Bayer), BETA ADALAT (Bayer).

Adcortyl
(Squibb)

A cream used as a steroid treatment for dermatitis, psoriasis, external ear infections, sunburn, insect bites and stings.

Dose: apply to the affected area 2-4 times a day.
Availability: NHS and private prescription.
Side effects: fluid retention, suppression of adrenal glands, thinning of the skin may occur.
Caution: use for short periods of time only.
Not to be used for: patients suffering from acne or any other skin infections caused by tuberculosis, ringworm, viruses, or fungi, or continuously especially in pregnant women.
Not to be used with:
Contains: TRIAMCINOLONE ACETONIDE.
Other preparations: Adcortyl Ointment.

Adcortyl in Orabase
(Squibb)

A paste used as a corticosteroid treatment for mouth ulcers, mouth infections, gingivitis, lesions.

Dose: apply the paste to the affected area 2-3 times a day without rubbing in.
Availability: NHS and private prescription.
Side effects:

Caution: in pregnant women. Do not use for infants over extended periods.
Not to be used for: patients suffering from untreated mouth infections.
Not to be used with:
Contains: TRIAMCINOLONE ACETONIDE.
Other preparations:

adrenal glands

the adrenal glands are organs situated above the kidneys which produce hormones, including steroids.

adrenaline *see* Brovon, Epifrin, Epinal, Eppy, Ganda, Medihaler-EPI, Rybarvin, Simplene

Aerolin Auto *see* Ventolin
(3M Riker)

Afrazine
(Kirby-Warrick)

A spray or nasal drops used as a SYMPATHOMIMETIC treatment for blocked nose.

Dose: adults and children over 5 years 2-3 sprays or drops in each nostril 2-3 times a day; children under 5 years use paediatric drops.
Availability: private prescription and over the counter.
Side effects: itching nose, headache, sleeplessness, rapid heart rate.
Caution: in patients suffering from overactive thyroid gland, diabetes, coronary disease. Do not use for extended periods.
Not to be used for:
Not to be used with: MAOIS.
Contains: OXYMETAZOLINE HYDROCHLORIDE.
Other preparations: Afrazine Paediatric.

Agarol
(Warner-Lambert)

An emulsion used as a lubricant and stimulant to treat constipation.

Dose: children 5-12 years 5 ml at bedtime, adults 5-15 ml at bedtime.
Availability: private prescription and over the counter.
Side effects: allergies to PHENOLPHTHALEIN, blood or protein in the urine.
Caution:
Not to be used for: children under 5 years.
Not to be used with:
Contains: LIQUID PARAFFIN, PHENOLPHTHALEIN, AGAR.
Other preparations:

Akineton
(Abbott)

A white, scored tablet supplied at a strength of 2 mg and used as an ANTI-CHOLINERGIC to treat Parkinson's disease.

Dose: 1/2 tablet twice a day at first, then increasing to a tablet 3 times a day, increasing again and then reducing.
Availability: NHS and private prescription.
Side effects: drowsiness, dry mouth, blurred vision.
Caution: in patients suffering from abnormal heart rhythm or heart attack.
Not to be used for: children or patients suffering from gastro-intestinal obstruction, glaucoma.
Not to be used with:
Contains: BIPERIDEN HYDROCHLORIDE.
Other preparations: Akineton Injection.

Albucid
(Nicholas)

Drops used as a sulphonamide antibiotic to treat eye infections.

Dose: 2-4 drops into the eye every 2-6 hours.
Availability: NHS and private prescription.
Side effects: temporary irritation.
Caution:
Not to be used for:
Not to be used with:
Contains: SODIUM SULPHACETAMIDE.
Other preparations: Albucid Ointment.

---

alclometasone diproprionate *see* Modrasone

---

alcohol *see* Glykola, Labiton, Verdiviton

Alcopar
(Wellcome)

Dispersible granules in a sachet of 2.5 g and used as an anti-worm treatment for worms.

Dose: adults and children over 2 years 1 sachet dispersed in water; children under 2 years half adult dose.
Availability: NHS, private prescription, over the counter.
Side effects: stomach upset.
Caution:
Not to be used for: patients who are continuously vomiting.
Not to be used with:
Contains: BEPHENIUM HYDROXY-NAPHTHOATE.
Other preparations:

Alcos-Anal
(Norgine)

An ointment used as a soothing antiseptic to treat haemorrhoids, anal itch.

Dose: apply night and morning after passing motions.

Availability: NHS and private prescription.
Side effects:
Caution:
Not to be used for:
Not to be used with:
Contains: SODIUM OLEATE, CHOROTHYMOL, LAURETH.
Other preparations:

Aldactide 50
(Gold Cross)

A buff tablet supplied at a strength of 50 mg and used as a DIURETIC to treat congestive heart failure.

Dose: adults 4 tablets a day; children 1.5-3 mg per kg bodyweight a day in divided doses.
Availability: NHS and private prescription.
Side effects: breast enlargement, stomach upset, drowsiness, rash, sensitivity to light, blood changes.
Caution: in pregnant women, young patients, and in patients suffering from liver or kidney disease, gout, or diabetes. Your doctor may advise regular blood tests.
Not to be used for: nursing mothers or for patients suffering from severe kidney failure, progressive kidney failure, raised potassium levels.
Not to be used with: potassium supplements, lithium, DIGITALIS, CARBENOXOLONE, anti-hypertensives, ACE INHIBITORS.
Contains: SPIRONOLACTONE, HYDROFLUMETHIAZIDE.
Other preparations: Aldactide 25.

Aldactone
(Searle)

A buff tablet or a white tablet according to strengths of 25 mg, 50 mg, 100 mg and used as a DIURETIC to treat congestive heart failure, cirrhosis of the liver, fluid retention.

Dose: adults congestive heart failure 100 mg a day increasing to 400 mg a day, then 75-200 mg a day with food; children 3 mg per kg bodyweight a day in divided doses. For other conditions as advised by physician.

Availability: NHS and private prescription.
Side effects: breast enlargement, stomach upset, rash, drowsiness, headache, confusion.
Caution: in pregnant women or young patients, and in patients suffering from kidney or liver disease. Your doctor may advise regular blood tests.
Not to be used for: nursing mothers or for patients suffering from kidney failure or raised potassium levels.
Not to be used with: potassium supplements, CARBENOXOLONE.
Contains: SPIRONOLACTONE.
Other preparations: LARACTONE (Lagap), SPIRETIC (DDSA), SPIROLONE (Berk).

Aldomet
(MSD)

A yellow tablet supplied at strengths of 125 mg, 250 mg, 500 mg and used as an anti-hypertensive to treat high blood pressure.

Dose: adults 250 mg 2-3 times a day at first, adjust to a maximum of 3 g a day at 2-day intervals; children 10 mg per kg bodyweight a day at first in 2-4 divided doses.
Availability: NHS and private prescription.
Side effects: sleepiness, headache, weakness, depression, slow heart rate, congestion of the nose, dry mouth, stomach upset, jaundice, blood changes.
Caution: in patients suffering from certain types of anaemia, history of liver disease, kidney disease, or patients undergoing anaesthesia. Your doctor may advise regular blood tests.
Not to be used for: patients suffering from liver disease, depression, phaeochromocytoma (a disease of the adrenal glands).
Not to be used with: TRICYCLICS, MAOIS, other anti-hypertensives.
Contains: METHLYDOPA.
Other preparations: DOPAMET (Berk), MEDOMET (DDSA).

---

alexitol sodium *see* Actal, Droxalin

---

alfacalcidol *see* One-Alpha

Algesal
(Duphar)

A cream used as an analgesic rub to treat rheumatic conditions.

Dose: massage into the affected area 3 times a day.
Availability: NHS, private prescription, over the counter.
Side effects:
Caution:
Not to be used for: children under 6 years.
Not to be used with:
Contains: DIETHYLAMINE SALICYLATE.
Other preparations:

Algicon
(Rorer)

A white tablet used as an antacid to treat heartburn, hiatus hernia, indigestion.

Dose: adults 1-2 tablets 4 times a day after meals and at night.
Availability: NHS, private prescription, and over the counter.
Side effects: few; constipation or diarrhoea.
Caution: diabetes owing to sucrose content.
Not to be used for: children, or in kidney failure or severe debilitation.
Not to be used with: TETRACYCLINE antibiotics.
Contains: MAGNESIUM ALGINATE, ALUMINIUM HYDROXIDE/MAGNESIUM CARBONATE, MAGNESIUM CARBONATE, POTASSIUM BICARBONATE.
Other preparations: Algicon Suspension.

alginic acid *see* Gastrocote, Gastron, Topal

Algitec *see* Tagamet
(S K B)

allantoin *see* Actinac, Alphosyl, Alphosyl HC

Allbee with C
(Robins)

A green/yellow capsule used as a multivitamin treatment for vitamin B and vitamin C deficiencies.

Dose: adults 1-3 capsules a day; children 1 capsule a day.
Availability: private prescription and over the counter.
Side effects:
Caution:
Not to be used for:
Not to be used with: LEVODOPA.
Contains: THIAMINE mononitrate, RIBOFLAVINE, PYRIDOXINE hydrochloride, NICOTINAMIDE, CALCIUM PANTOTHENATE, ASCORBIC ACID.
Other preparations:

Allegron
(Dista)

A white tablet or an orange, scored tablet according to strengths of 10 mg, 25 mg and used as an anti-depressant to treat depression, bedwetting in children.

Dose: adults 20-40 mg a day at first in divided doses increasing to up to 100 mg a day as needed and then reducing to 30-75 mg a day; elderly 10 mg 3 times a day at first; children over 6 years 10-30 mg half an hour before bed time. Reduced doses in the elderly.
Availability: NHS and private prescription.
Side effects: dry mouth, constipation, urine retention, blurred vision, palpitations, drowsiness, sleeplessness, dizziness, hands shaking, low blood presure, weight change, skin reactions, jaundice or blood changes. Loss of sexual desire may occur.
Caution: in nursing mothers or in patients suffering from heart disease, thyroid disease, epilepsy, diabetes, some other psychiatric conditions. Your doctor may advise regular blood tests.
Not to be used for: children under 6 years, pregnant women, or for patients suffering from heart attacks, liver disease, heart block.
Not to be used with: alcohol, ANTI-CHOLINERGICS, adrenaline, MAOIS, barbiturates, other anti-depressants, anti-hypertensives.
Contains: NORTRYPTILINE HYDROCHLORIDE.
Other preparations:

---

allopurinol *see* **Zyloric**

---

allyloestrenol *see* **Gestanin**

---

almasilate *see* **Malinal**

Almazine *see* **Ativan**
(Steinhard)

Almodan *see* **Amoxil**
(Berk)

---

aloin *see* **Alophen**

Alophen
(Warner-Lambert)

A brown pill used as a stimulant and ANTI-CHOLINERGIC to treat constipation.

Dose: adults 1-3 pills at bedtime.
Availability: over the counter and private prescription.
Side effects: allergy to PHENOLPHTHALEIN, skin rash, protein in the urine.
Caution:
Not to be used for: children or for patients suffering from glaucoma or inflammatory bowel disease.
Not to be used with:
Contains: ALOIN, PHENOLPHTHALEIN, IPECACUANHA, BELLADONNA EXTRACT.
Other preparations:

Aloral *see* **Zyloric**
(Lagap)

---

aloxiprin *see* **Palaprin Forte**

---

alpha-beta-pinenes *see* **Rowachol**

Alphaderm
(Norwich Eaton)

A cream used as a steroid and wetting agent to treat eczema, dermatitis.

Dose: wash and dry the affected area, and apply twice a day.
Availability: NHS and private prescription.
Side effects: fluid retention, suppression of adrenal glands. Thinning of the skin may occur.
Caution: use for short periods of time only.
Not to be used for: patients suffering from acne or any other skin infections caused by tuberculosis, ringworm, viruses, or fungi, or continuously especially in pregnant women.
Not to be used with:
Contains: HYDROCORTISONE, UREA.
Other preparations:

Alphosyl
(Stafford-Miller)
A cream used as an anti-psoriatic to treat psoriasis.
Dose: massage thoroughly into the affected area 2-4 times a day.
Availability: NHS, private prescription, over the counter.
Side effects: irritation, sensitivity to light.
Caution:
Not to be used for: patients suffering from acute psoriasis.
Not to be used with:
Contains: COAL TAR EXTRACT, ALLANTOIN.
Other preparations: Alphosyl Lotion, Alphosyl Shampoo.

Alphosyl HC
(Stafford-Miller)

A cream used as an anti-psoriatic and steroid treatment for psoriasis.

Dose: apply to the affected area 2-4 times a day.
Availability: NHS and private prescription.
Side effects: thinning of the skin, fluid retention, suppression of adrenal glands.
Caution: in pregnant women, and in patients on extended treatment — withdraw gradually.
Not to be used for: patients suffering from acne or other skin infections unless otherwise directed, or continuously especially in pregnancy.
Not to be used with:
Contains: COAL TAR EXTRACT, ALLANTOIN, HYDROCORTISONE.
Other preparations:

---

alprazolam *see* Xanax

Alrheumat *see* Orudis
(Bayer)

Altacite Plus
(Roussel)
A white liquid supplied in a 500 ml bottle and used as an antacid and anti-wind preparation to treat wind, indigestion, dyspepsia, and gastric ulcers.
Dose: adults 10 ml between meals and at bedtime; children 8-12 years half adult dose.
Availability: NHS, private prescription, over the counter.
Side effects: few; occasional diarrhoea and constipation.
Caution:
Not to be used for: children under 8 years.
Not to be used with: TETRACYCLINE antibiotics.
Contains: HYDROTALCITE, activated DIMETHICONE.
Other preparations: higher-strength suspension and tablets (some preparations are not available on NHS).

Alu-Cap
(3M-Riker)

A green/red capsule supplied at a strength of 475 mg and used as an antacid to treat hyperacidity.

Dose: adults 1 tablet 4 times a day and at bedtime.
Availability: over the counter and private prescription.
Side effects: few; occasional bowel disorders such as constipation.
Caution:
Not to be used for: children.
Not to be used with: TETRACYCLINE antibiotics.
Contains: ALUMINIUM HYDROXIDE GEL.
Other preparations:

Aludrox
(Wyeth)

A white gel supplied in a 200-500 ml bottle and used as an antacid to treat dyspepsia, hyperacidity.

Dose: 5-10 ml four times a day and at bedtime.
Availability: NHS (when described as a generic) and private prescription.
Side effects: few; occasionally constipation.
Caution:
Not to be used for: infants.
Not to be used with: TETRACYCLINE antibiotics.
Contains: ALUMINIUM HYDROXIDE GEL.
Other preparations: tablets and other combination preparations including Aludrox SA.

Aluhyde
(Sinclair)

A white, scored tablet used as an antispasmodic and antacid to treat hyperacidity and intestinal spasm.

Dose: 2 tablets after meals.
Availability: over the counter and private prescription.
Side effects: occasionally constipation and blurred vision.

Caution: in patients suffering from prostate enlargement.
Not to be used for: children or for patients suffering from glaucoma.
Not to be used with: TETRACYCLINE antibiotics.
Contains: ALUMINIUM HYDROXIDE GEL, MAGNESIUM TRISILICATE, BELLADONNA liquid extract.
Other preparations:

Aluline *see* **Zyloric**
(Stenhard)

---

aluminium acetate *see* **Xyloproct**

---

aluminium chlorhydroxide *see* **Medrone Lotion, Neo-Medrone Lotion**

---

aluminium hydroxide gel *see* **Alu-Cap, Aludrox, Aluhyde, Asilone, Diovol, Theodrox**

---

aluminium hydroxide *see* **Actonorm, APP, Caved-S, Gastrocote, Gastron, Genusil, Kolanticon, Loasid, Maalox, Mucaine, Polyalk, Topal,**

---

aluminium hydroxide/magnesium carbonate *see* **Algicon, Andursil**

---

aluminium oxide *see* **Andursil, Brasivol**

Alupent
(Boehringer Ingelheim)

An off-white, scored tablet supplied at a strength of 20 mg and used as an anti-asthma drug to treat bronchial spasm brought on by chronic bronchitis, asthma, emphysema.

Dose: adults 1 tablet 4 times a day; children use syrup.
Availability: NHS and private prescription.
Side effects: abnormal heart rhythm, heart tremor, nervous tension, headache, dilation of the veins, rapid heart rate.
Caution: in diabetics and patients suffering from high blood pressure.
Not to be used for: patients suffering from cardiac asthma, acute heart disease, overactive thyroid gland.
Not to be used with: MAOIS, TRICYCLICS, SYMPATHOMIMETICS.
Contains: ORCIPRENALINE SULPHATE.
Other preparations: Alupent Syrup, Alupent Aerosol.

Alupram *see* Valium
(Steinhard)

Aluzine *see* Lasix
(Steinhard)

alverine citrate *see* Spasmonal

amantadine *see* Symmetrel

Ambaxin
(Upjohn)

An off-white, oblong, scored tablet supplied at a strength of 400 mg and used as a broad-spectrum penicillin to treat respiratory, ear, nose, and throat, skin, and soft tissue infections.

Dose: adults 1-2 tablets 2-3 times a day; children over 5 years $^1/_2$ tablet 3 times a day.
Availability: NHS and private prescription.
Side effects: allergy, stomach disturbances.
Caution: in patients suffering from kidney disease, severe liver disease, glandular fever.
Not to be used for: children under 5 years.
Not to be used with:
Contains: BACAMPICILLIN hydrochloride.
Other preparations:

---

ambucetamide *see* **Femerital**

Amilco *see* **Amiloride**
(Norton)

Amiloride
(Morson)
A yellow, diamond-shaped tablet supplied at a strength of 5 mg and used as a potassium-sparing DIURETIC to maintain potassium level when used with other diuretics.
Dose: 1-2 tablets a day at first, then up to 4 tablets a day if needed.
Availability: NHS and private prescription.
Side effects: stomach upset, rash.
Caution: in pregnant women or nursing mothers and in patients suffering from diabetes with a predisposition to high potassium levels, gout, liver or kidney disease. Your doctor may advise blood tests for potassium levels.
Not to be used for: children or for patients suffering from high potassium levels or progressive kidney failure.
Not to be used with: potassium supplements, potassium-sparing diuretics, ACE INHIBITORS.
Contains: AMILORIDE hydrochloride.
Other preparations: AMILCO (Norton), BERKAMIL (Berk).

---

amiloride *see* Amiloride, Frumil, Hypertane, Kalten, Lasoride, Moducren, Normetic

---

aminoglutethimide *see* Orimeten

---

aminophylline *see* Phyllocontin Continus, Theodrox

---

amiodarone *see* Cordarone X

---

amitryptiline *see* Domical, Lentizol, Limbitrol 5, Triptafen,
Tryptizol

---

ammonium chloride *see* Benylin Expectorant, Guanor,
Histalix

---

amodiaquine *see* Camoquin

---

amoxapine *see* Asendis

Amoxidin *see* Amoxil
(Lagap)

Amoxil
(Bencard)

A maroon/gold capsule supplied at a strength of 250 mg, 500 mg and used as a broad-spectrum penicillin to treat respiratory, ear, nose, and throat, urinary, and soft tissue infections.

Dose: adults 250-500 mg 3 times a day; children half adult dose; infants under 6 months use Amoxyl Paediatric Suspension.
Availability: NHS and private prescription.
Side effects: stomach upset, allergy.
Caution: in patients suffering from glandular fever.
Not to be used for: patients suffering from penicillin allergy.
Not to be used with:
Contains: AMOXYCILLIN trihydrate.
Other preparations: Amoxil Dispersible, Amoxil Syrup SF, Amoxil Paediatric Suspension, Amoxil 3g Sachet SF, Amoxil 750 mg Sachet SF, AMOXIDIN (Lagap), ALMODAN (Berk).

---

amoxycillin *see* **Amoxil, Augmentin**

---

amphotericin *see* **Fungilin, Fungilin Cream, Fungilin Lozenges**

---

ampicillin

A red/grey capsule supplied at strengths of 250 mg, 500 mg and used as a broad-spectrum penicillin to treat respiratory, ear, nose, and throat, and soft tissue infections.

Dose: adults 250 mg-1 g 4 times a day; children half adult dose.
Availability: NHS and private prescription.
Side effects: stomach upset, allergy.
Caution: in patients suffering kidney disease, glandular fever.
Not to be used for: patients suffering from penicillin allergy.
Not to be used with:
Contains: AMPICILLIN.
Other preparations: Ampicillin Syrup, Ampicillin Injection, AMPILAR (Lagap).

---

ampicillin *see* **Ampicillin, Magnapen, Penbritin, Vidopen**

Ampilar *see* **ampicillin**
(Lagap)

A

---

amylobarbitone *see* Amytal, Sodium Amytal, Tuinal

Amytal
(Eli Lilly)

A white tablet supplied at strengths of 15 mg, 30 mg, 50 mg, 100 mg, 200 mg and used as a barbiturate to treat sleeplessness.

Dose: 100-200 mg before going to bed.
Availability: controlled drug.
Side effects: drowsiness, hangover, dizziness, allergies, headache, confusion, excitement.
Caution: in patients suffering from kidney or lung disease. Dependence (addiction) may develop.
Not to be used for: children, young adults, pregnant women, nursing mothers, the elderly, patients with a history of drug or alcohol abuse, or suffering from porphyria (a rare blood disorder), or in the management of pain.
Not to be used with: anti-coagulants (blood-thinning drugs), alcohol, other tranquillizers, steroids, the contraceptive pill, GRISEOFULVIN, RIFAMPICIN, PHENYTOIN, METRONIDAZOLE, CHLORAMPHENICOL.
Contains: AMYLOBARBITONE.
Other preparations:

Anacal
(Panpharma)

An ointment used as a soothing, antiseptic, steroid treatment for haemorrhoids, anal fissure, anal itch.

Dose: adults and children over 7 years apply one or more times a day as required.
Availability: NHS and private prescription.
Side effects: systemic corticosteroid effects.
Caution: do not use for prolonged periods; special care is required for pregnant women.

33

Not to be used for: children under 7 years or for patients suffering from tuberculous, fungal and viral infections.
Not to be used with:
Contains: HEPARINOID, PREDNISOLONE, LAUROMACROGOL, HEXACHLOROPHANE.
Other preparations: Anacal Suppositories.

Anaflex
(Geistlich)

A white lozenge supplied at a strength of 30 mg and used as an anti-bacterial and anti-fungal treatment for thrush and other bacterial infections of the mouth and throat.

Dose: adults 6-10 lozenges a day; children over 6 years half adult dose.
Availability: NHS, private prescription, over the counter.
Side effects:
Caution:
Not to be used for: children under 6 years.
Not to be used with:
Contains: POLYNOXYLIN.
Other preparations: Anaflex Cream, Anaflex Paste, Anaflex Powder.

Anaflex Cream
(Geistlich)

A cream used as an anti-bacterial and anti-fungal treatment for skin infections.

Dose: apply the cream to the affected area 1-2 times a day.
Availability: NHS, private prescription, over the counter.
Side effects:
Caution:
Not to be used for:
Not to be used with:
Contains: POLYNOXYLIN.
Other preparations: anaflex, Anaflex Paste, Anaflex Powder, Anaflex Aerosol.

Anafranil
(Geigy)

A yellow/caramel capsule, orange/caramel capsule, or blue/caramel capsule according to strengths of 10 mg, 25 mg, 50 mg and used as an anti-depressant to treat depression, obsessions, phobias.

Dose: adults 10 mg at first increasing to 30-150 mg a day ; elderly 10 mg a day at first up to a maximum of 75 mg a day.
Availability: NHS and private prescription.
Side effects: dry mouth, constipation, urine retention, blurred vision, palpitations, drowsiness, sleeplessness, dizziness, low blood pressure, weight change, skin reactions, jaundice or blood changes, loss of libido may occur.
Caution: in nursing mothers or in patients suffering from heart disease, liver disease, thyroid disease, epilepsy, diabetes, some other psychiatric conditions. Your doctor may advise regular blood tests.
Not to be used for: children, pregnant women, or for patients suffering from heart attacks, liver disease, heart block.
Not to be used with: alcohol, ANTI-CHOLINERGICS, adrenaline, MAOIS, barbiturates, other anti-depressants, anti-hypertensives.
Contains: CLOMIPRAMINE hydrochloride.
Other preparations: Anafranil SR, Anafranil Injection.

Androcur
(Schering)

A white, scored tablet supplied at a strength of 50 mg and used as an anti-androgen to treat severe hypersexuality and sexual deviation in men.

Dose: 1 tablet in the morning and 1 tablet in the evening.
Availability: NHS and private prescription.
Side effects: tiredness, depression, weight gain, breast enlargement, changes in hair pattern, osteoporosis.
Caution: in patients suffering from diabetes or liver disease. Patients must give consent to treatment. Your doctor may advise regular blood and sperm tests.
Not to be used for: men under 18 years or where bones and testes have not reached full development, or for patients suffering from acute liver disease, malignant or wasting disease, severe chronic depres-

sion, history of thrombosis or embolism.
Not to be used with: alcohol.
Contains: CYPROTERONE ACETATE.
Other preparations:

Andursil
(Geigy)

A white liquid supplied in a 100 ml bottle and used as an antacid and anti-wind preparation to treat dyspepsia, heartburn, peptic ulcer.

Dose: adults 5-10 ml 3 times a day and at bedtime.
Availability: private prescription and over the counter.
Side effects: few; possibly constipation or diarrhoea.
Caution:
Not to be used for: children.
Not to be used with: TETRACYCLINE antibiotics.
Contains: ALUMINIUM OXIDE, MAGNESIUM HYDROXIDE, ALUMINIUM HYDROXIDE/ MAGNESIUM CARBONATE, activated DIMETHICONE.
Other preparations: Andursil Tablets.

anethol *see* Rowatinex

Angilol *see* Inderal
(DDSA)

Anquil
(Janssen)

A white tablet supplied at a strength of 0.25 mg and used as an anti-psychotic drug for controlling unacceptable sexual behaviour.

Dose: 1-5 tablets a day in divided doses.
Availability: NHS and private prescription.
Side effects: muscle spasms, restlessness, hands shaking, dry mouth, urine retention, palpitations, low blood pressure, weight gain, changes in libido, low body temperature, breast swelling, menstrual

changes, jaundice, blood and skin changes, drowsiness, rarely fits. *Caution:* in pregnant women or nursing mothers. Your doctor may advise regular blood and liver tests.

Not to be used for: children or for patients suffering from Parkinson's disease.

Not to be used with: alcohol, tranquillizers, pain killers, anti-hypertensives, anti-depressants, anti-convulsants, anti-diabetic drugs, LEVODOPA.

Contains: BENPERIDOL.

Other preparations:

Antabuse
(CP Pharm)

A white, scored tablet supplied at a strength of 200 mg and used as an enzyme inhibitor, additional treatment for alcoholism.

Dose: 1 tablet a day.

Availability: NHS and private prescription.

Side effects: drowsiness, tiredness, nausea, bad breath, reduced sex drive, rarely mental disturbances.

Caution: in patients suffering from liver, kidney, or breathing diseases, diabetes, epilepsy.

Not to be used for: children, pregnant women, or patients suffering from heart failure, coronary artery disease, mental disorders, or drug addiction.

Not to be used with: alcohol, barbiturates, PARALDEHYDE, sedatives.

Contains: DISULFIRAM.

Other preparations:

---

antazoline phosphate *see* Vasocon-A

---

antazoline sulphate *see* Otrivine-Antistin

Antepar
(Wellcome)

An elixir used as an anti-worm agent for the treament of worms.

Dose: adults up to 30 ml as a single dose; children reduced doses.
Availability: NHS, private prescription, over the counter.
Side effects: stomach upset, changes in the central nervous system, hypersensitivity, bruising, blood changes, liver disorder.
Caution: in nursing mothers and in patients suffering from nervous disorders.
Not to be used for: patients suffering from epilepsy, or kidney or liver disease.
Not to be used with:
Contains: PIPERAZINE HYDRATE, PIPERAZINE CITRATE.
Other preparations:

Antepsin
(Wyeth)

A white, oblong tablet supplied at a strength of 1 g and used as a cell-surface protector in the treatment of gastritis and ulcers.

Dose: adults 2 tablets twice a day in water.
Availability: NHS and private prescription.
Side effects:
Caution: in kidney function impairment.
Not to be used for: children.
Not to be used with: TETRACYCLINE antibiotics, PHENYTOIN, DIGOXIN, CIMETIDINE.
Contains: SUCRALFATE.
Other preparations:

Anthranol
(Stiefel)

An ointment used as an anti-psoriatic treatment for psoriasis.

Dose: apply in small amounts once a day at first, and then wash off after 10 minutes, then allowing 30 minutes before washing off.
Availability: NHS and private prescription.
Side effects: irritation and burning, allergy.
Caution:
Not to be used for: patients suffering from acute or pustular psoriasis.

Not to be used with:
Contains: DITHRANOL.
Other preparations:

anthraquinone glycosides *see* Pyralvex

anti-cholinergic

a drug which blocks the action of acetyl choline, a nerve transmitter. Anti-cholinergics are used to reduce muscle spasm. The effects include dry mouth, difficulty passing urine, and possibly confusion. Example, HYOSCINE *see* Buscopan.

anti-cholinesterase

a drug which enhances the action of acetyl choline, a nerve transmitter. Example NEOSTIGMINE *see* Prostigmin.

Antipressan *see* Tenormin
(Berk)

Antoin
(Cox)

A white, scored tablet used as an analgesic for the relief of pain.

Dose: 1-2 tablets in water 3-4 times a day.
Availability: private prescription only.
Side effects: stomach upsets, allergy, asthma.
Caution: in the elderly, in pregnant women, and in patients with a history of allergy to aspirin or asthma, impaired kidney or liver function, indigestion.
Not to be used for: children, nursing mothers, or for patients suffering from haemophilia, or stomach ulcers.
Not to be used with: anti-coagulants (blood-thinning drugs), some

anti-diabetic drugs, anti-inflammatory agents, METHOTREXATE, SPIRONOLAC-TONE, steroids, some antacids, some uric acid-lowering drugs.
Contains: ASPIRIN, CODEINE phosphate, CAFFEINE citrate.
Other preparations:

Antraderm
(Brocades)

A waxy stick used as an anti-psoriatic treatment for psoriasis.

Dose: apply to the affected area and then wash off after $1/2$-1 hour, or apply at night and wash off in the morning.
Availability: NHS and private prescription.
Side effects: irritation, burning, allergy.
Caution:
Not to be used for: patients suffering from acute psoriasis.
Not to be used with:
Contains: DITHRANOL.
Other preparations: Antraderm Mild, Antraderm Forte.

Anturan
(Geigy)

A yellow tablet supplied at strengths of100 mg, 200 mg and used as a uric acid-lowering drug to treat gout, gouty arthritis, high uric acid levels.

Dose: 100-200 mg a day with food at first increasing to 600 mg a day over 2-3 weeks and then reduce to the minimum effective dose.
Availability: NHS and private prescription.
Side effects: acute gout, stones in the urinary tract, kidney colic, gastro-intestinal bleeding, kidney disease, rash, blood changes.
*Caution:*in pregnant women, in patients with a history of peptic ulcer, kidney disease, or who are suffering from anti-inflammatory drug induced allergy, latent heart failure. Drink plenty of fluids. Your doctor may advise blood and kidney tests.
Not to be used for: children, or patients suffering from peptic ulcer, severe liver disease, or sensitivity to pyrazones.
Not to be used with: salicylates, anti-coagulants, HYPOGLYCAEMICS, SULPHONAMIDES.

Contains: SULPHINPYRAZONE.
Other preparations:

Anugesic-HC
(Parke-Davis)

A cream used as a soothing, antiseptic, steroid treatment for haemorrhoids, anal itch, and other rectal disorders.

Dose: apply night and morning after passing motions.
Availability: NHS and private prescription.
Side effects: systemic corticosteroid effects.
Caution: do not use for prolonged periods; special care is required for pregnant women.
Not to be used for: children or for patients suffering from tuberculous, fungal, and viral infections.
Not to be used with:
Contains: PRAMOXINE HYDROCHLORIDE, HYDROCORTISONE acetate, ZINC OXIDE, PERU BALSAM, BENZYL BENZOATE, BISMUTH OXIDE, RESORCINOL.
Other preparations: Anugesic-HC suppositories.

Anusol
(Parke-Davis)

A suppository used as a soothing, antiseptic, astringent treatment for haemorrhoids, anal itch, and other rectal and anal disorders.

Dose: 1 suppository night and morning after passing motions.
Availability: NHS and private prescription.
Side effects:
Caution:
Not to be used for: children.
Not to be used with:
Contains: BISMUTH SUBGALLATE, BISMUTH OXIDE, PERU BALSAM.
Other preparations: Anusol cream, Anusol ointment.

Anusol HC
(Parke-Davis)

A suppository used as a steroid, antiseptic, astringent treatment for haemorrhoids and inflammation of the anus and rectum.

Dose: 1 suppository night and morning after passing motions.
Availability: NHS and private prescription.
Side effects: systemic corticosteroid effects.
Caution: in pregnant women; do not use for prolonged periods.
Not to be used for: children or for patients suffering from tuberculous, fungal, and viral infections.
Not to be used with:
Contains: HYDROCORTISONE acetate, BENZYL BENZOATE, BISMUTH SUBGALLATE, BISMUTH OXIDE, RESORCINOL, PERU BALSAM, ZINC OXIDE.
Other preparations: Anusol HC ointment.

Anxon
(S K B)

A dark-pink/light-pink capsule supplied at strengths of 15 mg, 30 mg and used as a tranquillizer for short-term relief of anxiety, muscle spasm.

Dose: elderly 15 mg a day at first then 15-60 mg a day; adults 30 mg at night then 15-60 mg a day as needed.
Availability: private prescription only.
Side effects:
Caution: in pregnant women, nursing mothers, and in patients suffering from chronic lung disease, liver or kidney disease. Avoid long-term treatment and withdraw gradually.
Not to be used for: children or for patients suffering from acute lung disease.
Not to be used with: alcohol, other sedatives, anti-convulsants.
Contains: KETAZOLAM.
Other preparations:

Apisate
(Wyeth)

A yellow tablet used as an appetite suppressant to treat obesity.

Dose: 1 tablet a day.

Availability: controlled drug.
Side effects: tolerance, addiction, mental disturbances, sleeplessness, nervousness, agitation.
Caution: in women during the first three months of pregnancy, and in
patients suffering from high blood pressure, angina, abnormal heart
rhythm, peptic ulcer.
Not to be used for: children, the elderly, or patients suffering from
arteriosclerosis, overactive thyroid, severe high blood pressure, glau-
coma, or with a history of alcoholism, drug addiction, or mental illness.
Not to be used with: MAOIS, SYMPATHOMIMETICS, METHYLDOPA, GUANETHID-
INE, psychotropics, or obesity drugs.
Contains: DIETHYLPROPION HYDROCHLORIDE, THIAMINE, RIBOFLAVINE, PYRI-
DOXINE, NICOTINAMIDE.
Other preparations:

APP
(Consolidated)

A powder used as an antacid to treat ulcers, indigestion, nausea,
acidity.

Dose: adults 5 ml 3-4 times a day.
Availability: private prescription only.
Side effects: few; occasionally constipation.
Caution: in patients suffering from prostate enlargement.
Not to be used for: infants or for patients suffering from glaucoma.
Not to be used with:
Contains: PAPAVERINE, CALCIUM CARBONATE, ALUMINIUM HYDROXIDE, HOMA-
TROPINE, MAGNESIUM CARBONATE, BISMUTH CARBONATE.
Other preparations: APP tablets.

Apresoline
(Ciba)

A yellow tablet or pink tablet according to strengths of 25 mg, 50 mg
and used as a vasodilator in addition to DIURETICS and glycosides for the
treatment of moderate to severe chronic heart failure, moderate to
severe high blood pressure.

Dose: 25 mg 3 or 4 times a day at first increasing every second day

to 50-75 mg 3 or 4 times a day if necessary; hypertension 25 mg 2-3 times a day at first with a ß-BLOCKER and DIURETIC.
Availability: NHS and private prescription.
Side effects: rapid heart rate, headache, flushes, especially if more than 100 mg a day are taken; rarely liver damage, kidney disorders, changes in blood count, nerve disorders.
Caution: in nursing mothers and in patients suffering from coronary or cerebrovascular disease, kidney failure, liver disease.
Not to be used for: children, for patients suffering from certain heart diseases, or during the first half of pregnancy
Not to be used with: TRICYCLIC anti-depressants, MAOIS, anti-hypertensives, anxiolytics.
Contains: HYDRALAZINE HYDROCHLORIDE.
Other preparations: Apresoline Injection.

Aprinox
(Boots)

A white tablet supplied at strengths of 2.5 mg, 5 mg and used as a DIURETIC to treat fluid retention, high blood pressure.

Dose: 5-10 mg each morning or each alternate day at first then 5-10 mg once or twice a week. High blood pressure 2.5-5 mg a day.
Availability: NHS and private prescription.
Side effects: low potassium levels, rash, sensitivity to light, blood changes, gout, tiredness.
Caution: in pregnant women, nursing mothers, the elderly and for patients suffering from diabetes, severe kidney or liver disease, or gout.
Not to be used for: children or for patients suffering from urine failure or severe or progressive kidney failure.
Not to be used with: LITHIUM, DIGITALIS, blood pressure-lowering drugs.
Contains: BENDROFLUAZIDE.
Other preparations:

Apsifen *see* Brufen
(APS)

Apsin VK *see* **penicillin**
(APS)

Apsolol *see* **Inderal**
(APS)

Apsolox *see* **Trasicor**
(APS)

Aquasept
(Hough, Hoseason)

A solution used as a disinfectant for skin and body cleansing and disinfecting.

Dose: use as a soap.
Availability: NHS, private prescription, over the counter.
Side effects:
Caution: keep out of the eyes.
Not to be used for:
Not to be used with:
Contains: TRICLOSAN.
Other preparations:

---

arachis oil *see* **Cerumol, Fletcher's Arachis Oil, Polytar
Liquid**

Aradolene
(Fisons)

A cream used as an analgesic rub to treat rheumatic conditions.

Dose: massage into the affected area 2-3 times a day.
Availability: NHS, private prescription , over the counter.

Side effects: may be irritant.
Caution:
Not to be used for: areas such as near the eyes, on broken or inflamed skin, or on membranes (such as the mouth).
Not to be used with:
Contains: DIETHYLAMINE SALICYLATE, CAPSICUM OLEORESIN, CAMPHOR OIL, MENTHOL.
Other preparations:

Arelix
(Hoechst/Albert)

A green/orange capsule supplied at a strength of 6 mg and used as a DIURETIC to treat high blood pressure.

Dose: 1-2 a day as a single morning dose.
Availability: NHS and private prescription.
Side effects: electrolyte imbalance.
Caution: in pregnant women, nursing mothers, or in patients suffering from liver or kidney disease, gout, diabetes, enlarged prostate, or impaired urination. Your doctor may advise regular bood tests.
Not to be used for: for children or for patients suffering from cirrhosis of the liver.
Not to be used with: DIGITALIS, LITHIUM, aminoglycosides, cephalosporin antibiotics, blood pressure-lowering drugs, NON-STEROID ANTI-INFLAMMATORY DRUGS.
Contains: piretanide.
Other preparations:

Arobon
(Nestle)
A powder used as an adsorbent to treat diarrhoea, dysentery, enteritis, colitis, coeliac disease.
Dose: 20-40 g a day in water; infants 2-5 g per 100 ml feed.
Availability: NHS and private prescription.
Side effects:
Caution:
Not to be used for:
Not to be used with:

Contains: CERATONIA, STARCH.
Other preparations:

aromatic oils *see* **Pavacol-D**

Arpicolin
(RP Drugs)

A syrup supplied at strengths of 2.5 mg/5 ml, 5 mg/5 ml and used as an ANTI-CHOLINERGIC treatment for Parkinson's disease.

Dose: 2.5-5 mg 3 times a day at first increasing every 2-3 days by 2.5-5 mg a day to a maximum of 30 mg a day.
Availability: NHS and private prescription.
Side effects: anti-cholinergic effects, confusion at high doses.
Caution: in patients suffering from heart problems, gastro-intestinal obstruction, glaucoma, enlarged prostate. The dosage should be reduced gradually.
Not to be used for: children or patients suffering from tardive dyskinesia (a movement disorder).
Not to be used with: PHENOTHIAZINES, antihistamines, anti-depressants.
Contains: PROCYCLIDINE hydrochloride.
Other preparations:

Arpimycin *see* Erythrocin
(RP Drugs)

Artane
(Lederle)
A white, scored tablet supplied at strengths of 2 mg, 5 mg and used as an ANTI-CHOLINERGIC treatment for Parkinson's disease, drug-induced Parkinson's disease.
Dose: 1 mg on the first day, 2 mg second day, then increased by 2 mg a day every 3-5 days usually to 5-15 mg a day.
Availability: NHS and private prescription.

Side effects: anti-cholinergic effects, confusion and agitation at high doses.
Caution: in patients suffering from heart, kidney, or liver disease, enlarged prostate, glaucoma, or gastro-intestinal obstruction. Dose should be reduced gradually.
Not to be used for: children.
Not to be used with: PHENOTHIAZINES, antihistamines, anti-depressants.
Contains: benzhexol.
Other preparations: BENTEX (Steinhard), BROFLEX (Bio-Medical).

Artracin *see* Indocid
(DDSA)

Arythmol
(Knoll)

A white tablet supplied in strengths of 50 mg, 300 mg and used as an anti-arrhythmic drug to treat heart rhythm disturbances

Dose: 150-300 mg 3 times a day.
Availability: NHS and private prescription.
Side effects: nausea, vomiting, dizziness, diarrhoea, constipation, headache, tiredness, skin rash, slow heart rate.
Caution: in the elderly, patients with pace makers, and in patients suffering from heart failure, liver and kidney disorders.
Not to be used for: pregnant women, or for patients suffering from uncontrolled heart failure, obstructive lung disease, electrolyte disturbances, some heart rhythm disturbances.
Not to be used with: other anti-arrhythmics, DIGOXIN, WARFARIN, CIMETIDINE, PROPANOLOL, METOPROLOL.
Contains: PROPAFERONE.
Other preparations:

Asacol
(S K B)

A red, coated, oblong tablet supplied at a strength of 400 mg and used as a salicylate to treat ulcerative colitis.

Dose: 3-6 tablets a day in divided doses.
Availability: NHS and private prescription.
Side effects: stomach disturbances, headache.
Caution: in patients suffering from kidney disease, raised blood urea, protein in the urine, and in pregnant women.
Not to be used for: children.
Not to be used with: lactulose or any preparations that increase the acidity of the motions.
Contains: MESALAZINE.
Other preparations:

Ascabiol
(M & B)

An emulsion used as an insect-destroying drug to treat scabies, pediculosis.

Dose:
Availability: NHS, private prescription, over the counter.
Side effects: irritation.
Caution: keep out of the eyes.
Not to be used for:
Not to be used with:
Contains: BENZYL BENZOATE.
Other preparations:

---

ascorbic acid *see* **Abidec, Allbee with C, BC 500, BC 500 with Iron, Concavit, Fefol-Vit Spansule, Ferrograd C, Fesovit Spansule, Fesovit Z Spansule, Galfervit, Givitol, Irofol C, Ketovite, Lipoflavonoid, Multivite, Octovit, Oralcer, Orovite, Orovite 7, Polyvite, Pregnavite Forte F, Redoxon, Surbex T, Tonivitan, Uniflu and Gregovite C, Villescon**

Asendis
(Lederle)

A white, orange, blue, or white, hexagonal tablet according to strengths of 25 mg, 50 mg, 100 mg, 150 mg and used as a TRICYCLIC anti-depressant to treat depression.

Dose: 100-150 mg a day increasing to 300 mg a day.
Availability: NHS and private prescription.
Side effects: ANTI-CHOLINERGIC effects, drowsiness, impotence, nausea, vomiting, breast enlargement, convulsions at high doses.
Caution: in the elderly, and in patients who are a suicide risk, or who are suffering from epilepsy, glaucoma, urine retention, confusion, agitation.
Not to be used for: pregnant women, nursing mothers, or for patients suffering from recent heart attack, heart block, heart rhythm disturbances, severe liver disease, mania.
Not to be used with: MAOIS, SYMPATHOMIMETICS, barbiturates, alcohol, anti-hypertensives, anaesthetics.
Contains: AMOXAPINE.
Other preparations:

Aserbine
(Bencard)

A cream used as a wound cleanser to treat varicose ulcers, burns, bed sores, and for cleansing of wounds.

Dose: wash the wound with the solution and apply cream twice a day.
Availability: NHS, private prescription, over the counter.
Side effects:
Caution:
Not to be used for:
Not to be used with:
Contains: MALIC ACID, BENZOIC ACID, SALICYLIC ACID, PROPYLENE GLYCOL.
Other preparations:

Asilone
(Rorer)

A white liquid used as an antacid, anti-wind preparation to treat gastritis, ulcers, dyspepsia, wind.

Dose: adults 5-10 ml before meals and at bedtime; for children use infant suspension or half adult dose.

Availability: NHS, private prescription, over the counter.
Side effects: few; occasionally constipation.
Caution:
Not to be used for: infants.
Not to be used with:
Contains: activated DIMETHICONE, ALUMINIUM HYDROXIDE GEL, MAGNESIUM OXIDE.
Other preparations: Asilone gel, infant suspension, and tablets. INFACOL (Pharmax), POLYCROL gel and tablets, POLYCROL FORTE gel (Nicholas), UNIGEST (Unigreg) — private and over the counter only. SILOXYL (Martindale) — private and over the counter only.

Asmaven *see* Ventolin
(APS)

Aspav
(Cox)

A buff, dispersible tablet used as analgesic to relieve pain after operations and pain associated with cancers for which surgery is inappropriate.

Dose: 1-2 tablets dispersed in water every 4-6 hours up to a maximum of 8 tablets in 24 hours.
Availability: NHS and private prescription.
Side effects: allergies, asthma, gastro-intestinal bleeding, constipation, nausea.
Caution: in pregnant women, women in labour, nursing mothers, the elderly, and in patients suffering from head injury, underactive thyroid gland, a history of bronchospasm or anti-inflammatory induced allergies, kidney or liver disease.
Not to be used for: children, unconscious patients, or patients suffering from respiratory depression, blocked airways, gastric ulcer, haemophilia.
Not to be used with: MAOIS, sedatives, anti-coagulants, anti-diabetic drugs, NON-STEROID ANTI-INFLAMMATORY DRUGS, uric acid-lowering drugs, METHOTREXATE, SULPHONAMIDES.
Contains: ASPIRIN, PAPAVERETUM.
Other preparations:

Aspellin
(Fisons)

A liniment or a spray used as a topical analgesic to treat muscular rheumatism, sciatica, lumbago, fibrositis, chilblains.

Dose: massage gently into the affected area every 3-4 hours.
Availability: NHS, private prescription , over the counter.
Side effects: may be irritant.
Caution:
Not to be used for: areas near the eyes, or where the skin is broken or inflamed, or on membranes (such as the mouth).
Not to be used with:
Contains: ASPIRIN, MENTHOL, CAMPHOR, METHYL SALICYLATE.
Other preparations:

---

aspirin *see also* Antoin, Aspav, Aspellin, Claradin, Co-Codaprin Dispersibe, Codis, Doloxene Co., Equagesic, Hypon, Migravess Forte, Nu-Seals Aspirin, Paynocil, Platet 300, Robaxisal Forte, Solprin, Trancoprin

A white tablet supplied at a strength of 300 mg and used as an analgesic to relievepain and reduce fever.

Dose: 1-3 tablets every 4-6 hours as needed to a maximum of 12 tablets a day.
Availability: NHS, private prescription, over the counter.
Side effects: stomach upsets, allergy, asthma.
Caution: in pregnant women, the elderly, or in patients with a history of allergy to aspirin, asthma, impaired kidney or liver function, indigestion.
Not to be used for: children, nursing mothers, or patients suffering from haemophilia, or ulcers.
Not to be used with: anti-coagulants (blood-thinning drugs), some anti-diabetic drugs, anti-inflammatory agents, METHOTREXATE, SPIRONOLACTONE, steroids, some antacids, some uric acid-lowering drugs.
Contains:
Other preparations: Dispersible Aspirin.

---

astemizole *see* Hismanal

AT 10
(Sterling Research Laboratories)

A

A solution used as a source of vitamin D to treat vitamin D deficiency.

Dose: 1-7 ml taken by mouth each week.
Availability: NHS, private prescription, over the counter.
Side effects: loss of appetite, listlessness, vertigo, stupor, nausea, urgent need to urinate.
Caution: in nursing mothers. Your doctor may advise that your calcium levels should be checked regularly.
Not to be used for: children.
Not to be used with:
Contains: DIHYDROTACHYSTEROL.
Other preparations:

Atarax
(Pfizer)

An orange tablet or a green tablet according to strengths of 10 mg, 25 mg and used as an antihistamine to treat anxiety.

Dose: 50-100 mg 4 times a day.
Availability: NHS and private prescription.
Side effects: drowsiness, ANTI-CHOLINERGIC effects, involuntary movements if a high dosage is taken.
Caution: in patients suffering from kidney disease. Patients should be warned of reduced judgement and abilities.
Not to be used for: children or pregnant women.
Not to be used with: alcohol and sedatives.
Contains: HYDROXYZINE HYDROCHLORIDE.
Other preparations: Atarax Syrup.

---

atenolol *see* Beta-Adalat, Kalten, Tenif, Tenoret 50, Tenoretic, Tenormin

---

Atensine *see* Valium
(Berk)

Ativan
(Wyeth)

A blue, oblong, scored tablet or a yellow, oblong, scored tablet according to strengths of 1 mg, 2.5 mg and used as a tranquillizer to treat anxiety.

Dose: elderly 0.5-2 mg a day; adults 1-4 mg a day.
Availability: NHS (when prescribed as a generic) and private prescription.
Side effects: drowsiness, confusion, unsteadiness, low blood pressure, rash, changes in vision, changes in libido, retention of urine. Risk of addiction increases with dose and length of treatment. May impair judgement.
Caution: in the elderly, pregnant women, nursing mothers, in women during labour, and in patients suffering from lung disorders, kidney or liver disorders. Avoid long-term use and withdraw gradually.
Not to be used for: children, or for patients suffering from acute lung diseases, some chronic lung diseases, some obsessional and psychotic diseases.
Not to be used with: alcohol, other tranquillizers, anti-convulsants.
Contains: LORAZEPAM.
Other preparations: ALMAZINE (Steinhard).

Atromid-S
(ICI)

A red capsule supplied at a strength of 500 mg and used as a lipid-lowering agent to treat elevated cholesterol.

Dose: 20-30 mg per kg body weight a day in 2-3 divided doses after meals.
Availability: NHS and private prescription.
Side effects: stomach upset, gallstones, muscle aches.
Caution: in patients with low serum proteins. Your doctor may advise diet and other changes in lifestyle as well as regular blood tests.
Not to be used for: children, pregnant women, or for patients with a history of gall bladder problems or kidney or liver disease.
Not to be used with: anti-coagulants, anti-diabetic drugs, phenytoin.
Contains: CLOFIBRATE.
Other preparations:

Atropine
(SNP)

Drops used as an ANTI-CHOLINERGIC preparation for pupil dilation.

Dose: 1 drop into the eye as needed.
Availability: NHS and private prescription.
Side effects: stinging in the eye, dry mouth, blurred vision, intolerance of light, rapid heart rate, rarely psychological changes.
Caution:
Not to be used for: patients suffering from narrow angle glaucoma.
Not to be used with:
Contains: ATROPINE SULPHATE.
Other preparations: OPULETS ATROPINE (Alcon)

---

atropine methonitrate *see* Brovon, Rybarvin

---

atropine sulphate *see* Atropine

Atrovent
(Boehringer Ingelheim)

An inhaler used as an ANTI-CHOLINERGIC preparation to relieve blocked airways especially as a result of bronchitis.

Dose: adults 1-2 metered doses 3-4 times a day; children under 6 years 1 dose 3 times a day; 6-12 years 1-2 doses 3 times a day.
Availability: NHS and private prescription.
Side effects: dry mouth, constipation, retention of urine.
Caution: in patients suffering from enlarged prostate, glaucoma.
Not to be used for:
Not to be used with:
Contains: IPRATROPIUM BROMIDE.
Other preparations: Atrovent Solution.

Audax
(Napp Consumer)

Drops used as an analgesic to relieve pain associated with acute inflammation of the outer or middle ear.

Dose: fill the ear with the liquid and plug it.
Availability: NHS, private prescription, over the counter.
Side effects:
Caution:
Not to be used for:
Not to be used with:
Contains: CHOLINE SALICYLATE.
Other preparations:

Audicort
(Lederle)

Drops used as an antibiotic, corticosteroid, and local anaesthetic treatment for inflammation and infection of the outer ear.

Dose: 2-5 drops into the ear 3-4 times a day.
Availability: NHS and private prescription.
Side effects: additional infection, local irritation.
Caution: in pregnant women and in patients suffering from a perforated ear drum. Do not use for extended periods on infants.
Not to be used for: patients suffering from viral lesions or tubercular skin diseases.
Not to be used with:
Contains: TRIAMCINOLONE ACETONIDE, NEOMYCIN, UNDECENOIC ACID.
Other preparations:

Augmentin
(S K B)

A white, oval tablet used as a broad-spectrum penicillin to treat respiratory, ear, nose, and throat, urinary tract, skin, and soft tissue infections.

Dose: 1-2 tablets 3 times a day for up to 14 days.
Availability: NHS and private prescription.
Side effects: penicillin allergy and stomach disturbances.
Caution: in patients suffering from kidney or liver disease, glandular fever.

Not to be used for: patients suffering from penicillin allergy.
Not to be used with:
Contains: CLAVULANIC ACID, AMOXYCILLIN.
Other preparations: Augmentin Dispersible, Augmentin Junior, Augmentin Paediatric, Augmentin Intravenous.

Auralgicin
(Fisons)

A liquid used as an anti-bacterial treatment for inflammation of the middle ear.

Dose: fill the ear with the liquid every hour and plug until the pain is relieved and then treat every 3 hours for 24 hours.
Availability: NHS, private prescription, over the counter.
Side effects:
Caution:
Not to be used for:
Not to be used with:
Contains: EPHEDRINE HYDROCHLORIDE, BENZOCAINE, CHLORBUTOL, POTASSIUM HYDROXYQUINOLONE SULPHATE, PHENAZONE, GLYCERIN.
Other preparations:

Auraltone
(Fisons)

Drops used as an analgesic, local anaesthetic treatment for acute inflammation of the ear drum or inner ear.

Dose: fill the ear with the drops and plug lightly, repeating every hour if needed.
Availability: NHS, private prescription, over the counter.
Side effects: skin eruptions.
Caution:
Not to be used for:
Not to be used with:
Contains: PHENAZONE, BENZOCAINE.
Other preparations:

Aureocort
(Lederle)

A cream used as a steroid, anti-bacterial treatment for skin disorders where there is also inflammation and infection.

Dose: apply a small quantity of the cream to the affected area 2-3 times a day.
Availability: NHS and private prescription.
Side effects: fluid retention, suppression of adrenal glands. Thinning of the skin may occur.
Caution: use for short periods of time only.
Not to be used for: patients suffering from acne or any other skin infections caused by tuberculosis, ringworm, viruses, or fungi, or continuously especially in pregnant women.
Not to be used with:
Contains: TRIAMCINOLONE ACETONIDE, CHLORTETRACYCLINE HYDROCHLORIDE.
Other preparations: Aureocort Ointment.

Aureomycin
(Lederle)

A yellow capsule supplied at a strength of 250 mg and used as a tetracycline to treat infections.

Dose: 1-2 capsules 4 times a day.
Availability: NHS and private prescription.
Side effects: stomach disturbances, allergies, further infections.
Caution: in patients suffering from liver or kidney disease.
Not to be used for: children, nursing mothers, or for women in the latter half of pregnancy.
Not to be used with: milk, antacids, mineral supplements, contraceptive pill.
Contains: CHLORTETRACYCLINE.
Other preparations: AUREOMYCIN OINTMENT.

Aureomycin Ointment
(Lederle)

An ointment used as an antibiotic to treat eye and skin infections.

Dose: apply ointment into the eye every 2 hours or on gauze to the affected area of skin once a day or as needed.
Availability: NHS and private prescription.
Side effects: additional infection.
Caution:
Not to be used for:
Not to be used with:
Contains: CHLORTETRACYCLINE hydrochloride.
Other preparations: Aureomycin Cream.

Aventyl
(Eli Lilly)

A white/yellow capsule supplied at a strength of 10 mg, 25 mg and used as an anti-depressant to treat depression, bed wetting in children.

Dose: adults 20-40 mg a day increasing to 100 mg a day if needed in divided doses, then usually 30-75 mg a day; elderly 10 mg 3 times a day at first; children over 6 years 10-35 mg $1/2$ hour before bedtime.
Availability: NHS and private prescription.
Side effects: dry mouth, constipation, urine retention, blurred vision, palpitations, drowsiness, sleeplessness, dizziness, hands shaking, low blood presure, weight change, skin reactions, jaundice or blood changes, loss of libido may occur.
Caution: in nursing mothers or in patients suffering from heart disease, thyroid disease, epilepsy, diabetes, some other psychiatric conditions. Your doctor may advise regular blood tests.
Not to be used for: children under 6 years, pregnant women, or for patients suffering from heart attacks, liver disease, heart block.
Not to be used with: alcohol, ANTI-CHOLINERGICS, adrenaline, MAOIS, barbiturates, other anti-depressants, anti-hypertensives.
Contains: NORTRYPTILINE hydrochloride.
Other preparations: Aventyl Liquid.

Avloclor
(ICI)

A white, scored tablet supplied at a strength of 250 mg and used as an anti-malarial, amoebicide preparation for the prevention of malaria, and the treatment of hepatitis, amoebiasis.

Dose: prevention of malaria adults 2 tablets on the same day once a week, children 5 mg per kg bodyweight once a week; treatment of hepatitis adults only 4 tablets a day for 2 days then 1 tablet twice a day for 2-3 weeks.
Availability: NHS and private prescription.
Side effects: headache, stomach upset, skin eruptions, hair loss, blurred vision, eye damage, blood disorders, loss of pigments.
Caution: in pregnant women, nursing mothers, and in patients suffering from porphyria (a rare blood disorder), kidney or liver disease, or psoriasis. Your doctor may advise regular eye tests before and during treatment.
Not to be used for:
Not to be used with:
Contains: CHLOROQUINE PHOSPHATE.
Other preparations:

Avomine
(M & B)

A white, scored tablet supplied at a strength of 25 mg and used as an antihistamine treatment for travel sickness, nausea, vomiting, vertigo.

Dose: adults travel sickness 1 at bedtime before long journeys or 1-2 hours before short journeys, nausea 1 tablet 1-3 times a day; children 5-10 years half adults dose.
Availability: NHS, private prescription, over the counter.
Side effects: drowsiness, reduced reactions, rarely skin eruptions.
Caution: in patients suffering from liver or kidney disease.
Not to be used for: children under 5 years.
Not to be used with: alcohol, sedatives, and some anti-depressants (MAOIS).
Contains: PROMETHAZINE THEOCLATE.
Other preparations:

Axid
(Eli Lilly)

A pale-yellow/ dark-yellow capsule supplied at a strength of150 mg and 300 mg and used as an anti-ulcer treatment for ulcers and for prevention of ulcers.

Dose: adult dose 300 mg in the evening or 150 mg twice a day. Prevention: 150 mg in the evening for up to a year.
Availability: NHS and private prescription.
Side effects: headache, chest pain, muscle ache, fatigue, dreams, runny nose, sore throat, cough, itch, sweating, changes in liver enzymes.
Caution: in patients suffering from impaired kidney and liver functions.
Not to be used for: children.
Not to be used with:
Contains: NIZATIDINE.
Other preparations:

---

azapropazone *see* **Rheumox**

---

azatadine maleate *see* **Optimine**

---

azatadine *see* **Congesteze**

---

bacampicillin hydrochloride *see* **Ambaxin**

---

bacitracin *see* **Cicatrin, Polybactrin, Polyfax, Tri-Cicatrin, Tribiotic**

---

baclofen *see* **Lioresal**

Bacticlens
(S & N)

A solution in a sachet used as a disinfectant to clean the skin, wounds, or broken skin.

Dose: use as needed.
Availability: NHS, private prescription, over the counter.
Side effects:
Caution: throw away any remaining solution straight away after use.
Not to be used for:
Not to be used with:
Contains: CHLORHEXIDINE gluconate.
Other preparations:

Bactrim *see* Septrin

Bactroban Nasal
(S K B)

An ointment used as an antibiotic to treat infections of the nose or skin.

Dose: apply 2-3 times a day for 5-7 days or up to 10 days for skin infections.
Availability: NHS and private prescription.
Side effects:
Caution: keep out of the eyes.
Not to be used for:
Not to be used with:
Contains: MUPIROCIN.
Other preparations:

Balmosa
(Pharmax)

A cream used as an analgesic rub to treat muscular rheumatism, fibrositis, lumbago, sciatica, unbroken chilblains.

Dose: massage into the affected area as needed.
Availability: NHS, private prescription , over the counter.
Side effects: may be irritant.
Caution:
Not to be used for: areas near the eyes, on broken or inflamed skin, or on membranes (such as the mouth).
Not to be used with:
Contains: MENTHOL, CAMPHOR, METHYL SALICYLATE, CAPSICUM OLEORESIN.
Other preparations:

Balneum with Tar
(Merck)

A bath oil used as an emolient and anti-psoriatic to treat eczema, itchy or thickening skin disorders, psoriasis.

Dose: adults add 4 5 ml teaspoonsful to the bath water; children over 2 years add 2 teaspoonsful and use for a maximum of 6 weeks.
Availability: NHS, private prescription, over the counter.
Side effects:
Caution:
Not to be used for: for children under 2 years or for patients suffering from wet or weeping skin problems or where the skin is badly broken.
Not to be used with:
Contains: COAL TAR, SOYA OIL.
Other preparations:

Baltar
(Merck)

A liquid used as an anti-psoriatic treatment for psoriasis, dandruff, eczema, dermatoses of the scalp.

Dose: shampoo the hair with the liquid 1-3 times a week.
Availability: NHS, private prescription, over the counter.
Side effects:
Caution: keep out of the eyes.

Not to be used for: children under 2 years or for patients suffering from wet or weeping dermatoses, or where the skin is badly broken.
Not to be used with:
Contains: COAL TAR.
Other preparations:

Banocide
(Wellcome)

A white, scored tablet supplied at a strength of 50 mg and used as an anti-worm agent to treat worms in the blood and lymph channels.

Dose: as advised by the physician.
Availability: NHS, private prescription, over the counter.
Side effects: itchy skin, eye disorders.
Caution: your doctor may advise regular eye tests.
Not to be used for: pregnant women.
Not to be used with:
Contains: DIETHYLCARBAMAZINE.
Other preparations:

Baratol
(Wyeth)

A blue tablet or a green, scored tablet according to strengths of 25 mg, 50 mg and used as an anti-hypertensive to treat high blood pressure.

Dose: 25 mg twice a day at first increasing by 25-50 mg a day at two-weekly intervals to a maximum of 200 mg a day if needed in 2-3 divided doses.
Availability: NHS and private prescription.
Side effects: drowsiness, dry mouth, blocked nose, increase in bodyweight, inability to ejaculate.
Caution: in patients suffering from kidney or liver weakness, Parkinson's disease, epilepsy, depression; patients with weak hearts should be treated with digitalis and DIURETICS.
Not to be used for: children or patients suffering from heart failure.
Not to be used with: MAOIS, anti-hypertensives.
Contains: INDORAMIN hydrochloride.
Other preparations:

Barquinol HC
(Fisons)

A cream used as a steroid, anti-bacterial, and anti-fungal preparation to treat infected skin disorders.

Dose: apply to the affected area 2-3 times a day.
Availability: NHS and private prescription.
Side effects: fluid retention, suppression of adrenal glands, thinning of the skin may occur.
Caution: use for short periods of time only.
Not to be used for: patients suffering from acne or any other skin infections caused by tuberculosis, ringworm, viruses, or fungi, or continuously especially in pregnant women.
Not to be used with:
Contains: HYDROCORTISONE acetate, CLIOQUINOL.
Other preparations:

Baxan
(Bristol-Myers)

A white capsule supplied at a strength of 500 mg and used as a cephalosporin antibiotic to treat respiratory, skin, and soft tissue infections, ear infections.

Dose: adults 1-2 capsules twice a day; children under 1 year 25 mg per kg body weight a day in divided doses, 1-6 years $1/2$ capsule twice a day, over 6 years 1 capsule twice a day.
Availability: NHS and private prescription.
Side effects: allergy, stomach disturbances.
Caution: in patients suffering from kidney disease or who are sensitive to penicillins.
Not to be used for:
Not to be used with: certain DIURETICS.
Contains: CEFADROXIL.
Other preparations:

Baycaron
(Bayer)

A white, scored tablet supplied at a strength of 25 mg and used as a

DIURETIC to treat high blood pressure, fluid retention.

Dose: 1-2 a day as a single dose in the morning for 10-14 days, then 1 a day or 1 every other day.
Availability: NHS and private prescription.
Side effects: dyspesia, nausea.
Caution: in pregnant women, nursing mothers, or in patients suffering from kidney or liver disease, diabetes, or gout.
Not to be used for: patients suffering from cirrhosis of the liver, severe kidney failure, Addison's disease, or severely raised calcium levels.
Not to be used with: DIGITALIS, LITHIUM, anti-hypertensives.
Contains: MEFRUSIDE.
Other preparations:

Bayolin
(Bayer)

A cream used as an analgesic rub to treat rheumatism, fibrositis, lumbago, sciatica.

Dose: massage gently into the affected area 2-3 times a day.
Availability: NHS, private prescription , over the counter.
Side effects: may be irritant.
Caution:
Not to be used for: areas near the eyes, broken or inflamed skin, or on membranes (such as the mouth).
Not to be used with:
Contains: HEPARINOID, GLYCOL SALICYLATE, BENZYL NICOTINATE.
Other preparations:

BC 500
(Wyeth)

An orange, oblong tablet used as a multivitamin preparation to treat vitamin B and vitamin C deficiency, and to aid recovery from illness, long-term alcoholism, long-term antibiotic treatment.

Dose: 1 tablet a day.
Availability: private prescription and over the counter.
Side effects:

Caution:
Not to be used for: children.
Not to be used with: LEVODOPA.
Contains: THIAMINE mononitrate, RIBOFLAVINE, NICOTINAMIDE, PYRIDOXINE hydrochloride, CALCIUM PANTOTHENATE, ASCORBIC ACID, CYANOCOBLAMIN.
Other preparations:

B

BC 500 with Iron
(Wyeth)

A red tablet used as vitamin and iron supplement to treat iron deficiency anaemia.

Dose: 1 tablet a day.
Availability: private prescription and over the counter.
Side effects: nausea, constipation.
Caution:
Not to be used for: children.
Not to be used with: TETRACYCLINES, LEVODOPA.
Contains: FERROUS FUMARATE, THIAMINE mononitrate, RIBOFLAVINE, NICOTINAMIDE, PYRIDOXINE hydrochloride, CALCIUM PANTOTHENATE, ASCORBIC ACID.
Other preparations:

Becloforte *see* Becotide
(A & H)

beclomethasone *see* Beconase, Becotide, Propaderm, Ventide

Becodisks *see* Becotide
(A & H)

Beconase
(A & H)

A powder in an aerosol or a suspension in an atomizer supplied at a strength of 50 micrograms and used as a corticosteroid to treat rhinitis, hay fever.

Dose: 2 sprays into each nostril twice a day.
Availability: NHS and private prescription.
Side effects:
Caution: in pregnant women, in patients with nasal infections, and in patients transferring from systemic steroids.
Not to be used for: children under 6 years.
Not to be used with:
Contains: BECLOMETHASONE DIPROPRIONATE.
Other preparations:

Becosym
(Roche)

A brown tablet used as a source of B vitamins to treat B vitamin deficiencies.

Dose: adults 1-3 tablets a day; children use syrup.
Availability: NHS (when prescribed as a generic), private prescription, over the counter.
Side effects:
Caution:
Not to be used for:
Not to be used with: LEVODOPA.
Contains: THIAMINE, RIBOFLAVINE, NICOTINAMIDE, PYRIDOXINE.
Other preparations: Becosym Syrup (not available on NHS), Becosym Forte Tablets (not available on NHS).

Becotide
(A & H)

An aerosol supplied at a strength of 50 micrograms, 100 micrograms and used as a corticosteroid to treat bronchial asthma.

Dose: adults 4 sprays of higher dose a day in 2-4 doses, up to 8 doses a day in severe cases; children 1-2 lower dose sprays a day.
Availability: NHS and private prescription.

Side effects: hoarseness, thrush.
Caution: in pregnant women, in patients transferring from systemic steroids, or in patients suffering from tubercular lungs.
Not to be used for:
Not to be used with:
Contains: BECLOMETHASONE.
Other preparations: BECLOFORTE (A & H), BECODISKS (A & H).

B

---

belladonna *see* Alophen, Aluhyde, Bellocarb, Carbellon

Bellocarb
(Sinclair)

A beige tablet used as an antacid and anti-spasm treatment for bowel spasm, ulcers, dyspepsia.

Dose: 1-2 tablets 4 times a day.
Availability: over the counter and private presecription.
Side effects: few; occasional constipation.
Caution: in patients with enlarged prostate, heart, kidney, or liver problems.
Not to be used for: patients suffering from glaucoma.
Not to be used with:
Contains: BELLADONNA, MAGNESIUM TRISILICATE, MAGNESIUM CARBONATE.
Other preparations:

Bendogen *see* Esbatal
(Lagap)

---

bendrofluazide *see also* Aprinox, Berkozide, Centyl, Centyl-K, Corgaretic 40, Inderetic, Neo-Naclex, Neo-Naclex-K, Prestim, Tenavoid

A white tablet or a white, scored tablet according to strengths of 2.5 mg, 5 mg used to treat fluid retention and high blood pressure.

Dose: heart failure 5-10 mg a day or every other day; high blood pressure 2.5-5 mg a day.
Availability: NHS
Side effects: low potassium levels, rash, sensitivity to light, blood changes, gout, tiredness
Caution: in pregnant women, nursing mothers, or in patients suffering from liver or kidney disease, diabetes, gout.
Not to be used for: for children or for patients suffering from kidney failure or severe kidney failure.
Not to be used with: DIGITALIS, LITHIUM, anti-hypertensives.
Contains:
Other preparations:

Benemid
(MSD)

A white, scored tablet supplied at a strength of 500 mg and used as a uric acid-lowering agent to to treat gout, hyperuricaemia.

Dose: $1/2$ tablet twice a day for the first 7 days then 1 tablet twice a day.
Availability: NHS and private prescription.
Side effects: headache, stomach upset, frequent urination, hypersensitivity, sore gums, flushes, acute gout, kidney stones, kidney colic.
Caution: in pregnant women and in patients with kidney disease or a history of peptic ulcer. Drink plenty of fluids.
Not to be used for: children, patients suffering from blood changes, kidney uric acid stones, or to start treatment during an acute attack.
Not to be used with: salicylates, PYRAZINAMIDE, sulphonylureas, sulphonamides, ß-lactam antibiotics, INDOMETHACIN, methotrexate.
Contains: PROBENECID.
Other preparations:

Benerva
(Roche)

A white tablet supplied in strengths of 25 mg, 50 mg, 100 mg, 300 mg and used as a source of vitamin B1 to treat beri-beri, neuritis.

Dose: 25-50 mg a day.
Availability: NHS (when prescribed as a generic), private prescription, over the counter.
Side effects:
Caution:
Not to be used for:
Not to be used with:
Contains: THIAMINE hydrochloride.
Other preparations: Benerva Compound.

Benoral
(Winthrop)

A white, oblong tablet supplied at a strength of 750 mg and used as an analgesic for the relief of pain, fever, rheumatoid arthritis, osteoarthritis, pain in bones or muscles.

Dose: 2 tablets 3 times a day.
Availability: NHS and private prescription.
Side effects: stomach upsets, allergy, asthma.
Caution: in the elderly, in pregnant women, and in patients with a history of allergy to aspirin or asthma, or who are suffering from impaired kidney or liver function, indigestion.
Not to be used for: children, nursing mothers, haemophiliacs, or patients suffering from ulcers.
Not to be used with: anti-coagulants (blood-thinning drugs), some anti-diabetic drugs, anti-inflammatory agents, METHOTREXATE, SPIRONOLACTONE, steroids, some antacids, some uric acid-lowering drugs.
Contains: BENORYLATE.
Other preparations: Benoral Suspension, Benoral Sachets.

---

benorylate *see* Benoral

Benoxyl 20
(Stiefel)

A lotion used as an anti-bacterial treatment for skin ulcers.

Dose: apply to the ulcers every 8-12 hours according to the size of the ulcer.
Availability: NHS and private prescription.
Side effects: allergic inflammation of the skin.
Caution: do not apply to the surrounding skin.
Not to be used for: treating the mucous membranes.
Not to be used with:
Contains: BENZOYL PEROXIDE.
Other preparations:

Benoxyl 5
(Stiefel)

A cream used as an anti-bacterial and skin softener to treat acne.

Dose: wash and dry the affected area, then apply once a day.
Availability: NHS, private prescription, over the counter.
Side effects: irritation, peeling.
Caution: keep out of the eyes, nose, and mouth.
Not to be used for:
Not to be used with:
Contains: BENZOYL PEROXIDE.
Other preparations: Benoxyl 5 with Sulphur, Benoxyl 10, Benoxyl 10 with Sulphur.

---

benperidol *see* Anquil

---

benserazide hydrochloride *see* Madopar

Bentex *see* Artane
(Steinhard)

---

benthiazide *see* Decaserpyl Plus

Benylin Expectorant
(Warner-Lambert)

A syrup used as an antihistamine, expectorant, and sputum softener to treat cough, bronchial congestion.

Dose: adults 1-2 5 ml teaspoonsful every 2-3 hours; children 1-5 years ½ teaspoonful every 3-4 hours, 6-12 years 1 teaspoonful every 3-4 hours.
Availability: private prescription and over the counter.
Side effects:
Caution:
Not to be used for: children under 1 year.
Not to be used with:
Contains: DIPHENHYDRAMINE HYDROCHLORIDE, AMMONIUM CHLORIDE, SODIUM CITRATE, MENTHOL.
Other preparations: Benylin Paediatric, Benylin Decongestant, Benylin with Codeine.

Benzagel
(Bioglan)

A white gel used as an anti-bacterial and skin softener to treat acne.

Dose: wash and dry the affected area, then apply 1-2 times a day.
Availability: NHS, private prescription, over the counter.
Side effects: irritation, peeling.
Caution: keep out of the eyes, nose, and mouth.
Not to be used for:
Not to be used with:
Contains: BENZOYL PEROXIDE.
Other preparations:

---

benzalkonium chloride *see* **Callusolve, Capitol, Conotrane, Drapolene, Ionax, Ionil T, Roccal, Timodine, Torbetol**

---

benzhexol *see* **Artane**

---

benzocaine *see* AAA Spray, Auralgicin, Auraltone, Intralgin, Medilave, Merocaine, Rybarvin, Transvasin, Tyrozets

B

benzoic acid *see* Aserbine, Malatex

benzoyl peroxide *see* Acetoxyl, Acnegel, Acnidazil, Benoxyl 20, Benoxyl 5, Benzagel, Nericur, Panoxyl, Quinoderm Cream, Quinoped, Theraderm

benzthiazide *see* Dytide

benztropine *see* Cogentin

benzydamine *see* Difflam, Difflam Oral Rinse

benzyl benzoate *see* Anugesic-HC, Anusol HC, Ascabiol

benzyl nicotinate *see* Bayolin, Salonair

bephenium hydroxy-naphthoate *see* Alcopar.

Berkamil *see* Amiloride
(Berk)

Berkatens *see* **Cordilox**

Berkmycen *see* **Tetracycline**
(Berk)

Berkolol *see* **Inderal**
(Berk)

Berkozide *see* **bendrofluazide**
(Berk)

Berotec
(Boehringer Ingelheim)

An aerosol supplied at a strength of 0.2 mg and used as a broncho-dilator to treat bronchial asthma, emphysema, bronchitis.

Dose: adults 1-2 sprays 3 times a day up to a maximum of 2 sprays every 4 hours; children 1 spray 3 times a day up to a maximum of 1 spray every 4 hours.
Availability: NHS and private prescription.
Side effects: headache, dilation of the blood vessels, nervous tension.
Caution: in pregnant women and in patients suffering from heart disease, angina, abnormal heart rhythms, high blood pressure, over-active thyroid gland.
Not to be used for:
Not to be used with: SYMPATHOMIMETICS.
Contains: FENOTEROL hydrobromide.
Other preparations: Berotec Solution.

Beta-Adalat
(Bayer)

A reddish-brown capsule used as an anti-hypertensive combination to treat high blood pressure, angina.

Dose: adults1 capsule a day increasing to 2 capsules a day if necessary; elderly no more than 1 capsule a day.
Availability: NHS and private prescription.
Side effects: flushing, headache, dizziness, dry eyes, skin rash, fluid retention, jaundice, gum swelling.
Caution: in patients under anaesthesia or those with weak heart, lung, kidney or liver disease, diabetes.
Not to be used for: children, pregnant women, nursing mothers, or for patients suffering from heart block, failure, or shock.
Not to be used with: CIMETIDINE, QUINIDINE, cardiodepressants.
Contains: ATENOLOL, NIFEDIPINE.
Other preparations: tenif (Stuart).

---

beta-blocker (ß-blocker)

a drug which blocks some of the effects of adrenaline in the body. Beta-blockers are used to treat angina, high blood pressure, and other conditions. Example PROPANOLOL *see* Inderal.

Beta-Cardone
(Duncan, Flockhart)

A green tablet, pink tablet, or white tablet according to strengths of 40 mg, 80 mg, 200 mg and used as a ß-blocker to treat angina, high blood pressure, and as an additional treatment for overactive thyroid.

Dose: 40 mg 3 times a day for 7 days, then 120-240 mg a day in single or divided doses. For angina 80 mg twice a day for 7-10 days, then 200-600 mg a day in single or divided doses. High blood pressure 80 mg twice a day for 7-10 days, then 200-600 mg a day. Overactive thyroid 120-240 mg a day.
Availability: NHS and private prescription.
Side effects: cold hands and feet, sleep disturbances, slow heart rate, tiredness, wheezing, heart failure, stomach upset.
Caution: in pregnant women, nursing mothers, and in patients suffering from diabetes, kidney or liver disorders, asthma. May need to be withdrawn before surgery. Withdraw gradually. Your doctor may

advise additional treatment with DIURETICS or digitalis.
Not to be used for: children or for patients suffering from heart block or failure, asthma.
Not to be used with: VERAPAMIL, CLONIDINE withdrawal, some anti-arrhythmic drugs and anaesthetics, some anti-hypertensives, ergot alkoloids, cimetidine, sedatives, SYMPATHOMIMETICS, INDOMETHACIN.
Contains: SOTALOL HYDROCHLORIDE.
Other preparations:

Betadine
(Napp)

A pessary and applicator supplied at a strength of 200 mg and used as an antiseptic to treat inflammation of the vagina.

Dose: 1 pessary to be inserted into the vagina night and morning for at least 14 days.
Availability: NHS, private prescription, over the counter.
Side effects: irritation and sensitivity.
Caution:
Not to be used for: children.
Not to be used with:
Contains: POVIDONE-IODINE.
Other preparations: Betadine Vaginal Gel, Betadine VC Kit.

Betadine Gargle and Mouthwash
(Napp)

A solution used as an antiseptic to treat inflammation of the mouth and pharynx brought on by thrush and other bacterial infections.

Dose: Wash out the mouth or gargle with the diluted or undiluted solution every 2-4 hours.
Availability: NHS, private prescription, over the counter.
Side effects: rarely local irritation and sensitivity.
Caution:
Not to be used for:
Not to be used with:
Contains: POVIDONE-IODINE.
Other preparations:

Betadine Ointment
(Napp)

An ointment used as an antiseptic to treat ulcers.

Dose: apply to the affected area and cover once a day.
Availability: NHS, private prescription, over the counter.
Side effects: rarely irritation.
Caution: in patients sensitive to iodine.
Not to be used for:
Not to be used with:
Contains: POVIDONE-IODINE.
Other preparations:

Betadine Scalp and Skin Cleanser
(Napp)

A solution used as an antiseptic and detergent to treat acne, seborrhoeic scalp and skin disorders.

Dose: use as a shampoo or apply directly ro the skin and then cleanse properly.
Availability: NHS, private prescription, over the counter.
Side effects: rarely irritation or sensitivity.
Caution:
Not to be used for:
Not to be used with:
Contains: POVIDONE-IODINE.
Other preparations: Betadine Skin Cleanser, Betadine Shampoo.

Betadine Spray
(Napp)

A spray used as an antiseptic to treat infected cuts, wounds, and burns.

Dose: spray on to the affected area once a day or as needed, and cover.
Availability: NHS, private prescription, over the counter.
Side effects:
Caution: keep out of the eyes.

Not to be used for: patients suffering from non-toxic colloid goitre.
Not to be used with:
Contains: POVIDONE-IODINE.
Other preparations: Betadine Dry Powder, Betadine Antiseptic Paint, Betadine Antiseptic Solution, Betadine Alcoholic Solution, Betadine Surgical Scrub.

B

betahistine dihydrochloride *see* Serc

betaine hydrochloride *see* Kloref

Betaloc
(Astra)

A white, scored tablet supplied at strengths of 50 mg, 100 mg and used as a ß-BLOCKER to treat angina, high blood pressure, and as additional treatment for overactive thyroid, migraine.

Dose: for angina 50-100 mg 2-3 times a day. High blood pressure 50 mg twice a day at first increasing to 400 mg a day if needed in 1 or 2 doses. Overactive thyroid 50 mg 4 times a day. Migraine 100-200 mg a day.
Availability: NHS and private prescription.
Side effects: cold hands and feet, sleep disturbances, slow heart rate, tiredness, wheezing, heart failure, stomach upset.
Caution: in pregnant women, nursing mothers, and in patients suffering from diabetes, kidney or liver disorders. May need to be withdrawn before surgery. Withdraw gradually. Your doctor may advise additional treatment with digitalis and DIURETICS.
Not to be used for: children or for patients suffering from heart block or failure, asthma.
Not to be used with: VERAPAMIL, CLONIDINE withdrawal, some anti-arrhythmic drugs and anaesthetics, some anti-hypertensives, ergot alkoloids, CIMETIDINE, sedatives, SYMPATHOMIMETICS, INDOMETHACIN.
Contains: METOPROLOL TARTRATE.
Other preparations: Betaloc injection, Betaloc-SA.

betamethasone *see* **Betnelan, Betnesol, Betnesol Drops, Betnovate, Betnovate Rectal, Bextasol, Diprosalic, Fucibet, Vista-Methasone**

betaxolol *see* **Betoptic, Kerlone**

bethanechol *see* **Myotonine**

Betim *see* **Blocadren**
(Leo)

Betnelan
(Glaxo)

A white, scored tablet supplied at a strength of 0.5 mg and used as a corticosteroid to treat severe asthma, allergies, rheumatoid arthritis, collagen diseases.

Dose: adults 1-10 tablets a day, then reduce as needed; children 1-7 years quarter to half adult dose, 7-12 years half to three-quarters adult dose.
Availability: NHS and private prescription.
Side effects: high blood sugar, thin bones, mood changes, ulcers.
Caution: in pregnant women, in patients who have had recent bowel surgery, or who are suffering from inflamed veins, psychiatric disorders, virus infections, some cancers, some kidney diseases, thinning of the bones, ulcers, tuberculosis, other infections, high blood pressure, glaucoma, epilepsy, diabetes, underactive thyroid, liver disease, stress. Withdraw gradually.
Not to be used for: infants under 1 year.
Not to be used with: PHENYTOIN, PHENOBARBITONE, EPHEDRINE, RIFAMPICIN, DIURETICS, ANTI-CHOLINESTERASES, DIGITALIS, anti-diabetic agents, anticoagulants, NON-STEROID ANTI-INFLAMMATORY DRUGS.
Contains: BETAMETHASONE.
Other preparations:

Betnesol
(Glaxo)

A pink, scored tablet supplied at a strength of 0.5 mg and used as a corticosteroid to treat severe asthma, allergies, rheumatoid arthritis, collagen diseases.

Dose: adults1-10 tablets a day, then reduce as needed; children 1-7 years quarter to half adult dose, 7-12 years half to three-quarters adult dose.
Availability: NHS and private prescription.
Side effects: high blood sugar, thin bones, mood changes, ulcers.
Caution: in pregnant women, in patients who have had recent bowel surgery, or who are suffering from inflamed veins, psychiatric disorders, virus infections, some cancers, some kidney diseases, thinning of the bones, ulcers, tuberculosis, other infections, high blood pressure, glaucoma, epilepsy, diabetes, underactive thyroid, liver disease, stress. Withdraw gradually.
Not to be used for: infants under 1 year.
Not to be used with: PHENYTOIN, PHENOBARBITONE, EPHEDRINE, RIFAMPICIN, DIURETICS, ANTI-CHOLINESTERASES, DIGITALIS, anti-diabetic agents, anticoagulants, NON-STEROID ANTI-INFLAMMATORY DRUGS.
Contains: BETAMETHASONE SODIUM PHOSPHATE.
Other preparations: Betnesol Injection, Betnesol-N, BETNESOL DROPS.

Betnesol Drops
(Glaxo)

Drops used as a corticosteroid to treat inflammation of the ear, nasal passages, or eyes where infection is not present.

Dose: 2-3 drops into each nostril 2-3 times a day, or 2-3 drops into the ear every 2-3 hours, or 1-2 drops into the eye every 1-2 hours.
Availability: NHS and private prescription.
Side effects: sensitivity, resistance to neomycin, thining of the cornea, cataract, rise in the eye pressure.
Caution: do not use for longer than is necessary especially in pregnancy.
Not to be used for: patients suffering from viral, tubercular, or fungal conditions of the nose, ear, or eye, dendritic ulcer, glaucoma, or where soft contact lenses are worn.
Not to be used with:

Contains: BETAMETHASONE SODIUM PHOSPHATE.
Other preparations: Betnesol-N, betnesol, Betnesol Ointment, Betnesol-N Ointment.

Betnovate
(Glaxo)

A cream used as a steroid to treat psoriasis, eczema, external ear and other skin disorders, dermatitis.

Dose: apply a small quantity of the cream to the affected area 2-3 times a day.
Availability: NHS and private prescription.
Side effects: fluid retention, suppression of adrenal glands, thinning of the skin may occur.
Caution: use for short periods of time only.
Not to be used for: patients suffering from acne or any other skin infections caused by tuberculosis, ringworm, viruses, or fungi, or continuously especially in pregnant women.
Not to be used with:
Contains: BETAMETHASONE valerate.
Other preparations: Betnovate RD, Betnovate Scalp Application, Betnovate-N, Betnovate-C, DIPROSONE (Kirby-Warrick), LOTRIDERM (Kirby-Warrick).

Betnovate Rectal
(Glaxo)

An ointment with applicator used as a steroid, local anaesthetic treatment for haemorrhoids and mild proctitis.

Dose: apply 2 or 3 times a day at first and then reduce.
Availability: NHS and private prescription.
Side effects: systemic corticosteroid effects.
Caution: do not use for prolonged periods; care for pregnant women.
Not to be used for: children or for patients suffering from tuberculous, bacterial, fungal, or viral infections.
Not to be used with:
Contains: BETAMETHASONE valerate, PHENYLEPHRINE hydrochloride, LIGNOCAINE hydrochloride.
Other preparations:

Betoptic
(Alcon)

Drops used as a ß-BLOCKER to treat hypertension of the eyes, glaucoma.

Dose: 1 drop into the eye twice a day.
Availability: NHS and private prescription.
Side effects: temporary discomfort, rarely reduction in the sensitivity of the cornea, reddening, staining, or inflammation of the cornea.
Caution: in patients with a history of blocked airways disease, diabetes, overactive thyroid, or who are under general anaesthetic.
Not to be used for: children, or for patients using soft contact lenses or suffering from some heart diseases.
Not to be used with:
Contains: BETAXOLOL hydrochloride.
Other preparations:

Bextasol
(Glaxo)

An aerosol supplied at a strength of100 micrograms and used as a corticosteroid to treat asthma.

Dose: 2 sprays 4 times a day at first, reducing if possible.
Availability: NHS and private prescription.
Side effects: thrush, hoarseness.
Caution: in pregnant women, in patients transferring from systemic steroids, and in patients suffering from fungal lung infections.
Not to be used for:
Not to be used with:
Contains: BETAMETHASONE valerate.
Other preparations:

---

bezafibrate *see* Bezalip-Mono

Bezalip-Mono
(MCP)

A white tablet supplied at a strength of 400 mg and used as a lipid-lowering drug to treat high blood lipids.

Dose: 1 tablet a day with or after evening meal.
Availability: NHS and private prescription.
Side effects: stomach upset, muscle aches.
Caution: in patients with kidney disease. Your doctor may advise change in diet or lifestyle.
Not to be used for: children, pregnant women, nusring mothers, or for patients suffering from severe kidney or liver disease.
Not to be used with: anti-coagulants.
Contains: BEZAFIBRATE.
Other preparations: Bezalip.

BiNovum
(Cilag)

A white tablet and a peach tablet used as a oestrogen, progestogen contraceptive.

Dose: 1 tablet a day for 21 days starting on day 1 of the period.
Availability: NHS and private prescription.
Side effects: enlarged breasts, bloating and fluid retention, cramps, leg pains, mood change, reduction in sexual desire, headaches, nausea, vaginal erosion, discharge, and bleeding, weight gain, skin changes.
Caution: in patients suffering from high blood pressure, diabetes, vascular disorders, asthma, depression, kidney disease, multiple sclerosis, womb diseases. Your doctor may advise you not to smoke, to have regular examinations. You should stop treatment at the first sign of serious symptoms such as severe headache or jaundice. Treatment should be stopped before surgery.
Not to be used for: pregnant women, or for patients suffering from sickle-cell anaemia, history of heart disease or thrombosis, liver disorders, some cancers, undiagnosed vaginal bleeding, some ear, skin, and kidney disorders.
Not to be used with: RIFAMPICIN, TETRACYCLINES, GRISEOFULVIN, BARBITU-RATES, PHENYTOIN, PRIMIDONE, CARBAMAZEPINE, ETHOSUXIMIDE, CHLORAL HYDRATE, DICHLORALPHENAZONE.
Contains: ETHINYLOESTRADIOL, NORETHISTERONE.
Other preparations:

Biogastrone
(Sterling Research Laboratories)

A white, scored tablet supplied at a strength of 50 mg and used as an anti-ulcer treatment for stomach ulcers.

Dose: 2 tablets 3 times a day after food for 7 days followed by reduced-dose maintenance therapy.
Availability: NHS and private prescription.
Side effects: fluid retention.
Caution: in the elderly or during pregnancy.
Not to be used for: patients with heart, kidney, or liver problems or low potassium levels.
Not to be used with: DIGITALIS.
Contains: CARBENOXOLONE.
Other preparations: Duogastrone for duodenal ulcers. Pyrogastrone containing ALUMINIUM HYDROXIDE, SODIUM ALGINATE, and POTASSIUM BICARBONATE, BIOPLEX (Thames) for mouth ulcers.

Biophylline
(Delandale)

A syrup used as a broncho-dilator to treat bronchial spasm.

Dose: adults 1-2 5 ml teaspoonsful every 6-8 hours; children 2-6 years $^{1}/_{2}$ 5 ml spoonful every 6-8 hours, 6-12 years $^{1}/_{2}$ -1 5 ml spoonful every 6-8 hours.
Availability: NHS, private prescription, over the counter.
Side effects: rapid heart rate, stomach upset, headache, sleeplessness, nausea, abnormal rhythms.
Caution: in the elderly, pregnant women, nursing mothers, and in patients suffering from heart or liver disease, or peptic ulcer.
Not to be used for:
Not to be used with: CIMETIDINE, ERYTHROMYCIN, CIPROFLOXACIN, INTERFERON.
Contains: THEOPHYLLINE hydrate.
Other preparations:

Bioplex *see* Biogastrone
(Thames)

Bioral
(Winthrop)

A gel used as a cell-surface protector to treat mouth ulcers.

Dose: apply after meals and at bed time.
Availability: NHS, private prescription, over the counter.
Side effects:
Caution:
Not to be used for:
Not to be used with:
Contains: CARBENOXOLONE sodium.
Other preparations:

Biorphen
(Bio-Medical)

A solution to be taken by mouth, supplied at a concentration of 25 mg/5 ml and used as an ANTI-CHOLINERGIC preparation to treat Parkinson's disease.

Dose: 6 5 ml spoonsful a day at first in divided doses increasing every 2-3 days by 1-2 spoonsful to up to 12 spoonsful a day.
Availability: NHS and private prescription.
Side effects: euphoria, anti-cholinergic effects, confusion, agitation, rash.
Caution: in patients with heart disorders or gastro-intestinal blockage. Dose should be reduced slowly.
Not to be used for: patients suffering from glaucoma, enlarged prostate, some movement disorders.
Not to be used with: PHENOTHIAZINES, antihistamines, anti-depressants.
Contains: ORPHENADRINE.
Other preparations:

---

biotin *see* Ketovite

---

biperiden hydrochloride *see* Akineton

bisacodyl *see* also Dulcolax

A tablet supplied at a strength of 5 mg and used as a stimulant to treat constipation.

Dose: children under 10 years 1 tablet at night, adults and children over 10 years 2 tablets at night.
Availability: NHS and private prescription.
Side effects:
Caution:
Not to be used for:
Not to be used with: no antacids should be taken within 1 hour.
Contains:
Other preparations: Bisacodyl Suppositories.

---

bismuth carbonate *see* APP

---

bismuth oxide *see* Anugesic-HC, Anusol, Anusol HC

---

bismuth subgallate *see* Anusol, Anusol HC

---

bismuth subnitrate *see* Roter

---

bisoprolol fumarate *see* Monocor

---

bisoprolol *see* Emcor

Blocadren
(MSD)

A blue, scored tablet supplied at a strength of 10 mg and used as a ß-BLOCKER to treat angina, high blood pressure, migraine.

Dose: $^1/_2$ tablet twice a day for 2 days, then 1 tablet twice a day. For angina $^1/_2$ tablet 2-3 times a day at first increasing if required by 1-1$^1/_2$ tablets a day every 3 days. For high blood pressure 1 tablet a day at first increasing to a maximum of 6 tablets a day if needed. For migraine 1-2 tablets twice a day.
Availability: NHS and private prescription.
Side effects: cold hands and feet, sleep disturbances, slow heart rate, tiredness, wheezing, heart failure, stomach upset.
Caution: in pregnant women, nursing mothers, and in patients suffering from diabetes, kidney or liver disorders. May need to be withdrawn before surgery. Withdraw gradually. Your doctor may advise additional treatment with digitalis and DIURETICS.
Not to be used for: children, or for patients suffering from heart block or failure, asthma.
Not to be used with: VERAPAMIL, CLONIDINE withdrawal, some anti-arrhythmic drugs and anaesthetics, some anti-hypertensives, ergot alkoloids, CIMETIDINE, sedatives, SYMPATHOMIMETICS, INDOMETHACIN.
Contains: TIMOLOL MALEATE.
Other preparations: BETIM (Leo).

Bocasan
(Oral-B)

A sachet of white granules used as a disinfectant to treat gingivitis, mouth infections.

Dose: dissolve a sachet of granules in warm water and rinse out the mouth 3 times a day after meals.
Availability: NHS, private prescription, over the counter.
Side effects:
Caution:
Not to be used for: patients suffering from kidney disease.
Not to be used with:
Contains: SODIUM PERBORATE MONOHYDRATE, SODIUM HYDROGEN TARTRATE.
Other preparations:

Bolvidon
(Organon)

A white tablet supplied at a strength of 10 mg and used as tetracyclic anti-depressant to treat depression.

Dose: adults 2-3 tablets a day at first, increasing gradually if needed to 3-9 tablets a day and up to a maximum of 20 tablets a day; elderly up to 3 tablets a day at first.
Availability: NHS and private prescription.
Side effects: drowsiness, bone marrow depression, possibility of jaudice, hypomania or convulsions when the drug should be withdrawn.
Caution: in pregnant women and in patients suffering from heart attacks. Your doctor may advise regular blood tests.
Not to be used for: children, nursing mothers, or for patients suffering from mania or severe liver disease.
Not to be used with: MAOIS, alcohol.
Contains: MIANSERIN HYDROCHLORIDE.
Other preparations:

---

boric acid *see* **Phytex**

---

borneol *see* **Rowachol, Rowatinex**

Bradilan
(Napp)

A white tablet supplied at a strength of 250 mg and used as a vasodilator to treat peripheral vascular problems including intermittent difficulty walking, night cramps, chilblains, Raynaud's phenomenon (spasm of the arteries), some brain disorders.

Dose: 2-4 tablets 3 times a day.
Availability: NHS and private prescription.
Side effects: flushes.
Caution:
Not to be used for: children.
Not to be used with:
Contains: NICOFURANOSE.
Other preparations:

Bradosol
(Ciba)

A white lozenge   supplied at a strength of 0.5 mg and used as a disinfectant to treat infections of the mouth and throat.

Dose: 1 lozenge to be sucked every 2-3 hours.
Availability: NHS, private prescription, over the counter.
Side effects:
Caution:
Not to be used for:
Not to be used with:
Contains: DOMIPHEN BROMIDE.
Other preparations: Bradosol Plus.

---

bran *see* Fybranta

Brasivol
(Stiefel)

A paste used as an abrasive to treat acne.

Dose: wet the area then rub in vigorously for 15-20 seconds, rinse and repeat 1-3 times a day.
Availability: NHS, private prescription, over the counter.
Side effects:
Caution:
Not to be used for: patients suffering from visible superficial arteries or veins on the skin.
Not to be used with:
Contains: ALUMINIUM OXIDE.
Other preparations:

Brevinor
(Syntex)

A white tablet used as an oestrogen, progestogen contraceptive.

Dose: 1 tablet a day for 21 days starting on day 5 of the period.
Availability: NHS and private prescription.

Side effects: enlarged breasts, bloating and fluid retention, cramps, leg pains, mood change, reduction in sexual desire, headaches, nausea, vaginal erosion, discharge, and bleeding, weight gain, skin changes.

Caution: in patients suffering from high blood pressure, diabetes, vascular disorders, asthma, depression, kidney disease, multiple sclerosis, womb diseases. Your doctor may advise you not to smoke, to have regular examinations. You should stop treatment at the first sign of serious symptoms such as severe headache or jaundice. Treatment should be stopped before surgery.

Not to be used for: pregnant women, or for patients suffering from sickle-cell anaemia, history of heart disease or thrombosis, liver disorders, some cancers, undiagnosed vaginal bleeding, some ear, skin, and kidney disorders.

Not to be used with: RIFAMPICIN, TETRACYCLINES, GRISEOFULVIN, barbiturates, PHENYTOIN, PRIMIDONE, CARBAMAZEPINE, ETHOSUXIMIDE, CHLORAL HYDRATE, DICHLORALPHENAZONE.

Contains: ETHINYLOESTRADIOL, NORETHISTERONE.

Other preparations:

Bricanyl
(Astra)

A white, scored tablet supplied at a strength of 5 mg and used as a broncho-dilator to treat bronchial spasm brought on by asthma, bronchitis, or emphysema.

Dose: adults 1 tablet twice a day or every 8 hours; children under 7 years use syrup, 7-15 years half adult dose.

Availability: NHS and private prescription.

Side effects: shaking of the hands, dilation of the blood vessels, tension, headache.

Caution: in pregnant women and in diabetics, or in patients suffering from high blood pressure, abnormal heart rhythms, heart muscle disorders, overactive thyroid gland, angina.

Not to be used for:

Not to be used with: SYMPATHOMIMETICS.

Contains: TERBUTALINE SULPHATE.

Other preparations: Bricanyl SA, Bricanyl Syrup, Bricanyl Inhaler, Bricanyl Spacer Inhaler, Bricanyl Refill Canister, Bricanyl Turboinhaler, Bricanyl Respirator Solution, Bricanyl Resules, Bricanyl Injection.

Bricanyl Expectorant
(Astra)

A solution used as a broncho-dilator and expectorant to treat bronchial spasm, congestion.

Dose: 2-3 5 ml teaspoonsful every 8 hours.
Availability: private prescription only.
Side effects: shaking of hands, dilation of the blood vessels, tension, headache.
Caution: in patients with impaired cardiovascular system, or suffering from high blood pressure.
Not to be used for: children.
Not to be used with: MAOIS, TRICYCLICS, SYMPATHOMIMETICS.
Contains: TERBUTALINE SULPHATE, GUAIPHENESIN.
Other preparations: Bricanyl Compound.

---

brilliant green *see* Variclene

Britiazim
(Thames)

A white tablet supplied at a strength of 60 mg and used as a calcium antagonist to treat angina.

Dose: 1 tablet 3 times a day increasing if required to up to 6 a day in divided doses; elderly 1 twice a day at first.
Availability: NHS and private prescription.
Side effects: slow heart rate, fluid retention, nausea, rash, headache.
Caution: your doctor may advise regular monitoring of heart rate, especially in elderly patients or in patients suffering from kidney or liver problems.
Not to be used for: for children or for pregnant women, or in patients suffering from severe heart conduction defects.
Not to be used with: ß-BLOCKERS, DIGITALIS.
Contains: DILTIAZEM HYDROCHLORIDE.
Other preparations:

Brocadopa *see* **Larodopa**
(Brocades)

Broflex *see* **Artane**
(Bio-Medical)

bromazepam *see* **Lexotan**

bromocriptine mesylate *see* **Parlodel**

brompheniramine *see* **Dimotane Expectorant, Dimotane Plus, Dimotapp LA**

Bronchilator
(Sterling Research Laboratories)

An aerosol used as a broncho-dilator to treat bronchial spasm brought on by chronic bronchitis or bronchial asthma.

Dose: 1-2 sprays then again after 30 minutes if required up to a maximum of 16 sprays in 24 hours.
Availability: NHS and private prescription.
Side effects: abnormal heart rhythms, rapid heart rate, headache, dilation of the blood vessels.
Caution: in patients suffering from diabetes.
Not to be used for: children or for patients suffering from cardiac asthma, heart disease, high blood pressure, overactive thyroid gland.
Not to be used with: MAOIS, TRICYCLICS.
Contains: ISOETHARINE MESYLATE, PHENYLEPHRINE HYDROCHLORIDE.
Other preparations:

Bronchodil
(Degussa)

An aerosol supplied at a strength of 0.5 mg and used as a broncho-dilator to treat bronchial asthma, bronchitis, emphysema.

Dose: adults 1-2 sprays every 3-6 hours; children over 6 years 1 spray every 3-6 hours.
Availability: NHS and private prescription.
Side effects: shaking of hands, nervous tension, headache, dilation of the blood vessels.
Caution: in pregnant women and in patients suffering from heart muscle disorders, angina, high blood pressure, abnormal heart rhythms, overactive thyroid gland.
Not to be used for: children under 6 years.
Not to be used with: SYMPATHOMIMETICS.
Contains: REPROTEROL HYDROCHLORIDE.
Other preparations: Bronchodil Tablets, Bronchodil Respirator Solution.

Brovon
(Torbet)

A solution used as a broncho-dilator to treat bronchial spasm brought on by chronic bronchitis, bronchial asthma, emphysema.

Dose: inhale 1-2 times a day and once at night.
Availability: NHS, private prescription, over the counter.
Side effects: nervousness, tremor, dry mouth, abnormal heart rhythms.
Caution: in patients suffering from diabetes.
Not to be used for: children or for patients suffering from heart disease, high blood pressure, overactive thyroid gland.
Not to be used with: SYMPATHOMIMETICS.
Contains: ADRENALINE, ATROPINE METHONITRATE, PAPAVERINE HYDROCHLORIDE.
Other preparations:

Broxil
(S K B)

An ivory/black capsule supplied at a strength of 250 mg and used as a penicillin treatment for infections.

Dose: adults 1 capsule 4 times a day $1/2$-1 hour before meals; children (using syrup) under 2 years quarter adult dose, over 2 years half adult dose.
Availability: NHS and private prescription.
Side effects: allergy, stomach disturbances.
Caution:
Not to be used for: for patients suffering from penicillin allergy.
Not to be used with:
Contains: PHENETHICILLIN POTASSIUM.
Other preparations: Broxil Syrup.

Brufen
(Boots)

A magenta-coloured, oval tablet supplied at strengths of 200 mg, 400 mg, 600 mg and used as a NON-STEROID ANTI-INFLAMMATORY DRUG to treat pain, rheumatoid arthritis, ankylosing spondylitis, osteoarthritis, sero-negative arthritis, peri-articular disorders, soft tissue injuries.

Dose: adults 1200-1800 mg a day in divided doses, to a maximum of 2400 mg a day; children 20 mg per kg body weight a day.
Availability: NHS and private prescription.
Side effects: dyspepsia, stomach bleeding, rash, rarely low blood platelet levels.
Caution: in pregnant women, or in patients suffering from asthma or allergy to aspirin or anti-inflammatory drugs.
Not to be used for: patients suffering from peptic ulcer.
Not to be used with:
Contains: IBUPROFEN.
Other preparations: APSIFEN (APS), EBUFAC (DDSA), LIDIFEN (Berk), MOTRIN (Upjohn), PAXOFEN (Steinhard).

Buccastem
(Reckitt & Colman)

A pale-yellow tablet supplied at a strength of 3 mg and used as an antihistamine treatment for vertigo as a result of Ménière's disease or labyrinthitis, nausea, vomiting, migraine.

Dose: 1-2 tablets twice a day allowed to dissolve between the upper lip and gum.
Availability: NHS and private prescription.
Side effects: low blood pressure especially in elderly or dehydrated patients, drowsiness, ANTICHOLINERGIC effects, sleeplessness, skin reactions.
Caution: in pregnant women or nursing mothers.
Not to be used for: children or for patients suffering from kidney or liver disease, blood changes, epilepsy, Parkinson's disease, prostate enlargement, glaucoma.
Not to be used with: alcohol, sedatives, alpha-blockers.
Contains: PROCHLORPERAZINE MALEATE.
Other preparations:

---

buclizine hydrochloride *see* Migraleve

---

budesonide *see* Pulmicort, Rhinocort

---

bumetanide *see* Burinex, Burinex K

---

buprenorphine *see* Temgesic

Burinex
(Leo)

A white, scored tablet supplied at strengths of 1 mg, 5 mg and used as a DIURETIC to treat fluid retention associated with congestive heart failure, liver and kidney disease, including the nephrotic syndrome.

Dose: 1 mg a day according to patient's response.
Availability: NHS and private prescription.
Side effects: low blood potassium, stomach discomfort, rash, cramps,

blood changes, breast enlargement.

Caution: in pregnant women, nursing mothers, and in patients suffering from kidney or liver damage, diabetes, gout, enlarged prostate, or impaired urination. Your doctor may advise that potassium supplements may be needed.

Not to be used for: children or patients suffering from cirrhosis of the liver.

Not to be used with: LITHIUM, DIGITALIS, anti-hypertensives, aminoglycosides.

Contains: BUMETANIDE.

Other preparations: Burinex Liquid, Burinex Injection, BURINEX K.

Burinex K
(Leo)

A white, egg-shaped tablet used as a DIURETIC/potassium supplement to treat fluid retention associated with congestive heart failure, liver disease, and kidney disease where potassium supplement is required.

Dose: 1-4 tablets a day.

Availability: NHS and private prescription.

Side effects: rash, cramps, stomach discomfort, blood changes, breast enlargement.

Caution: in pregnant women, nursing mothers, and in patients suffering from enlarged prostate, or impaired urination, kidney or liver disease, gout, diabetes.

Not to be used for: children, or for patients suffering from raised potassium levels, Addison's disease, liver cirrhosis.

Not to be used with: LITHIUM, DIGITALIS, anti-hypertensives, aminoglycosides

Contains: BUMETANIDE, POTASSIUM CHLORIDE.

Other preparations:

Buscopan
(Boehringer Ingelheim)

A white tablet supplied at a strength of 10 mg and used as an anti-spasm treatment for bowel spasm, painful periods.

Dose: adults painful periods 2 tablets 4 times a day for 5 days starting 2 days before the period begins; children bowel spasm 6-12 years 1 tablet 3 times a day, adults 2 tablets 4 times a day.
Availability: NHS and private prescription.
Side effects: blurred vision, confusion, dry mouth.
Caution:
Not to be used for: patients with glaucoma, inflammatory bowel disease, intestinal obstruction, or enlarged prostate.
Not to be used with:
Contains: HYOSCINE BUTYLBROMIDE.
Other preparations: Buscopan Injection.

---

buserelin *see* Suprefact

Buspar
(Bristol-Myers)

A white, oval tablet supplied at a strength of 5 mg and used as a tranquillizer for the short-term treatment of anxiety.

Dose: 1 tablet 2-3 times a day increasing every 2-3 days to a maximum of 9 tablets a day.
Availability: NHS and private prescription.
Side effects: dizziness, headache, nervousness, rarely rapid heart rate, chest pain, confusion, dry mouth, tiredness.
Caution: in patients with a history of kidney or liver disease.
Not to be used for: children, pregnant women, nursing mothers, or for patients suffering from severe kidney or liver disease, epilepsy.
Not to be used with:
Contains: BUSPIRONE HYDROCHLORIDE.
Other preparations:

---

buspirone *see* Buspar

---

butethamate citrate *see* CAM

---

butobarbitone *see* **Soneryl**

---

butoxethyl nicontinate *see* **Actinac**

C

butoxyethyl nicotinate *see* **Finalgon**

---

butryptiline *see* **Evadyne**

---

cade oil *see* **Polytar Liquid**

---

cadexomer iodine *see* **Iodosorb**

Cafadol
(Typharm)

A yellow, scored tablet used as an analgesic to relieve pain including period pain.

Dose: adults 2 tablets every 3-4 hours; children 5-12 years half adult dose.
Availability: private prescription and over the counter.
Side effects:
Caution: in patients with liver or kidney disease.
Not to be used for: children under 5 years.
Not to be used with:
Contains: PARACETAMOL, CAFFEINE.
Other preparations:

Cafergot
(Sandoz)

99

A white tablet used as an ergot preparation to treat migraine.

Dose: 1-2 tablets at the beginning of a migraine attack to a maximum of 4 tablets a day or 10 tablets a week.
Availability: NHS and private prescription.
Side effects: nausea, muscular pain, reduced circulation, weak legs.
Caution:
Not to be used for: children, pregnant women, nursing mothers, or in patients suffering from coronary, peripheral, or occlusive vascular disease, severe high blood pressure, kidney or liver disease, sepsis.
Not to be used with: ERYTHROMYCIN, ß-BLOCKERS.
Contains: ERGOTAMINE tartrate, CAFFEINE.
Other preparations:

---

caffeine *see* **Antoin, Cafadol, Cafergot, Doloxene Co., Glykola, Hypon, Labiton, Migril, Parahypon, Pardale, Propain, Solpadeine, Syndol, Uniflu and Gregovite C**

Calabren *see* **Daonil**
(Berk)

Calcichew
(Shire)

A white, chewable tablet supplied at a strength of 500 mg and used as a calcium supplement to treat calcium deficiency.

Dose: 1 tablet chewed 3 times a day.
Availability: NHS, private prescription, over the counter.
Side effects: constipation, wind.
Caution:
Not to be used for: children or for patients suffering from overactive parathyroid glands, severe kidney disease, decalcifying tumours.
Not to be used with: TETRACYCLINES.
Contains: CALCIUM CARBONATE.
Other preparations:

---

calciferol *see* **Abidec, Calcimax, Chocovite, Concavit, Multivite, Orovite 7, Polyvite, Pregnavite Forte F, Tonivitan**

Calcimax
(Wallace)

A brown syrup used as a calcium and vitamin supplement to treat calcium deficiency where vitamins are also needed.

Dose: adults 4 5 ml teaspoonsful 2-3 times a day; children 1-2 5 ml teaspoonsful 3 times a day.
Availability: private prescription and over the counter.
Side effects:
Caution:
Not to be used for: children or for patients suffering from overactive parathyroid glands, severe kidney disease, decalcifying tumours.
Not to be used with:
Contains: CALCIUM GLYCINE HYDROCHLORIDE, CALCIFEROL, THIAMINE, RIBOFLAVINE, PYRIDOXINE, CYANOCOBALAMIN, NICOTINAMIDE, CALCIUM PANTOTHENATE.
Other preparations:

Calcisorb
(3M Riker)

A powder in a sachet of 4.7 g and used as an ion-exchange compound to treat raised calcium levels in the urine, recurring kidney stones, osteopetrosis.

Dose: adults 1 sachet dispersed in water with meals or sprinkled on to food 3 times a day; children 2 sachets a day in 3 divided doses with food.
Availability: NHS, private prescription, over the counter.
Side effects: diarrhoea.
Caution: treatment of children should be monitored, and the treatment should be accompanied by a low-calcium diet with foods rich in oxalates.
Not to be used for: pregnant women, nursing mothers, or for patients suffering from kidney disease, congestive heart disease, or any other conditions in which a low-sodium diet is needed.
Not to be used with:

Contains: SODIUM CELLULOSE PHOSPHATE.
Other preparations:

calcitriol *see* **Rocaltrol**

calcium carbonate *see* **APP, Citrical, Calcichew, Gaviscon, Titralac**

calcium chloride *see* **Glandosane**

calcium folinate *see* **Refolinon, Rescufolin**

calcium gluconate *see* **Chocovite**

calcium glycerophosphate *see* **Glykola, Metatone, Tonivitan A & D, Tonivitan B, Verdiviton**

calcium glycine hydrochloride *see* **Calcimax**

calcium hydrogen phosphate *see* **Octovit**

calcium lactate gluconate *see* **Sandocal**

calcium oxytetracycline *see* **Trimovate**

calcium pantothenate *see* **Allbee with C, BC 500, BC 500 with Iron, Calcimax, Concavit, Ketovite, Polyvite**

calcium phosphate *see* **Pregnavite Forte F**

calcium polystyrene *see* **Calcium Resonium**

Calcium Resonium
(Winthrop)

A powder used as an ion-exchange resin to treat raised potassium levels.

Dose: adults 15 g 3-4 times a day; children 1 g per kg body weight a day in divided doses.
Availability: NHS, private prescription, over the counter.
Side effects: hypercalcaemia (raised calcium levels).
Caution: potassium and calcium levels should be checked.
Not to be used for: for patients suffering from overactive parathyroid glands, multiple myeloma (a bone marrow tumour), sarcoidosis (a disease causing raised calcium levels), certain forms of cancer with kidney failure and hypercalcaemia (raised calcium levels).
Not to be used with:
Contains: CALCIUM POLYSTYRENE SULPHONATE.
Other preparations:

calcium sulphaloxate *see* **Enteromide**

Callusolve
(Dermal)

A paint used as a skin softener to treat warts.

Dose: apply 4-5 drops of the paint to the wart, cover for 24 hours, rub

away the treated part, and repeat the process.
Availability: NHS, private prescription, over the counter.
Side effects:
Caution: apply only to warts and avoid healthy skin.
Not to be used for: for treating warts on the face or anal and genital areas.
Not to be used with:
Contains: BENZALKONIUM CHLORIDE-BROMINE.
Other preparations:

Calmurid HC
(Pharmacia)

A cream used as a steroid, wetting agent and skin softener to treat dry hyperkeratotic eczema and other skin disorders.

Dose: wash and dry the affected area, and apply twice a day.
Availability: NHS and private prescription.
Side effects: fluid retention, suppression of adrenal glands, thinning of the skin may occur.
Caution: use for short periods of time only.
Not to be used for: patients suffering from acne or any other skin infections caused by tuberculosis, ringworm, viruses, or fungi, or continuously especially in pregnant women.
Not to be used with:
Contains: HYDROCORTISONE, UREA, LACTIC ACID.
Other preparations:

Calpol Infant
(Calmic)

A suspension supplied at a strength of 120 mg/ 5 ml teaspoonful and used as an analgesic to relieve pain.

Dose: 3 months- 1 year $^1/_2$-1 5 ml teaspoonful 4 times a day; 1-6 years 1-2 5 ml teaspoonsful 4 times a day.
Availability: NHS and private prescription.
Side effects:
Caution: in patients suffering from kidney or liver disease.
Not to be used for: infants under 3 months.

Not to be used with:
Contains: PARACETAMOL.
Other preparations: Calpol Six Plus (prescribed as a generic), PALDESIC (RP Drugs), PANALEVE (Leo).

Calthor
(Wyeth)

A white, scored tablet supplied at strengths of 250 mg, 500 mg and used as a broad-spectrum penicillin to treat respiration and skin infections, ear infections, urinary infections.

Dose: adults 1-2 g a day in 3-4 divided doses; children over 2 months (using suspension) 50-100 mg a day in 3-4 divided doses.
Availability: NHS and private prescription.
Side effects: allergy, stomach disturbances.
Caution: in patients suffering from kidney disease.
Not to be used for: patients suffering from penicillin allergy.
Not to be used with:
Contains: CICLACILLIN.
Other preparations: Calthor Suspension.

CAM
(Rybar)

A syrup used as a broncho-dilator to treat bronchial spasm.

Dose: adults 4 5 ml teaspoonsful 3-4 times a day; children under 2 years $1/2$ teaspoonful 3-4 times a day, 2-4 years 1 teaspoonful 3-4 times a day, over 4 years 2 teaspoonsful 3-4 times a day.
Availability: NHS, private prescription, over the counter.
Side effects: nervousness, sleeplessness, restlessness, dry mouth, cold hands and feet, abnormal heart rhythms.
Caution: in patients suffering from diabetes.
Not to be used for: patients suffering from heart disease, high blood pressure, overactive thyroid gland.
Not to be used with: MAOIS
Contains: EPHEDRINE HYDROCHLORIDE, BUTETHAMATE CITRATE.
Other preparations:

Camcolit
(Norgine)

A white, scored tablet supplied at strengths of 250 mg, 400 mg and used as a lithium salt to treat mania, manic depression, aggressive and self-injuring behaviour.

Dose: your doctor may advise a blood test to check correct dose.
Availability: NHS and private prescription.
Side effects: nausea, diarrhoea, shaking hands, muscular weakness, brain and heart disturbances, weight gain, fluid retention, overactive or underactive thyroid gland, thirst, frequent urination, skin reactions.
Caution: patients should be treated in hospital at first.
Not to be used for: children, pregnant women, nursing mothers, or for patients suffering from kidney or heart disease, Addison's disease, underactive thyroid gland, disturbed sodium balance.
Not to be used with: DIURETICS, NON-STEROID ANTI-INFLAMMATORY DRUGS, CARBAMAZEPINE, FLUPENTHIXOL, METHYLDOPA, PHENYTOIN, HALOPERIDOL.
Contains: LITHIUM CARBONATE.
Other preparations:

Camoquin
(Parke-Davis)

A yellow, scored tablet supplied at a strength of 200 mg and used as an anti-malarial treatment for acute malaria.

Dose: adults one dose of 3 tablets, or 3 tablets once a day for 3 days according to immunity; children under 15 years 10 mg per kg body weight as one dose, or 10 mg per kg body weight once a day for 3 days according to immunity.
Availability: NHS and private prescription.
Side effects: blood changes, liver disease, nausea, diarrhoea. lethargy, eye disorders, nerve changes, colouring of skin and nails.
Caution: your doctor may advise that eyes, blood, and liver function should be checked regularly.
Not to be used for:
Not to be used with: other malaria drugs.
Contains: AMODIAQUINE HYDROCHLORIDE.
Other preparations:

---

camphene *see* Rowachol, Rowatinex

---

camphor oil *see* Aradolene, Aspellin, Balmosa, Salonair

Canesten
(Baypharm)

A solution used as an anti-fungal treatment for fungal inflammation and infection of the outer ear, skin, and nails.

Dose: 2-3 applications a day until 14 days after the symptoms have gone.
Availability: NHS, private prescription, over the counter.
Side effects: local irritation.
Caution:
Not to be used for:
Not to be used with:
Contains: CLOTRIMAZOLE, POLYETHYLENE GLYCOL SOLUTION.
Other preparations: Canesten Spray, Canesten Powder.

Canesten 1
(Baypharm)

A white, vaginal tablet plus applicator supplied at a strength of 500 mg and used as an anti-fungal, anti-bacterial treatment for vaginal infections.

Dose: 1 tablet inserted into the vagina at night.
Availability: NHS and private prescription
Side effects: mild burning or irritation.
Caution:
Not to be used for: children.
Not to be used with:
Contains: CLOTRIMAZOLE.
Other preparations: Canesten 10% VC, Canesten Vaginal Tablets, Canesten Cream, Canesten Duopak, Canesten Vaginal Cream.

Canesten-HC
(Bayer)

A cream used as a steroid, anti-fungal, anti-bacterial treatment for fungal skin infections where there is also inflammation.

Dose: apply to the affected area twice a day.
Availability: NHS and private prescription.
Side effects: fluid retention, suppression of adrenal glands, thinning of the skin may occur.
Caution: use for short periods of time only.
Not to be used for: patients suffering from acne or any other skin infections caused by tuberculosis, ringworm, viruses, or fungi, or continuously especially in pregnant women.
Not to be used with:
Contains: CLOTRIMAZOLE, HYDROCORTISONE.
Other preparations:

Cantil
(MCP)

A yellow tablet supplied at a strength of 25 mg and used as an anti-spasm treatment for bowel spasm.

Dose: children 6-12 years 5 ml 3 or 4 times a day; adults 1-2 tablets 3 or 4 times a day.
Availability: NHS and private prescription.
Side effects: blurred vision.
Caution: enlarged prostate gland.
Not to be used for: patients suffering from glaucoma.
Not to be used with:
Contains: MEPENZOLATE BROMIDE.
Other preparations: Cantil Elixir (liquid).

Capitol
(Dermal)

A gel used as an anti-bacterial treatment for dandruff and other similar scalp disorders.

Dose: use as a shampoo.

Availability: NHS, private prescription, over the counter.
Side effects:
Caution:
Not to be used for:
Not to be used with:
Contains: BENZALKONIUM CHLORIDE.
Other preparations:

Caplenal *see* Zyloric
(Berk)

Capoten
(Squibb)

A mottled white, scored tablet, a mottled white, square tablet, or a mottled white, oval tablet according to strengths of 12.5 mg, 25 mg, 50 mg and used as an ACE INHIBITOR in addition to DIURETICS and digitalis in the treatment of severe congestive heart failure, high blood pressure.

Dose: adults 6.25 mg or 12.5 mg at first then 25 mg 3 times a day up to a maximum of 150 mg a day; children as advised by physician. For moderate to mild high blood pressure 12.5 mg a day then 25 mg twice a week increasing to 50 mg twice a day at 2-4 week intervals if needed. Severe high blood pressure 12.5 mg twice a day at first, then 50 mg 3 times a day if needed.
Availability: NHS and private prescription.
Side effects: rash, loss of taste, rarely a cough, blood changes, protein in the urine.
Caution: in patients suffering from kidney disease, auto-immune diseases, or patients undergoing anaesthesia, immune suppressant treatment, or who are taking leucopenic drugs. Your doctor may advise regular blood tests.
Not to be used for: pregnant women, nursing mothers, or for patients suffering from some heart valve diseases , kidney disease.
Not to be used with: potassium-sparing diuretics, potassium supplements, NON-STEROID ANTI-INFLAMMATORY DRUGS, vasodilators, CLO-NIDINE, ALLOPURINOL, PROCAINAMIDE, PROBENECID, immunosuppressants.
Contains: CAPTOPRIL.
Other preparations: ACEPRIL (Duncan, Flockhart).

Capozide
(Squibb)

A white, scored tablet used as a DIURETIC/ACE INHIBITOR combination to treat high blood pressure.

Dose: 1-2 tablets a day.
Availability: NHS and private prescription.
Side effects: protein in the urine, low blood pressure, rash, loss of taste, blood changes, sensitivity to light, tiredness, rarely a cough.
Caution: in patients undergoing anaesthesia, immune suppressant treatment, or leucopenic drugs and those suffering from kidney disease, auto-immune diseases, diabetes, gout, liver disease.
Not to be used for: children, pregnant women, nursing mothers or for patients suffering from some heart valve diseases, kidney disease.
Not to be used with: LITHIUM, sulphonamides, NON-STEROID ANTI-INFLAMMATORY DRUGS, ALLOPURINOL, PROCAINAMIDE, PROBENECID, immunosuppressants, vasodilators, CLONIDINE, potassium-sparing diuretics, potassium supplements, anti-hypertensives.
Contains: CAPTOPRIL, HYDROCHLOROTHIAZIDE.
Other preparations:

Caprin
(Sinclair)

A pink tablet supplied at a strength of 324 mg and used as an analgesic to treat rheumatic and associated conditions.

Dose: 3 tablets 3-4 times a day.
Availability: NHS, private prescription, over the counter.
Side effects: stomach upsets, allergy, asthma.
Caution: in the elderly, pregnant women, patients with a history of allergy to aspirin or asthma, or who are suffering from impaired liver or kidney function.
Not to be used for: children, nursing mothers, or patients suffering from haemophilia or ulcers.
Not to be used with: anti-coagulants, some anti-diabetic drugs, anti-inflammatory drugs, METHOTREXATE, SPIRONOLACTONE, steroids, some antacids, some uric acid lowering drugs.
Contains: ASPIRIN.
Other preparations:

---

capsicum oleoresin *see* **Aradolene, Balmosa, Cremalgin**

captopril *see* **Capoten, Capozide**

Carace
(Morson)

A blue, oval tablet, a white, oval, scored tablet, a yellow, oval, scored tablet, or an orange, oval, scored tablet according to strengths of 2.5 mg, 5 mg, 10 mg, 20 mg and used as an ACE INHIBITOR to treat congestive heart failure in addition to DIURETICS and/or digitalis; high blood pressure.

Dose: 2.5 mg once a day at first, increasing to 5-20 mg a day over 2-4 weeks. For high blood pressure 2.5 mg once a day at first, increasing to 10-20 mg once a day and a maximum of 40 mg a day.
Availability: NHS and private prescirption.
Side effects: low blood pressure, kidney failure, swelling, rash, dizziness, headache, diarrhoea, cough, tiredness, palpitations, chest pains, weakness.
Caution: in nursing mothers and in patients suffering from kidney disease.
Not to be used for: children, pregnant women, or for patients suffering from some heart valve or lung diseases.
Not to be used with: potassium-sparing diuretics, potassium supplements, INDOMETHACIN.
Contains: LISINOPRIL.
Other preparations:

Carbachol
(Alcon)

Drops used as a cholinergic and lubricant treatment for glaucoma.

Dose: 2 drops into the eye 3 times a day.
Availability: NHS and private prescription.
Side effects:
Caution:

Not to be used for: children or for patients suffering from damaged cornea, acute iritis, or who wear soft contact lenses.
Not to be used with:
Contains: CARBACHOL, HYPROMELLOSE.
Other preparations:

C Carbalax
(Pharmax)

A suppository used to treat constipation, local anal conditions.

Dose: 1 suppository 30 minutes before evacuation required.
Availability: NHS and private prescription.
Side effects:
Caution:
Not to be used for: children.
Not to be used with:
Contains: SODIUM BICARBONATE, ANYHDROUS SODIUM ACID PHOSPHATE.
Other preparations:

---

carbamazepine *see* Tegretol

---

carbaryl *see* Carylderm, Derbac Shampoo, Suleo-C

---

carbaryl *see* Clinicide

Carbellon
(Torbet)

A black tablet used as an anti-spasm, anti-wind, antacid preparation to treat acidity, ulcers, food poisoning.

Dose: children 1-3 tablets a day; adults 2-4 tablets 3 times a day.
Availability: over the counter and private prescription.

Side effects: few; occasionally constipation.
Caution:
Not to be used for: glaucoma, pyloric stenosis, enlarged prostate.
Not to be used with:
Contains: BELLADONNA, MAGNESIUM HYDROXIDE, CHARCOAL, PEPPERMINT OIL.
Other preparations:

carbenoxolone *see* Biogastrone, Bioplex, Bioral

carbidopa monohydrate *see* Sinemet

carbimazole *see* Neo-Mercazole

carbinoxamine *see* Davenol

Carbo-Cort
(Lagap)

A cream used as a steroid, anti-psoriatic treatment for eczema, lichen planus (a rare skin disorder).

Dose: apply to the affected area 2-3 times a day.
Availability: NHS and private prescription.
Side effects: fluid retention, suppression of adrenal glands, thinning of the skin may occur.
Caution: use for short periods of time only
Not to be used for: patients suffering from acne or any other skin infections caused by tuberculosis, ringworm, viruses, or fungi, or continuously especially in pregnant women.
Not to be used with:
Contains: HYDROCORTISONE, COAL TAR solution.
Other preparations:

Carbo-Dome
(Lagap)

A cream used as an anti-psoriatic treatment for psoriasis.

Dose: apply to the affected area 2-3 times a day.
Availability: NHS, private prescription, over the counter.
Side effects: irritation, sensitivity to light.
Caution:
Not to be used for: patients suffering from acute psoriasis.
Not to be used with:
Contains: COAL TAR.
Other preparations:

---

carbocisteine *see* Mucodyne

Carbomix
(Penn)

Granules used as an adsorbent to treat acute poisoning, overdose of drugs.

Dose: adults dissolve the contents of the bottle in water and take by mouth as soon as possible after poisoning; children usually half adult dose.
Availability: NHS, private prescription, over the counter.
Side effects:
Caution: your doctor may advise additional treatment for certain over-doses.
Not to be used for:
Not to be used with: antidotes or emetics taken by mouth.
Contains: ACTIVATED CHARCOAL.
Other preparations:

---

carboxymethylcellulose *see* Glandosane

Cardene
(Syntex)

A blue/white or blue/pale-blue capsule according to strengths of 20 mg, 30 mg and used as an anti-anginal, anti-hypertensive drug to treat chronic stable angina, high blood pressure.

Dose: 20 mg 3 times a day increasing after not less than 3 day intervals to 30 mg 3 times a day as required. Not more than 120 mg a day.
Availability: NHS and private prescirption.
Side effects: chest pain, dizziness, headache, swelling of lower limbs, flushing, feeling warm, palpitations and nausea.
Caution: in patients suffering from weak heart, congestive heart failure, or liver or kidney disease.
Not to be used for: children, pregnant women, nursing mothers, or for patients suffering from some heart valve diseases.
Not to be used with: DIGOXIN, CIMETIDINE.
Contains: NICARDIPINE hydrochloride.
Other preparations:

Cardiacap
(Consolidated)

A blue/yellow capsule supplied at a strength of 30 mg and used as a NITRATE treatment for angina.

Dose: 1 capsule every 12 hours.
Availability: NHS and private prescription.
Side effects: headache, flushes.
Caution:
Not to be used for: children.
Not to be used with:
Contains: PENTAERYTHRITOL TETRANITRATE.
Other preparations:

Cardura
(Invicta)

A white tablet supplied at strengths of 1 mg, 2 mg, 4 mg and used as an alpha-blocker to treat high blood pressure.

Dose: usually 1-4 mg a day, occasionally up to 16 mg.
Availability: NHS and private prescription.
Side effects: headache, tiredness, weakness, swelling, low blood pressure on standing, dizziness.
Caution: in pregnant women.
Not to be used for: nursing mothers.
Not to be used with:
Contains: DOXAZOSIN.
Other preparations:

Cardura
(Pfizer)

A white five-sided tablet, a white egg-shaped tablet, or a white square tablet according to strengths of 1 mg, 2 mg, 4 mg and used as a selective alpha-blocker to treat high blood pressure.

Dose: 1 mg once a day at first increasing after 1-2 weeks if needed to 2 mg once a day and then 4 mg once a day, up to a maximum of of 16 mg a day.
Availability: NHS, private prescription.
Side effects: low blood pressure on standing, vertigo, dizziness, headache, tiredness, weakness, fluid retention.
Caution: pregnant women.
Not to be used for: children or nursing mothers.
Not to be used with:
Contains: DOXAZOSIN.
Other preparations:

carfecillin *see* Uticillin

Carisoma
(Pharmax)

A white tablet supplied at strengths of 125 mg, 350 mg and used as a sedative to treat muscle and bone problems associated with muscle spasm.

Dose: elderly 125 mg 3 times a day; adults 350 mg 3 times a day.
Availability: NHS and private prescription.
Side effects: drowsiness, dizziness, nausea, lassitude, flushes, headache, constipation, rash.
Caution: in patients suffering from kidney or liver disease, or a history of alcoholism or drug addiction. Avoid long-term treatment and withdraw gradually.
Not to be used for: children, pregnant women, nursing mothers, or for patients suffering from acute intermittent porphyria (a rare blood disorder).
Not to be used with: sedatives, anti-coagulants, steroids, the contraceptive pill, PHENYTOIN, GRISEOFULVIN, RIFAMPICIN, PHENOTHIAZINES, TRICYCLICS.
Contains: carisoprodol.
Other preparations:

---

carisoprodol *see* **Carisoma**

---

carmellose sodium *see* **Orabase**

Carpine
(Alcon)

Drops used as a cholinergic, lubricant treatment for glaucoma.

Dose: 2 drops into the eye 3 times a day.
Availability: NHS and private prescription.
Side effects:
Caution:
Not to be used for: patients suffering from acute iritis or who wear soft contact lenses.
Not to be used with:
Contains: PILOCARPINE, HYPROMELLOSE.
Other preparations:

Carylderm
(Napp Consumer)

A lotion used as a pediculicide to treat lice in the head and pubic areas.

Dose: rub into the hair and allow to dry, then shampoo.
Availability: NHS, private prescription, over the counter.
Side effects:
Caution: keep out of the eyes.
Not to be used for:
Not to be used with:
Contains: CARBARYL.
Other preparations: Cerylderm Liquid Shampoo.

Catapres
(Boehringer Ingelheim)

A white tablet scored on one side supplied at strengths of 0.1 mg, 0.3 mg and used to treat high blood pressure.

Dose: 0.05-0.1 mg 3 times a day increasing every second or third day.
Availability: NHS and private prescription.
Side effects: drowsiness, dry mouth, dizziness, fluid retention.
Caution: in nursing mothers, in patients suffering from depression or peripheral vascular disease, and where ß-BLOCKERS are being withdrawn.
Not to be used for: children.
Not to be used with: tricyclics, some alpha-blockers, other anti-hypertensives, sedatives.
Contains: *clonidine* hydrochloride.
Other preparations: Catapres Perlongets, Catapres Injection.

Caved-S
(Tillotts)

A brown tablet used as a cell-surface protector and antacid to treat peptic ulcer.

Dose: adults 2 tablets chewed between meals; children 10-14 years half adult dose.
Availability: over the counter and private prescription.
Side effects: few; occasionally constipation.
Caution:
Not to be used for: infants.
Not to be used with: tetracycline antibiotics.
Contains: LIQUORICE EXTRACT, ALUMINIUM HYDROXIDE, MAGNESIUM CARBONATE, SODIUM BICARBONATE.
Other preparations: Rabro (Sinclair).

C

Ce-Cobalin
(Paines & Byrne)

A syrup used as a multivitamin preparation for anorexia, recovery from illness.

Dose: adults 1-2 5 ml teaspoonsful 3 times a day; children 1 teaspoonful 3 times a day.
Availability: private prescription, over the counter.
Side effects:
Caution:
Not to be used for:
Not to be used with:
Contains: CYANOCOBALAMIN.
Other preparations:

Ceanel Concentrate
(Quinoderm)

A liquid used as an anti-bacterial, anti-fungal treatment for psoriasis, seborrhoeic inflammation of the scalp.

Dose: use as a shampoo 3 times a week at first and then twice a week or apply directly to other areas of skin as needed.
Availability: NHS, private prescription, over the counter.
Side effects:
Caution: keep out of the eyes.
Not to be used for:
Not to be used with:

Contains: PHENYLETHYL ALCOHOL.
Other preparations:

Cedilanid
(Sandoz)

A white, scored tablet supplied at a strength of 0.25 mg and used as a heart muscle stimulator to treat heart failure.

Dose: adults 6-8 a day for 3-5 days, 1-6 a day thereafter; children 10-30 micrograms a day per kg of body weight in 3 doses.
Availability: NHS and private prescription.
Side effects: anorexia, nausea, heart rhythm changes, rash.
Caution: in elderly patients, and in patients suffering from heart attacks, heart block, electrolyte changes, severe heart, liver, or kidney disease, thyroid failure.
Not to be used for: patients suffering from rapid heart rate, a complete heart block, or during planned defibrillation (electrical shock to the heart), or raised calcium levels.
Not to be used with: calcium supplements, psychotropics, potassium-depleting drugs, other similar drugs.
Contains: LANATOSIDE C.
Other preparations:

Cedocard
(Tillotts)

A blue, scored tablet or a green, scored tablet according to strengths of 20 mg, 40 mg and used as a NITRATE treatment for severe congestive heart failure.

Dose: 10-40 mg 3-4 times a day.
Availability: NHS and private prescription.
Side effects: headache, flushes, dizziness.
Caution:
Not to be used for: children or for patients suffering from severe low blood pressure, heart shock, severe anaemia, brain haemorrhage.
Not to be used with:
Contains: ISOSORBIDE DINITRITE.
Other preparations: Cedocard I.V.

Cedocard Retard
(Tillotts)

A yellow, scored tablet or an orange, scored tablet according to strengths of 20 mg, 40 mg and used as a NITRATE treatment for angina.

Dose: 20-80 mg morning and evening.
Availability: NHS and private prescription.
Side effects: headache, flushes, dizziness.
Caution:
Not to be used for: children.
Not to be used with:
Contains: ISOSORBIDE DINITRATE.
Other preparations:

---

cefaclor *see* Distaclor

---

cefadroxil *see* Baxan

---

cefuroxime axetil *see* Zinnat

Celevac
(Boehringer Ingelheim)

A pink tablet supplied at a strength of 500 mg and used as an adsorbent and bulking agent to treat constipation, colostomy control, diarrhoea, ulcerative colitis, diverticular disease, obesity.

Dose: adults 3-6 tablets night and morning with at least 300 ml liquid, or 3 tablets with liquid 30 minutes before a meal or when hungry; children in proportion to the dosage for a 70 kg adult.
Availability: NHS (when prescribed as a generic) and private prescription.
Side effects:
Caution: do not drink for 30 minutes before and after each dose.
Not to be used for: treating obesity in children or for patients suffering

from blocked intestine.
Not to be used with:
Contains: METHYLCELLULOSE.
Other preparations: Celevac granules.

---

cellulose *see* Nilstim

Centyl
(Leo)

A white tablet or a white, scored tablet according to strengths of 2.5 mg, 5 mg and used as a DIURETIC to treat fluid retention, high blood pressure, toxaemia of pregnancy.

Dose: adults 5-10 mg every morning at first, then 2.5-10 mg a day; children in proportion to dose for 70 kg adult.
Availability: NHS and private prescription.
Side effects: low blood potassium, rash, sensitivity to light, blood changes, gout, tiredness.
Caution: in pregnant women, nursing mothers, and in patients suffering from liver or kidney disease, gout, diabetes. Potassium supplements may be necessary. Your doctor may advise blood tests.
Not to be used for: patients suffering from severe kidney failure.
Not to be used with: LITHIUM, DIGITALIS, anti-hypertensives, other diuretics.
Contains: BENDROFLUAZIDE.
Other preparations:

Centyl-K
(Leo)

A green, egg-shaped tablet used as a DIURETIC to treat fluid retention, high blood pressure, toxaemia of pregnancy, where a potassium supplement is needed; also prevention of recurring calcium kidney stones.

Dose: 2-4 tablets a day in the morning at first, then 1-4 a day or every other day; for kidney stones 2-3 tablets a day.

Availability: NHS and private prescription.
Side effects: rash, sensitivity to light, blood changes, gout, tiredness.
Caution: in pregnant women, nursing mothers, and in patients suffering from diabetes, kidney or liver disease, and gout.
Not to be used for: children or for patients suffering from severe kidney failure, Addison's disease, or raised potassium levels.
Not to be used with: LITHIUM, DIGITALIS, anti-hypertensives, some other diuretics.
Contains: BENDROFLUAZIDE, POTASSIUM CHLORIDE.
Other preparations:

---

cephalexin *see* **Ceporex, Keflex**

---

cephradine *see* **Velosef**

Ceporex
(Glaxo)

A pink tablet supplied at strengths of 250 mg, 500 mg, 1 g and used as a cephalosporin antibiotic to treat respiratory, skin, and soft tissue infections, ear infections, urinary infections, gonorrhoea.

Dose: adults and children over 7 years 1-2 g a day in 2-4 divided doses; children under 3 months 62.5-125 mg twice a day, 4 months-2 years 250-500 mg a day, 3-6 years 500 mg-1 g a day, in 2-4 divided doses.
Availability: NHS and private prescription.
Side effects: allergy,stomach disturbances.
Caution: in patients suffering from kidney disease or who are very sensitive to penicillins.
Not to be used for:
Not to be used with: loop DIURETICS (such as FRUSEMIDE).
Contains: CEPHALEXIN.
Other preparations: Ceporex Capsules, Ceporex Syrup, Ceporex Suspension, Ceporex Paediatric Drops.

ceratonia *see* Arobon

Cerumol
(LAB)

Drops used as a wax softener to remove wax from the ears.

Dose: 5 drops into the ear twice a day for 3 days may enable syringing to be avoided.
Availability: NHS, private prescription, over the counter.
Side effects:
Caution:
Not to be used for: inflammation of the outer ear, dermatitis, eczema.
Not to be used with:
Contains: PARADICHLOROBENZENE, CHLORBUTOL, ARACHIS OIL.
Other preparations:

Cesamet
(Eli Lilly)

A blue/white capsule supplied at a strength of 1 mg and used as an anti-emetic drug to treat nausea and vomiting brought on by cytotoxic drugs.

Dose: 1-2 capsules the night before and again 1-3 hours before taking the first dose of the cytotoxic drug, up to a maximum of 6 capsules a day.
Availability: NHS and private prescription.
Side effects: drowsiness, reduced reactions, confusion, blurred vision, brain disturbances, low blood pressure, rapid heart rate, dry mouth, loss of appetite, stomach cramps.
Caution: in pregnant women, patients with a history of mental disorders, or patients suffering from severe liver disease.
Not to be used for:
Not to be used with: sedatives, alcohol, narcotic analgesics.
Contains: NABILONE.
Other preparations:

cetalkonium chloride *see* **AAA Spray, Teejel**

Cetavlex
(Care)

A cream used as an antiseptic to treat minor cuts and wounds, nappy rash.

Dose: apply as needed.
Availability: NHS, private prescription, over the counter.
Side effects:
Caution:
Not to be used for:
Not to be used with:
Contains: CETRIMIDE.
Other preparations:

Cetavlon PC
(Care)

A liquid used as a disinfectant to treat dandruff.

Dose: use as a shampoo, diluting 1 5 ml teaspoonful in 50 ml of water, once a week or more frequently if needed.
Availability: NHS, private prescription, over the counter.
Side effects:
Caution: keep out of the eyes.
Not to be used for:
Not to be used with:
Contains: CETRIMIDE.
Other preparations:

cetirizine dihydrochloride *see* **Zirtek**

Cetriclens
(S & N)

A solution in a sachet used as a disinfectant for cleansing broken skin and dirty wounds.

Dose: use as needed.
Availability: NHS, private prescription, over the counter.
Side effects:
Caution: throw away any unused solution straight away after use.
Not to be used for:
Not to be used with:
Contains: CHLORHEXIDINE GLUCONATE, CETRIMIDE.
Other preparations: Cetriclens Forte.

---

cetrimide *see* **Cetavlex, Cetavlon PC, Cetriclens, Crado-cap, Drapolene,Savloclens, Savlodil, Savlon Hospital Concentrate, Tisept, Torbetol, Travasept 100**

---

cetyl alcohol/coal tar distillate *see* **Pragmatar**

---

cetylpyridinium *see* **Medilave, Merocaine, Merocet**

---

charcoal *see* **Carbellon, Carbomix, Medicoal**

Chemotrim Paediatric *see* **Septrin**

Chendol Tablets
(CP Pharmaceuticals)

An orange, scored tablet supplied at a strength of 250 mg and used as a bile acid to dissolve non-calcified gallstones.

Dose: 3-4 tablets a day.
Availability: NHS and private prescription.

Side effects: diarrhoea, itch.
Caution: monitor effects on liver function.
Not to be used for: children, women who are not taking contraceptive precautions, or for patients suffering from chronic liver disease or inflammatory intestinal disease.
Not to be used with: oral contraceptives.
Contains: CHENODEOXYCHOLIC ACID.
Other preparations: Chendol Capsules. chenofalk (Thames).

C

chenodeoxycholic acid *see* Chendol Tablets

Chenofalk *see* Chendol Tablets
(Thames)

Chloramphenicol
(SNP)

Drops used as an antibiotic to treat bacterial infections of the eye.

Dose: adults 1 or more drops into the eye as needed; children 1 drop into the eye as needed.
Availability: NHS and private prescription.
Side effects: local allergy, bone marrow suppression.
Caution:
Not to be used for:
Not to be used with:
Contains: CHLORAMPHENICOL.
Other preparations:

chloramphenicol *see* **Actinac, Chloramphenicol, Chloromycetin, Chloromycetin Hydrocortisone, Chloromycetin Ointment**

Chlorasept 2000
(Baxter)

A solution in a sachet used as a disinfectant for cleansing wounds.

Dose: use as needed.
Availability: NHS and private prescription.
Side effects:
Caution:
Not to be used for:
Not to be used with:
Contains: CHLORHEXIDINE ACETATE.
Other preparations:

Chloraseptic
(Richardson-Vick)

A solution supplied with a spray and used as a disinfectant to treat sore throat, mouth ulcers, minor mouth and gum infections.

Dose: adults 5 sprays every 2 hours as needed or gargle or rinse mouth with solution diluted with equal amount of water; children 6-12 years 3 sprays every 2 hours as needed or rinse out mouth.
Availability: NHS, private prescription, over the counter.
Side effects:
Caution:
Not to be used for: children under 6 years.
Not to be used with:
Contains: PHENOL, SODIUM PHENOLATE.
Other preparations:

Chlorasol
(Seton-Prebbles)

A solution in a sachet used as a disinfectant for cleaning and removing dead skin from ulcers.

Dose: apply to the affected areas as needed.
Availability: NHS, private prescription, over the counter.
Side effects: irritation.
Caution: keep away from the eyes and the clothes; throw away any

remaining solution immediately.
Not to be used for: internal use.
Not to be used with:
Contains: SODIUM HYPOCHLORITE.
Other preparations:

---

chlorbutol *see* Auralgicin, Cerumol, Eludril, Monphytol

---

chlordiazepoxide *see* Librium, Limbitrol 5

---

chlorform *see* Eludril

---

chlorhexidine *see* Bacticlens, Cetriclens, Chlorasept 2000, Corsodyl, CX Powder, Eludril, Hibiscrub, Hibisol, Hibitane, Naseptin, Nystaform, Nystaform-HC, pHiso-Med, Rotersept, Savloclens, Savlodil, Savlon Hospital Concentrate, Tisept, Travasept 100, Unisept

---

chlormethiazole edisylate *see* Heminevrin.

---

chlormezanone *see* Lobak, Trancopal,Trancoprin

---

chloroform suspension *see* Glykola

Chloromycetin
(Parke-Davis)

A white/grey capsule supplied at a strength of 250 mg and used as an antibiotic to treat typhoid, influenzae meningitis, severe infections.

Dose: adults and children over 2 weeks 50 mg per kg body weight a day in divided doses every 6 hours; children under 2 weeks half adult dose.
Availability: NHS and private prescription.
Side effects: blood changes, stomach disturbances, allergies.
Caution: your doctor may advise regular blood tests.
Not to be used for: minor infections or for prevention.
Not to be used with: anti-coagulants, anti-convulsants, PARACETAMOL.
Contains: CHLORAMPHENICOL.
Other preparations: Chloromycetin Palmitate Suspension, CHLORO-MYCETIN OINTMENT, SNO PHENICOL (SNP).

Chloromycetin Hydrocortisone
(Parke-Davis)

An ointment used as an antibiotic, corticosteroid to treat eye infections.

Dose: apply into the eye up to once an hour depending on the severity of the infection.
Availability: NHS and private prescription.
Side effects: rise in eye pressure, thinning cornea, cataract, rarely bone marrow suppression.
Caution: in infants and pregnant women; do not use for extended periods.
Not to be used for: patients suffering from glaucoma, viral, fungal, or weeping infections.
Not to be used with:
Contains: CHLORAMPHENICOL, HYDROCORTISONE.
Other preparations:

Chloromycetin Ointment
(Parke-Davis)

An ointment used as an antibiotic to treat bacterial conjunctivitis.

Dose: apply the ointment into the eye every 3 hours or more often if needed and continue until 2 days after the symptoms have gone.

Availability: NHS and private prescription.
Side effects: rarely bone marrow suppression.
Caution:
Not to be used for:
Not to be used with:
Contains: CHLORAMPHENICOL.
Other preparations:

C

chlorophenoxyethanol *see* **Phytocil**

chloroquine *see* **Avloclor, Nivaquine**

chlorothalidone *see* **Kalspare**

chlorothiazide *see* **Saluric**

chlorpheniramine hydrochloride *see* **Expulin**

chlorpheniramine maleate *see* **Expulin, Expurhin, Haymine, Piriton**

chlorpromazine *see* **Largactil**

chlorpropamide *see* **Diabinese**

chlortetracycline *see* **Aureocort, Aureomycin, Aureomycin Ointment**

---

chlorthalidone *see* **Hygroton, Hygroton K, Lopresoretic, Tenoret 50, Tenoretic**

Chlorthymol *see* **Alcos-Anal**

Chocovite
(Torbet)

A buff-coloured tablet used as a calcium and vitamin D_2 supplement to treat calcium deficiency.

Dose: 1-3 tablets sucked 3 times a day.
Availability: private prescription and over the counter.
Side effects:
Caution:
Not to be used for:
Not to be used with:
Contains: CALCIUM GLUCONATE, CALCIFEROL.
Other preparations:

---

cholecalciferol *see* **Octovit**

Choledyl
(Parke-Davis)

A pink tablet or a yellow tablet according to strengths 100 mg, 200 mg and used as a broncho-dilator to treat bronchial spasm brought on by chronic bronchitis or asthma.

Dose: adults 100-400 mg 4 times a day; children 3-6 years use syrup, 6-12 years 100 mg 3-4 times a day.
Availability: NHS, private prescription , over the counter.

Side effects: rapid heart rate, sleeplessness, nausea, change in heart rhythms, stomach upset.
Caution: in pregnant women, nursing mothers, and in patients suffering from heart or liver disease or peptic ulcer. Diabetics should avoid syrup.
Not to be used for: children under 3 years.
Not to be used with: CIMETIDINE, ERYTHROMYCIN, CIPROFLOXACIN, INTERFERON.
Contains: CHOLINE THEOPHYLLINATE.
Other preparations: Choledyl Syrup.

C

---

cholestyramine *see* **Questran**

---

choline bitartrate *see* **Lipoflavonoid, Lipotriad**

---

choline chloride *see* **Ketovite**

---

choline magnesium trisalicylate *see* **Trilisate**

---

choline salicylate *see* **Audax, Teejel**

---

choline theophyllinate *see* **Choledyl**

---

choral hydrate *see* **Noctec**

Chymocyclar *see* **Tetracycline**
(Rorer)

Chymoral Forte
(Rorer)

An orange tablet supplied at a strength of 100 000 units and used as an enzyme to treat acute inflammatory swelling.

Dose: 1 tablet 4 times a day before meals.
Availability: NHS, private prescription, over the counter.
Side effects: stomach disturbance.
Caution:
Not to be used for: children.
Not to be used with:
Contains: TRYPSIN, CHYMOTRYPSIN.
Other preparations: Chymoral.

---

chymotrypsin *see* Chymoral Forte

Cicatrin
(Calmic)

A cream used as an aminoglycoside antibiotic to treat skin infections.

Dose: apply to the affected area up to 3 times a day.
Availability: NHS and private prescription.
Side effects: hearing damage, sensitization.
Caution: where there are large areas of damaged skin.
Not to be used for:
Not to be used with:
Contains: NEOMYCIN SULPHATE, BACITRACIN ZINC, L-CYSTEINE, GLYCINE, DL-THREONINE.
Other preparations: Cicatrin Powder.

---

ciclacillin *see* Calthor

Cidomycin Cream
(Roussel)

A cream used as an aminoglycoside antibiotic to treat burns, wounds, and skin infections including impetigo.

Dose: apply to the affected area 3-4 times a day.
Availability: NHS and private prescription.
Side effects: hearing damage, sensitization.
Caution: where there are large areas of damaged skin.
Not to be used for:
Not to be used with:
Contains: GENTAMICIN sulphate.
Other preparations: Cidomycin Ointment.

C

Cidomycin Drops
(Roussel)

Drops used as an antibiotic to treat infections of the outer ear or eye.

Dose: 2-4 drops into the ear 3-4 times a day and at night, or 1-3 drops into the eye 3-4 times a day.
Availability: NHS and private prescription.
Side effects: additional infection.
Caution:
Not to be used for: patients suffering from perforated ear drum.
Not to be used with:
Contains: GENTAMICIN sulphate.
Other preparations: Cidomycin Eye Ointment, GARAMYCIN (Kirby-Warrick), GENTICIN (Nicholas).

cimetidine *see* Tagamet

cinchocaine *see* Proctosedyl, Scheriproct, Ultraproct, Uniroid

cineole *see* Copholco, Copholcoids, Rowachol, Rowatinex, Tercoda, Terpoin

cinnarizine *see* **Stugeron, Stugeron Forte**

Cinobac
(Eli Lilly)

A green/orange capsule supplied at a strength of 500 mg and used as a quinolone antibiotic to treat infections of the urinary tract.

Dose: 1 capsule twice a day for 7-14 days.
Availability: NHS and private prescription.
Side effects: allergy, brain and stomach disturbances.
Caution: in patients suffering from kidney disease.
Not to be used for: children, pregnant women, nursing mothers or for patients suffering from severe kidney disease.
Not to be used with:
Contains: CINOXACIN.
Other preparations:

cinoxacin *see* **Cinobac**

ciprofloxacin *see* **Ciproxin**

Ciproxin
(Baypharm)

A white tablet supplied at a strength of 250 mg and used as an antibiotic to treat ear, nose, and throat, and urinary infections, respiratory, skin, and soft tissue infections, bone, joint, and stomach infections, gonorrhoea, severe and major infections.

Dose: 1-3 tablets twice a day.
Availability: NHS and private prescription.
Side effects: stomach disturbances, dizziness, headache, tiredness, confusion, convulsions, rash, pain in the joints.
Caution: in patients suffering from severe kidney disease or with a history of convulsions. Plenty of liquid should be drunk.

Not to be used for: children, growing youngsters unless absolutely necessary, and pregnant women or nursing mothers.
Not to be used with: THEOPHYLLINE, antacids.
Contains: CIPROFLOXACIN.
Other preparations: Ciproxin Infusion.

---

cisapride *see* **Prepulsid**

---

citric acid *see* **Effercitrate, Mictral, Rehidrat**

Citrical
(Shire)

Orange-flavoured granules supplied in sachets of 500 mg and used as a calcium supplement to treat calcium deficiency.

Dose: 1 sachet dissolved in water 3 times a day.
Availability: NHS, private prescription, over the counter.
Side effects: constipation, wind.
Caution:
Not to be used for: children or for patients suffering from overactive parathyroid gland, decalcifying tumours, severe kidney failure.
Not to be used with: TETRACYCLINES.
Contains: CALCIUM CARBONATE.
Other preparations:

---

citrus fibre *see* **Proctofibe**

Claradin
(Nicholas)

A white, scored, effervescent tablet supplied at a strength of 300 mg and used as an analgesic to treat pain, fever, rheumatoid arthritis, osteoarthritis, Still's disease.

Dose: 2-3 tablets in water every 4 hours.
Availability: private prescription only.
Side effects: stomach upsets, allergy, asthma.
Caution: in the elderly, pregnant women, or patients with a history of allergy to aspirin or asthma, or who are suffering from impaired kidney or liver functions.
Not to be used for: children, nursing mothers, or for patients suffering from haemophilia, or ulcers.
Not to be used with: anti-coagulants (blood-thinning drugs), some anti-diabetic drugs, anti-inflammatory agents, METHOTREXATE, SPIRONOLAC-TONE, steroids, some antacids, some uric acid-lowering drugs.
Contains: ASPIRIN.
Other preparations:

Clarityn
(Kirby-Warrick)

A white, oval, scored tablet supplied at a strength of 10 mg and used as an antihistamine treatment for allergic rhinitis and other allergies.

Dose: 1 tablet a day.
Availability: NHS and private prescription.
Side effects: tiredness, headache, nausea.
Caution:
Not to be used for: children, the elderly, pregnant women, or nursing mothers.
Not to be used with:
Contains: LORATADINE.
Other preparations:

---

clavulanic acid *see* Augmentin

---

clemastine *see* Tavegil

---

clindamycin *see* Dalacin C, Dalacin T

Clinicide
(De Witt)

A liquid used as a pediculicide to treat lice of the head and pubic areas.

Dose: apply to the hair and allow to dry, then shampoo the following day.
Availability: NHS, private prescription, over the counter.
Side effects:
Caution: keep out of the eyes.
Not to be used for:
Not to be used with:
Contains: CARBARYL.
Other preparations:

Clinitar Cream
(SNP)

A cream used as an antipsoriatic treatment for psoriasis, eczema.

Dose: apply to the affected area 1-2 times a day.
Availability: NHS, private prescription, over the counter.
Side effects: sensitivity to light.
Caution:
Not to be used for: patients suffering from pustular psoriasis.
Not to be used with:
Contains: COAL TAR EXTRACT.
Other preparations: Clinitar Gel, Clinitar Shampoo.

Clinium
(Janssen)

A white tablet supplied at a strength of 120 mg and used as a calcium antagonist to treat angina.

Dose: 1 tablet a day at first with food, increasing by 1 tablet a day at 7-day intervals to 1 tablet 3 times a day.
Availability: NHS and private prescription.
Side effects: stomach upset, dizziness, buzzing in the ears, headache.
Caution: patients susceptible to palpitations.

Not to be used for: children or pregnant women.
Not to be used with:
Contains: LIDOFLAZINE.
Other preparations:

Clinoril
(MSD)

A hexagonal, yellow, scored tablet supplied at strengths of 100 mg, 200 mg and used as a NON-STEROIDAL ANTI-INFLAMMATORY DRUG to treat rheumatoid arthritis, osteoarthritis, ankylosing spondylitis, acute gouty arthritis, other joint disorders.

Dose: 200 mg twice a day with drink or food.
Availability: NHS and private prescription.
Side effects: stomach pain, dyspepsia, rash, dizziness, buzzing in the ears, withdraw if fever or liver disorders occur.
Caution: in patients with a history of stomach haemorrhage or ulcer, kidney or liver disease.
Not to be used for: children, pregnant women, nursing mothers, or for patients suffering from anti-inflammatory or aspirin induced allergy, peptic ulcer, or stomach bleeding.
Not to be used with: DIMETHYL SULPHOXIDE, ASPIRIN, ANTI-COAGULANTS, HYPOGLYCAEMICS.
Contains: SULINDAC.
Other preparations:

---

clioquinol *see* **Barquinol HC, Oralcer, Vioform-Hydrocortisone**

---

clioquinol *see* **Lorocorten-Vioform**

---

clobazam *see* **Frisium**

---

clobetasol propionate *see* **Dermovate**

---

clobetasone butyrate *see* **Trimovate**

---

clobetasone *see* **Eumovate, Eumovate Cream**

---

clofazimine *see* **Lamprene**

---

clofibrate *see* **Atromid-S**

Clomid
(Merrell Dow)

A pale-yellow, scored tablet supplied at a strength of 50 mg and used as an anti-oestrogen treatment for sterility caused by failure of ovulation.

Dose: 1 tablet a day for five days starting on the fifth day of the period.
Availability: NHS and private prescription.
Side effects: enlargement of the ovaries, hot flushes, uncomfortable abdomen, blurred vision.
Caution:
Not to be used for: children, pregnant women, or for patients suffering from liver disease, large ovarian cyst, womb cancer.
Not to be used with:
Contains: CLOMIPHENE CITRATE.
Other preparations:

---

clomiphene citrate *see* **Clomid, Serophene**

---

clomipramine hydrochloride *see* **Anafranil**

---

ciomocycline *see* **Megaclor**

---

clonazepam *see* **Rivotril**

---

clonidine *see* **Catapres, Dixarit**

---

clopamide *see* **Viskaldix**

Clopixol
(Lundbeck)

A pink tablet, light-brown tablet, or brown tablet according to strengths of 2 mg, 10 mg, 25 mg and used as a tranquillizer to treat mental disorders especially schizophrenia.

Dose: 20-30 mg a day at first, then usually 20-50 mg a day up to a maximum of 150 mg a day.
Availability: NHS and private prescription.
Side effects: muscle spasms, restlessness, hands shaking, dry mouth, urine retention, palpitations, low blood pressure, weight gain, changes in libido, low body temperature, breast swelling, menstrual changes, jaundice, blood and skin changes, drowsiness, rarely fits.
Caution: in pregnant women and in the elderly who should take smaller dosage.
Not to be used for: children or for patients suffering from acute opiate, alcohol, or barbiturate poisoning, advanced kidney, liver, or heart disease, senility, apathy, or withdrawal, Parkinson's disease, severe arteriosclerosis, or for anyone who is intolerant of these drugs taken by mouth.
Not to be used with:
Contains: ZUCLOPENTHIXOL hydrochloride.
Other preparations: Clopixol Injection, Clopixol-Conc.

clorazepate potassium *see* **Tranxene**

---

clotrimazole *see* **Canesten, Canesten 1, Canesten-HC**

---

cloxacillin *see* **Orbenin**

C

Co-Betaloc
(Astra)

A white, scored tablet used as a ß-BLOCKER and DIURETIC combination to treat high blood pressure.

Dose: 1-3 tablets a day in single or divided doses.
Availability: NHS and private prescription.
Side effects: cold hands and feet, sleep disturbances, slow heart rate, tiredness, wheezing, heart failure, stomach upset.
Caution: in pregnant women, nursing mothers, or patients suffering from asthma, diabetes, kidney or liver disorders. May need to be withdrawn before surgery. Withdraw gradually. Your doctor may advise addititional treatment with diuretics and digitalis.
Not to be used for: children or patients suffering from heart block or failure.
Not to be used with: VERAPAMIL, CLONIDINE withdrawal, some anti-arrhythmic drugs and anaesthetics, RESERPINE, some anti-hypertensives, ergot alkaloids, CIMETIDINE, sedatives, SYMPATHOMIMETICS, INDOMETHACIN.
Contains: METOPROLOL tartrate, HYDROCHLOROTHIAZIDE.
Other preparations: Co-Betaloc SA.

Co-Codamol

A tablet used as an analgesic to relieve pain.

Dose: adults 1-2 tablets every 4-6 hours to a maximum of 8 tablets a day; children 7-12 years $1/2$-1 tablet every 4-6 hours to a maximum of 4 tablets a day.

Availability: NHS, private prescription, over the counter
Side effects:
Caution: in patients suffering from kidney or liver disease.
Not to be used for: children under 7 years.
Not to be used with:
Contains: CODEINE phosphate, PARACETAMOL.
Other preparations: Co-Codamol Dispersible.

Co-Codaprin Dispersible

A dispersible tablet used as an analgesic to relieve pain.

Dose: 1-2 tablets in water every 4-6 hours as needed.
Availability: NHS, private prescription, over the counter.
Side effects: stomach upsets, allergy, asthma.
Caution: in the elderly, pregnant women, in patients with a history of allergy to aspirin or asthma, or who are suffering from impaired kidney or liver function.
Not to be used for: children, nursing mothers, or for patients suffering from haemophilia, ulcers.
Not to be used with: anti-coagulants (blood-thinning drugs), some anti-diabetic drugs, anti-inflammatory agents, METHOTREXATE, SPIRONOLAC-TONE, steroids, some antacids, some uric acid-lowering drugs.
Contains: ASPIRIN, CODEINE phosphate.
Other preparations: Co-Codaprin.

Co-Danthrusate

Capsules used as a stimulant and faecal softener to treat constipation.

Dose: adults 1-3 capsules at night; children over 6 years 1 capsule at night.
Availability: NHS and private prescription.
Side effects: obstruction of the intestine.
Caution: nursing mothers.
Not to be used for: children uner 6 years.
Not to be used with:
Contains: DANTHRON, DOCUSATE sodium.
Other preparations:

co-dydramol

A tablet used as an opiate analgesic to control pain.

Dose: 1-2 tablets every 4-6 hours up to a maximum of 8 tablets a day.
Availability: NHS and private prescription.
Side effects: constipation, nausea, headache.
Caution: in pregnant women, the elderly, and in patients suffering from allergies, kidney or liver disease, or underactive thyroid.
Not to be used for: children or patients suffering from respiratory depression or blocked airways.
Not to be used with: alcohol, sedatives.
Contains: DIHYDROCODEINE tartrate, PARACETAMOL.
Other preparations:

co-proxamol

A tablet used as an opiate analgesic to control pain.

Dose: 2 tablets 3-4 times a day.
Availability: NHS and private prescription.
Side effects: tolerance, dependence, drowsiness, constipation, dizziness, nausea, rash.
Caution: in pregnant women and in patients suffering from liver or kidney disease.
Not to be used for: children.
Not to be used with: alcohol, sedatives, anti-convulsant drugs, anti-coagulants.
Contains: DEXTROPROPOXYPHENE hydrochloride, PARACETAMOL.
Other preparations: DISTALGESIC (Dista).

coal tar extract *see* **Alphosyl, Alphosyl HC, Clinitar Cream, Polytar, T Gel, Tarcortin**

coal tar *see* **Balneum with Tar, Baltar, Carbo-Cort, Carbo-Dome, Gelcosal, Gelcotar, Genisol, Ionil T, Meditar, Polytar, Psoriderm, Psorigel, Psorin**

Cobadex
(Cox)

A cream used as a steroid treatment for skin disorders, itch of the anus and vulva.

Dose: apply a small quantity to the affected area 2-3 times a day.
Availability: NHS and private prescription.
Side effects: fluid retention, suppression of adrenal glands, thinning of the skin may occur.
Caution: use for short periods of time only.
Not to be used for: patients suffering from acne or any other skin infections caused by tuberculosis, ringworm, viruses, or fungi, or continuously especially in pregnant women.
Not to be used with:
Contains: HYDROCORTISONE.
Other preparations:

Cobutolin
(Cox)

A pink tablet supplied at strengths of 2 mg, 4 mg and used as a broncho-dilator to treat bronchial spasm brought on by chronic bronchitis, asthma, emphysema.

Dose: adults 2-4 mg 3-4 times a day; elderly 2 mg 3-4 times a day at first; children 2-6 years 1-2 mg 3-4 times a day, 6-12 years 2 mg 3-4 times a day.
Availability: NHS and private prescription.
Side effects: headache, dilation of the blood vessels, nervous tension, shaking of the hands.
Caution: in pregnant women and in patients suffering from overactive thyroid, angina, abnormal heart rhythms, high blood pressure, heart muscle disease.
Not to be used for: children under 2 years.
Not to be used with: SYMPATHOMIMETICS.
Contains: SALBUTAMOL sulphate.
Other preparations: Cobutolin Inhaler, VENTOLIN (A & H).

---

codeine phosphate *see* also Antoin, Co-Codamol, Co-Codaprin Dispersible, Codis, Diarrest, Galcodine, Medoc-

odene, Migraleve, Panadeine, Paracodol, Parahypon, Parake, Pardale, Phensedyl, Propain, Solpadeine, Syndol, Tercoda, Terpoin, Tylex, Uniflu and Gregovite C

A tablet supplied at strengths of 15 mg, 30 mg, 60 mg and used as an opiate analgesic to treat pain.

Dose: adults 10-60 mg every 4 hours as needed to a maximum of 200 mg a day; children 1-12 years 3 mg per kg body weight a day in divided doses.
Availability: NHS and private prescription.
Side effects: tolerance, dependence, drowsiness, dry mouth, blurred vision, constipation.
Caution: in women in labour, the elderly, or in patients suffering from overactive thyroid gland or liver disease.
Not to be used for: infants under 1 year or for patients suffering from respiratory depression or blocked airways.
Not to be used with: MAOIS, sedatives.
Contains:
Other preparations:

---

codergocrine mesylate *see* Hydergine

Codis
(Reckitt & Colman)

A white, dispersible tablet used as an opiate analgesic to control pain and reduce fever.

Dose: 1-2 tablets dispersed in water every 4 hours to a maximum of 8 tablets in 24 hours.
Availability: NHS (when prescribed as a generic) and private prescription.
Side effects: stomach upsets, allergy, asthma.
Caution: in the elderly, pregnant women, and in patients with a history of allergy to aspirin or asthma, or who are suffering from impaired liver or kidney function, indigestion.
Not to be used for: children, nursing mothers, or patients suffering from haemophilia, ulcers.
Not to be used with: anti-coagulants (blood-thinning drugs), some

anti-diabetic drugs, anti-inflammatory agents, METHOTREXATE, SPIRONOLAC-
TONE, steroids, some antacids, some uric acid-lowering drugs.
Contains: ASPIRIN, CODEINE PHOSPHATE.
Other preparations:

Cogentin
(MSD)

A white, quarter-scored tablet supplied at a strength of 2 mg and used
as an ANTI-CHOLINERGIC treatment for Parkinson's disease.

Dose: adults ¹/₄ tablet a day at first increasing by ¹/₄ tablet a day every
5-6 days to a maximum of 3 tablets a day; children 3-12 years as
advised by physician.
Availability: NHS and private prescription.
Side effects: anti-cholinergic effects, confusion, agitation, and rash
at high doses.
Caution: in patients suffering from rapid heart rate, glaucoma, stom-
ach blockage. Dose should be reduced gradually.
Not to be used for: infants under 3 years or for patients suffering from
certain movement disorders.
Not to be used with: phenothiazines, antihistamines, anti-depres-
sants.
Contains: BENZTROPINE MESYLATE.
Other preparations: Cogentin Injection.

Colestid
(Upjohn)

Granules in sachets used as a lipid-lowering agent to reduce lipids.

Dose: 15-30 g a day in 2-4 divided doses in fluid.
Availability: NHS and private prescription.
Side effects: constipation.
Caution: in pregnant women, nursing mothers. Vitamin A, D, and K
supplements should be taken.
Not to be used for: patients suffering from complete biliary blockage.
Not to be used with: DIGITALIS, antibiotics, DIURETICS. Allow 1 hour
between taking this and any other drug.
Contains: COLESTIPOL.
Other preparations:

colestipol *see* **Colestid**

Colifoam
(Stafford-Miler)

Foam supplied in an aerosol and used as a steroid treatment for ulcerative colitis and other bowel inflammations.

Dose: 1 application once or twice a day for 2 or 3 weeks followed by reduced applications.
Availability: NHS and private prescription.
Side effects: high blood sugar, thin bones, mood changes, ulcers.
Caution: in pregnant women and in patients suffering from severe ulcerative disease. Do not use for prolonged periods.
Not to be used for: children or for patients suffering from obstruction, abscess, fresh intestinal surgery, tuberculous, fungal or viral infections.
Not to be used with:
Contains: HYDROCORTISONE acetate.
Other preparations:

Colofac
(Duphar)

A white tablet supplied at a strength of 135 mg and used as an anti-spasm treatment for bowel spasm.

Dose: adults 1 tablet 3 times a day, children over 10 years only adult dose.
Availability: NHS and private prescription.
Side effects:
Caution:
Not to be used for:
Not to be used with:
Contains: MEBEVERINE hydrochloride.
Other preparations: Colofac liquid.

Cologel
(Eli Lilly)

A liquid used as a bulking agent to treat constipation.

Dose: adults 5-15 ml with water; children in proportion to dosage for 70 kg adult.
Availability: NHS (when prescribed as a generic) and private prescription.
Side effects: may cause dehydration in children.
Caution:
Not to be used for:
Not to be used with:
Contains: METHYLCELLULOSE.
Other preparations:

Colpermin
(Tillotts)

A blue capsule used as an anti-spasm treatment for irritable bowel syndrome.

Dose: adults 1-2 tablets 3 times a day.
Availability: over the counter.
Side effects:
Caution:
Not to be used for: children.
Not to be used with:
Contains: PEPPERMINT OIL.
Other preparations:

Colven
(Rekitt & Colman)

Sachets used as an anti-spasmodic and bulking agent to treat irritable bowel syndrome.

Dose: 1 sachet twice a day before meals.
Availability: NHS and private prescription.
Side effects:
Caution:
Not to be used for: children or for patients suffering from bowel obstruction, or kidney or heart disorders.

Not to be used with:
Contains: MEBEVERINE hydrochloride, ISPAGHULA husk.
Other preparations:

Combantrin
(Pfizer)

An orange tablet supplied at a strength of 125 mg and used as an anti-worm agent to treat worms.

Dose: adults and children over 6 months 10 mg per kg body weight in one dose.
Availability: NHS and private prescription.
Side effects: stomach and brain disturbances.
Caution: in patients suffering from liver disease.
Not to be used for:
Not to be used with:
Contains: PYRANTEL EMBONATE.
Other preparations:

Comox *see* Septrin
(Norton)

Comploment Continus
(Napp)

A yellow tablet supplied at a strength of 100 mg and used as a source of vitamin B_6 to treat vitamin B_6 deficiency including that developed by the contraceptive pill.

Dose: 1 tablet a day.
Availability: private prescription, over the counter.
Side effects:
Caution:
Not to be used for: children.
Not to be used with: LEVODOPA.
Contains: PYRIDOXINE hydrochloride.
Other preparations:

Comprecin
(Parke-Davis)

A blue, oval tablet supplied at a strength of 200 mg and used as an antibiotic to treat general and urinary infections.

Dose: 1-2 tablets twice a day for up to 14 days.
Availability: NHS and private prescription.
Side effects: nausea, vomiting, dizziness, altered taste, headache, indigestion, rash, stomach pain, tiredness, rapid heart rate, sleeplessness, seizures, shaking of the hands.
Caution: in patients with a history of epilepsy or impaired circulation to the brain, or suffering from kidney disease.
Not to be used for: pregant women, nursing mothers.
Not to be used with: THEOPHYLLINE, WARFARIN, FENBUFEN.
Contains: ENOXACIN.
Other preparations:

Concavit
(Wallace)

A capsule used as a multivitamin treatment for vitamin deficiencies.

Dose: 1 capsule a day.
Availability: private prescription, over the counter.
Side effects:
Caution:
Not to be used for:
Not to be used with: LEVODOPA.
Contains: VITAMIN A, THIAMINE, RIBOFLAVINE, PYRIDOXINE, CYANOCOBALAMIN, ASCORBIC ACID, CALCIFEROL, VITAMIN E, NICOTINAMIDE, CALCIUM PANTOTHENATE.
Other preparations: Concavit Drops, Concavit Syrup.

Concordin
(MSD)

A pink tablet or a white tablet according to strengths of 5 mg, 10 mg and used as an anti-depressant to treat depression.

Dose: adults 15-60 mg a day in divided doses at first; elderly 5 mg 3 times a day at first.

Availability: NHS and private prescription.
Side effects: dry mouth, constipation, urine retention, blurred vision, palpitations, drowsiness, sleeplessness, dizziness, hands shaking, low blood presure, weight change, skin reactions, jaundice or blood changes, loss of libido may occur.
Caution: in nursing mothers or in patients suffering from heart disease, thyroid disease, epilepsy, diabetes, some other psychiatric conditions. Your doctor may advise regular blood tests.
Not to be used for: children, pregnant women, or for patients suffering from heart attacks, liver disease, heart block.
Not to be used with: alcohol, ANTI-CHOLINERGICS, ADRENALINE, MAOIS, barbiturates, other anti-depressants, anti-hypertensives.
Contains: PROTRYPTILINE hydrochloride.
Other preparations:

Congesteze
(Kirby-Warrick)

A white tablet used as an antihistamine, SYMPATHOMIMETIC treatment for allergic rhinitis.

Dose: 1 tablet twice a day.
Availability: NHS and private prescription.
Side effects: drowsiness.
Caution: in the elderly and in patients suffering from raised eye pressure, enlarged prostate.
Not to be used for: children, pregnant women, nursing mothers, or for patients suffering from overactive thyroid gland, coronary artery disease, severe high blood pressure.
Not to be used with: MAOIS, alcohol.
Contains: AZATADINE MALEATE, PSEUDOEPHEDRINE sulphate.
Other preparations:

---

conjugated oestrogens *see* Premarin, Prempak-C

Conotrane
(Boehringer Ingelheim)

A cream used as an antiseptic for protecting the skin from water, nappy rash, bed sores.

Dose: apply to the affected area several times a day.
Availability: NHS, private prescription, over the counter.
Side effects:
Caution:
Not to be used for:
Not to be used with:
Contains: BENZALKONIUM CHLORIDE, DIMETHICONE.
Other preparations:

Conova 30
(Gold Cross)

A white tablet used as an oestrogen, progestogen contraceptive.

Dose: 1 tablet a day for 21 days starting on day 5 of the period.
Availability: NHS and private prescription.
Side effects: enlarged breasts, bloating and fluid retention, cramps, leg pains, mood change, reduction in sexual desire, headaches, nausea, vaginal erosion, discharge, and bleeding, weight gain, skin changes.
Caution: in patients suffering from high blood pressure, diabetes, vascular disorders, asthma, depression, kidney disease, multiple sclerosis, womb diseases. Your doctor may advise you not to smoke, to have regular examinations. You should stop treatment at the first sign of serious symptoms such as severe headache or jaundice. Treatment should be stopped before surgery.
Not to be used for: pregnant women, or for patients suffering from sickle-cell anaemia, history of heart disease or thrombosis, liver disorders, some cancers, undiagnosed vaginal bleeding, some ear, skin, and kidney disorders.
Not to be used with: RIFAMPICIN, TETRACYCLINES, GRISEOFULVIN, barbiturates, PHENYTOIN, PRIMIDONE, CARBAMAZEPINE, ETHOSUXIMIDE, CHLORAL HYDRATE, DICHLORALPHENAZONE.
Contains: ETHINYLOESTRADIOL, ETHYNODIOL diacetate.
Other preparations:

Controvlar
(Schering)

A pink tablet used as an oestrogen, progestogen treatment for menstrual problems.

Dose: 1 tablet a day for 21 days starting on the fifth day of the period, then 7 days without tablets.
Availability: NHS and private prescription.
Side effects: enlarged breasts, bloating and fluid retention, cramps, leg pains, mood change, reduction in sexual desire, headaches, nausea, vaginal erosion, discharge, and bleeding, weight gain, skin changes.
Caution: in patients suffering from high blood pressure, diabetes, vascular disorders, asthma, depression, kidney disease, multiple sclerosis, womb diseases. Your doctor may advise you not to smoke, to have regular examinations. You should stop treatment at the first sign of serious symptoms such as severe headache or jaundice. Treatment should be stopped before surgery.
Not to be used for: pregnant women, or for patients suffering from sickle-cell anaemia, history of heart disease or thrombosis, liver disorders, some cancers, undiagnosed vaginal bleeding, some ear, skin, and kidney disorders.
Not to be used with: RIFAMPICIN, TETRACYCLINES, GRISEOFULVIN, barbiturates, PHENYTOIN, PRIMIDONE, CARBAMAZEPINE, ETHOSUXIMIDE, CHLORAL HYDRATE, DICHLORALPHENAZONE.
Contains: ETHINYLOESTADIOL, NORETHISTERONE acetate.
Other preparations:

Copholco
(Fisons)

A linctus used as an opiate, expectorant to treat laryngitis, inflammation of the windpipe.

Dose: adults 2 5 ml teaspoonsful 4-5 times a day; children over 5 years ¹/₂-1 teaspoonful 3 times a day.
Availability: private prescription, over the counter.
Side effects: constipation.
Caution: patients suffering from asthma.
Not to be used for: children under 5 years, or for patients suffering from liver disease.
Not to be used with: MAOIS.
Contains: PHOLCODINE, MENTHOL, CINEOLE, TERPIN HYDRATE.
Other preparations:

Copholcoids
(Fisons)

A black pastille used as an opiate, expectorant to treat dry cough.

Dose: adults 1-2 pastilles sucked 3-4 times a day; children over 5 years 1 pastille sucked 3 times a day.
Availability: NHS, private prescription , over the counter.
Side effects: constipation.
Caution: in patients suffering from asthma.
Not to be used for: children under 5 years or for patients suffering from liver disease.
Not to be used with: MAOIS.
Contains: PHOLCODINE, MENTHOL, CINEOLE, TERPIN HYDRATE.
Other preparations:

---

copper acetate *see* Cuplex

---

copper sulphate *see* Folicin, Tonivitan A & D

Cordarone X
(Sanofi)

A white, scored tablet supplied at strengths of 100 mg, 200 mg and used as an anti-arrhythmic drug to treat heart rhythm disturbances.

Dose: adults 200 mg 3 times a day for 7 days, then 200 mg twice a day for 7 days, and 200 mg a day thereafter; children as advised by the physician.
Availability: NHS and private prescription.
Side effects: corneal deposits, sensitivity to light, pulmonary alveolitis, kidney, nervous system, and thyroid effects.
Caution: in pregnant women and in patients suffering from heart failure. Your doctor may advise thyroid, eyes, heart, and liver tests.
Not to be used for: nursing mothers or for patients suffering from cardiac shock, some types of heart block, thyroid disease.
Not to be used with: calcium antagonists, anti-coagulants taken by mouth, ß-BLOCKERS, DIGOXIN.

Contains: AMIODARONE hydrochloride.
Other preparations: Cordarone X Intravenous.

Cordilox
(Abbott)

A yellow tablet supplied at strengths of 40 mg, 80 mg, 120 mg and used as a calcium antagonist to treat angina, high blood pressure, heart rhythm disturbances.

Dose: adults 40-120 mg 3 times a day; children under 2 years 20 mg 2-3 times a day; children over 2 years 40-120 mg 2-3 times a day. For angina 120 mg 3 times a day. For high blood pressure 240 mg once a day.
Availability: NHS and private prescription.
Side effects: constipation, flushes.
Caution: in patients suffering from some types of heart conduction block or failure, liver disease, slow heart rate.
Not to be used for: patients suffering from severe heart conduction block, very slow heart rates.
Not to be used with: ß-BLOCKERS, QUINIDINE, DIGOXIN.
Contains: VERAPAMIL hydrochloride.
Other preparations: Cordilox I.V., SECURON (Knoll), UNIVER (Rorer), BERKATENS (Berk).

Cordilox 160
(Abbott)

A yellow tablet supplied at a strength of 160 mg and used as a calcium antagonist to treat high blood pressure.

Dose: adults1 tablet twice a day; children up to 10 mg per kg body weight a day in divided doses.
Availability: NHS and private prescription.
Side effects: constipation, flushes.
Caution: in patients suffering from some types of heart conduction block or failure, liver disease, slow heart rate.
Not to be used for: patients suffering from severe heart conduction block, very slow heart rates.
Not to be used with: ß-BLOCKERS, QUINIDINE, DIGOXIN.

Contains: VERAPAMIL hydrochloride.
Other preparations:

Corgard
(Squibb)

A pale-blue tablet supplied at strengths of 40 mg, 80 mg and used as a ß-BLOCKER to treat heart rhythm disturbances, angina, high blood pressure, additional treatment in thyroid disease, migraine.

Dose: 40 mg a day at first increasing to 160 mg a day as required. A maximum of 240 mg a day is used in the treatment of angina. High blood pressure 80 mg a day at first, then 80-240 mg a day. Thyroid disease 80-160 mg once a day. Migraine 40 mg once a day at first, increasing to 80-160 mg a day as needed.
Availability: NHS and private prescription.
Side effects: cold hands and feet, sleep disturbances, slow heart rate, tiredness, wheezing, heart failure, stomach upset.
Caution: in pregnant women, nursing mothers, and in patients suffering from diabetes, kidney or liver disorders, asthma. May need to be withdrawn before surgery. Withdraw gradually. Your doctor may advise additional treatment with diuretics or digitalis.
Not to be used for: children or for patients suffering from heart block or failure.
Not to be used with: VERAPAMIL, CLONIDINE withdrawal, some anti-arrhythmic drugs and anaesthetics, RESERPINE, some anti-hyperten-sives, ergot alkaloids, CIMETIDINE, sedatives, SYMPATHOMIMETICS, IN-DOMETHACIN.
Contains: NADOLOL.
Other preparations:

Corgaretic 40
(Squibb)

A white, mottled, scored tablet used as a ß-BLOCKER/thiazide DIURETIC combination drug to treat high blood pressure.

Dose: 1-2 tablets a day.
Availability: NHS and private prescription.
Side effects: cold hands and feet, sleep disturbances, slow heart

rate, tiredness, wheezing, heart failure, stomach upset, low blood potassium, rash, sensitivity to light, blood changes, gout.
Caution: in pregnant women or nursing mothers, or patients suffering from asthma, gout, diabetes, kidney or liver disorders. May need to be withdrawn before surgery. Withdraw gradually. Your doctor may advise additional treatment with digitalis or diuretics.
Not to be used for: children or for patients suffering from heart block or failure, severe kidney failure.
Not to be used with: VERAPAMIL, CLONIDINE withdrawal, some anti-arrhythmic drugs and anaesthetics, RESERPINE, some anti-hypertensives, ergot alkaloids, CIMETIDINE, sedatives, SYMPATHOMIMETICS, INDOMETHACIN, LITHIUM, DIGITALIS, anti-hypertensives, other diuretics.
Contains: NADOLOL, BENDROFLUAZIDE.
Other preparations: Corgaretic 80.

Corlan
(Glaxo)

A pellet supplied at a strength of 2.5 mg and used as a corticosteroid to treat mouth ulcers.

Dose: 1 pellet allowed to dissolve in the mouth touching the ulcer.
Availability: NHS and private prescription.
Side effects:
Caution: in pregnant women.
Not to be used for: patients suffering from untreated mouth infections.
Not to be used with:
Contains: HYDROCORTISONE.
Other preparations:

Coro-Nitro
(MCP)

An aerosol used as a NITRATE for the treatment and prevention of angina.

Dose: 1-2 sprays on to or close to the tongue before exertion or when an attack begins to a maximum of 3 doses per attack.
Availability: NHS and private prescription.

Side effects: headache, flushes, dizziness.
Caution: do not inhale spray.
Not to be used for: children.
Not to be used with:
Contains: GLYCERYL TRINITRATE.
Other preparations:

Corsodyl
(ICI)

A solution used as an anti-bacterial treatment for gingivitis, mouth ulcers, thrush, and for mouth hygiene.

Dose: rinse with 2 5 ml teaspoonsful for 1 minute twice a day.
Availability: NHS, private prescription, over the counter.
Side effects: local irritation, stained tongue or teeth, may affect taste.
Caution:
Not to be used for:
Not to be used with:
Contains: CHLORHEXIDINE GLUCONATE.
Other preparations: Corsodyl Gel.

Cortelan
(Glaxo)

A white, scored tablet supplied at a strength of 25 mg and used as a corticosteroid for replacement treatment in Addison's disease and following removal of the adrenal gland.

Dose: 25-50 mg a day in 2 divided doses. A lower dose may be needed for children.
Availability: NHS and private prescription.
Side effects: high blood sugar, thin bones, mood changes, ulcers.
Caution: in pregnant women, in patients who have had recent bowel surgery, or who are suffering from inflamed veins, psychiatric disorders, virus infections, some cancers, some kidney diseases, thinning of the bones, ulcers, tuberculosis, other infections, high blood pressure, glaucoma, epilepsy, diabetes, underactive thyroid, liver disease, stress. Withdraw gradually.
Not to be used for: infants under 1 year.

Not to be used with: PHENYTOIN, PHENOBARBITONE, EPHEDRINE, RIFAMPICIN, diuretics, ANTI-CHOLINESTERASES, DIGITALIS, anti-diabetic agents, anti-coagulants, NON-STEROID ANTI-INFLAMMATORY DRUGS.
Contains: CORTISONE ACETATE.
Other preparations: CORTISTAB (Boots), CORTYSIL (Roussel).

Cortenema
(Bengue)

An enema supplied at a strength of 100 mg and used as a steroid treatment for ulcerative colitis.

Dose: 1 enema at bedtime for 2-3 weeks followed by every other day.
Availability: NHS and private prescription.
Side effects: systemic corticosteroid effects.
Caution: in pregnant women; do not use for prolonged periods.
Not to be used for: children or for patients suffering from obstruction, abscess, perforation, peritonitis, extensive fistulas.
Not to be used with:
Contains: HYDROCORTISONE.
Other preparations:

cortisone *see* Cortelan

Cortistab *see* Cortelan
(Boots)

Cortucid
(Nicholas)

A cream used as a sulphonamide and corticosteroid treatment for inflamation of the eyes.

Dose: insert 1 drop of cream into the eye every 3-6 hours.
Availability: NHS and private prescription.
Side effects: rise in eye pressure, thinning cornea, cataract, fungal

infection.

Caution: in pregnant women and infants; avoid using over extended periods.

Not to be used for: patients suffering from glaucoma, viral, fungal, tubercular, or weeping infections.

Not to be used with:

Contains: SODIUM SULPHACETAMIDE, HYDROCORTISONE acetate.

Other preparations:

Corwin
(Stuart)

A yellow tablet supplied at a strength of 200 mg and used as a heart muscle stimulant to treat heart failure.

Dose: 1 tablet twice a day.

Availability: NHS and private prescription.

Side effects: stomach upset, headache, dizziness, muscle cramp, palpitations, rash.

Caution: in patients suffering from some lung and kidney disease, heart muscle and valve disease.

Not to be used for: children, pregnant women, nursing mothers, or patients suffering from sudden heart failure.

Not to be used with:

Contains: XAMOTEROL fumate.

Other preparations:

Cosuric *see* Zyloric
(DDSA)

Cosylan
(Warner-Lambert)

A cough syrup used to treat dry cough.

Dose: adults 1 5 ml teaspoonful 3-4 times a day; children 1-5 years quarter adult dose, 6-12 years half adult dose.

Availability: private prescription and over the counter.

Side effects: drowsiness, dizziness, stomach upset.
Caution: in patients suffering from liver disease.
Not to be used for: infants under 1 year.
Not to be used with:
Contains: DEXTROMETHORPHAN HYDROBROMIDE.
Other preparations:

Cotazym
(Organon)

A green capsule used to supply pancreatic enzymes in the treatment of fibrocystic disease, steatorrhoea, diseases of the pancreas.

Dose: sprinkle the powder on to food from up to 6 capsules a day depending on diet.
Availability: NHS and private prescription.
Side effects: buccal and perianal irritation.
Caution:
Not to be used for: pregnant women or for patients particularly sensitive to pork.
Not to be used with:
Contains: PANCREATIN.
Other preparations:

Cradocap
(Napp Consumer)

A shampoo used as an antiseptic treatment for cradle cap, scurf cap.

Dose: shampoo twice a week.
Availability: NHS, private prescription, over the counter.
Side effects:
Caution:
Not to be used for:
Not to be used with:
Contains: CETRIMIDE.
Other preparations:

Cremalgin
(Rorer)

A balm used as an analgesic rub to treat rheumatism, fibrositis, lumbago, sciatica.

Dose: massage into the affected area 2-3 times a day.
Availability: NHS, private prescription, over the counter.
Side effects: may be irritant.
Caution:
Not to be used for: areas near the eyes, or on broken or inflamed skin, or on membranes (such as the mouth).
Not to be used with:
Contains: METHYL NICOTINATE, GLYCOL SALICYLATE, CAPSICUM OLEORESIN.
Other preparations:

Creon
(Duphar)

A brown/yellow capsule used to supply pancreatic enzymes in the treatment of pancreatic exocrine insufficiency.

Dose: 1-2 capsules with meals.
Availability: NHS and private prescription.
Side effects: perianal irritation.
Caution:
Not to be used for:
Not to be used with:
Contains: PANCREATIN.
Other preparations:

---

crotamiton *see* Eurax, Eurax-Hydrocortisone

Cuplex
(SNP)

A gel used as a skin softener to treat warts, corns, and callouses.

Dose: at night apply 1-2 drops of gel to the wart after soaking in water

and drying, remove the film in the morning and repeat the process, rubbing the area with a pumice stone between treatments.
Availability: NHS, private prescription, over the counter.
Side effects:
Caution: do not apply to healthy skin.
Not to be used for: warts on the anal or genital areas.
Not to be used with:
Contains: SALICYLIC ACID, LACTIC ACID, COPPER ACETATE.
Other preparations:

CX Powder
(Bio-Medical)

A powder used as a disinfectant to clean and disinfect the skin and prevent infection.

Dose: apply to the affected area 3 times a day.
Availability: NHS, private prescription, over the counter.
Side effects:
Caution:
Not to be used for:
Not to be used with:
Contains: CHLORHEXIDINE ACETATE.
Other preparations:

cyanocobalamin *see* **Calcimax, Cobalin, Concavit, Cytacon, Ketovite, Octovit, Verdiviton**

cyanocoblamin *see* **BC 500**

cyclandelate *see* **Cyclobral, Cyclospasmol**

cyclizine *see* **Diconal, Migril, Valoid**

Cyclo-Progynova 1 mg
(Schering)

A beige tablet and a brown tablet used as an oestrogen and progesto-gen treatment for senile vaginitis, post-menopausal osteoporosis.

Dose: 1 beige tablet a day for 11 days then 1 brown tablet a day for 10 days followed by 7 days without tablets. Begin on the fifth day of the period if present.

Availability: NHS and private prescription.

Side effects: enlarged breasts, bloating and fluid retention, cramps, leg pains, mood change, reduction in sexual desire, headaches, nausea, vaginal erosion, discharge, and bleeding, weight gain, skin changes.

Caution: in patients suffering from high blood pressure, diabetes, vascular disorders, asthma, depression, kidney disease, multiple sclerosis, womb diseases. Your doctor may advise you not to smoke, to have regular examinations. You should stop treatment at the first sign of serious symptoms such as severe headache or jaundice. Treatment should be stopped before surgery.

Not to be used for: pregnant women, or for patients suffering from sickle-cell anaemia, history of heart disease or thrombosis, liver disorders, some cancers, undiagnosed vaginal bleeding, some ear, skin, and kidney disorders.

Not to be used with: diuretics, anti-hypertensives, and drugs that change liver enzymes.

Contains: OESTRADIOL valerate; OESTRADIOL valerate and LEVONORGESTREL.

Other preparations: Cyclo-Progynova 2 mg.

---

cyclobarbitone *see* Phanodorm

Cyclobral
(Norgine)

A pink/brown capsule supplied at a strength of 400 mg and used as a vaso-dilator to treat hardening of the arteries, peripheral vascular disorders including intermittent claudication and Raynaud's phe-nomenon (spasm of the arteries in the hands).

Dose: 1 capsule 3-4 times a day.

Availability: NHS and private prescription.
Side effects: flushes, stomach upset.
Caution:
Not to be used for: children or for patients suffering from recent strokes or heart attacks.
Not to be used with:
Contains: CYCLANDELATE.
Other preparations:

---

cyclofenil *see* **Rehibin**

Cyclogest
(Hoechst)

A suppository supplied at strengths of 200 mg, 400 mg and used as a progesterone treatment for premenstrual syndrome, puerperal depression.

Dose: 200-400 mg 1-2 times a day in the rectum or the vagina from the twelfth or fourteenth day of the cycle until the period begins.
Availability: NHS and private prescription.
Side effects:
Caution: in patients suffering from liver disease.
Not to be used for: children or for patients suffering from abnormal vaginal bleeding or a history of thromboembolic conditions.
Not to be used with:
Contains: PROGESTERONE.
Other preparations:

Cyclokapron
(KabiVitrum)

A white, oblong, scored tablet supplied at a strength of 500 mg and used as a blood-clotting agent to treat menorrhagia and other heavy bleeding states.

Dose: 2-3 tablets 3-4 times a day for 3-4 days for a maximum of 3 cycles.

Availability: NHS and private prescription.
Side effects: stomach upset.
Caution: in patients with kidney disease, haematuria in haemophilia, history of thrombosis. Your doctor may advise some patients to have regular eye tests.
Not to be used for: patients suffering from multiple attacks of thrombosis.
Not to be used with:
Contains: TRANEXAMIC ACID.
Other preparations: Cyclokapron Injection, Cyclokapron Syrup.

---

cyclopenthiazide *see* Navidrex, Navidrex-K

Cyclopentolate
(SNP)

Drops used as an ANTI-CHOLINERGIC agent in ophthalmic procedures.

Dose: 1 or more drops into the eye as needed.
Availability: NHS and private prescription.
Side effects:
Caution:
Not to be used for: patients suffering from narrow angle glaucoma.
Not to be used with:
Contains: CYCLOPENTOLATE HYDROCHLORIDE.
Other preparations:

---

cyclopentolate hydrochloride *see* Cyclopentolate Mydri-late, Opulets Cyclopentonate

---

Cyclospasmol
(Brocades)

A pink tablet supplied at a strength of 400 mg and used as a vaso-dilator to treat impaired mental ability caused by cerebrovascular disease, peripheral vascular disorders, intermittent claudication (poor blood supply to the legs), Raynaud's syndrome (spasm of the arteries in the hands).

Dose: 4 tablets a day in 2 or 4 doses.
Availability: NHS and private prescription.
Side effects: flushes, stomach upset.
Caution:
Not to be used for: children or for patients suffering from recent strokes or heart attacks.
Not to be used with:
Contains: CYCLANDELATE.
Other preparations: Cyclospasmol Capsules, Cyclospasmol Suspension.

---

cyproheptadine hydrochloride *see* Periactin

---

cyproterone acetate *see* Androcur, Dianette

Cytacon
(Duncan, Flockhart)

A white tablet supplied at a strength of 50 micrograms as a source of vitamin B_{12} to treat undernourishment, vitamin deficiencies, some types of anaemia, vitamin B_{12} deficiency after stomach surgery.

Dose: adults 1-3 tablets a day up to a maximum of six tablets a day for pernicious anaemia; children use liquid.
Availability: private prescription and over the counter.
Side effects: rarely allergy.
Caution:
Not to be used for:
Not to be used with: PARA-AMINOSALICYLIC ACID, METHYLDOPA, COLCHICINE, CHOLESTYRAMINE, NEOMYCIN, BIGUANIDES, POTASSIUM CHLORIDE, CIMETIDINE.
Contains: CYANOCOBALAMIN.
Other preparations: Cytacon Liquid.

Cytotec
(Searle)

A white, hexagonal tablet supplied at a strength of 200 micrograms and used as a prostaglandin for the prevention and treatment of ulcers caused by anti-inflammatory drugs.

Dose: 4 tablets a day with meals and at bedtime for 4-8 weeks; prevention 1 tablet 2-4 times a day.
Availability: NHS and private prescription.
Side effects: diarrhoea.
Caution: circulatory disorders of the brain, heart, or peripheral vessels.
Not to be used for: women of child-bearing age.
Not to be used with:
Contains: MISOPROSTOL.
Other preparations:

---

d-alpha-tocopheryl acetate *see* Vita-E

---

d-panthenol *see* Verdiviton

Daktacort
(Janssen)

A cream used as a steroid, anti-fungal, and anti-bacterial treatment for skin infections where there is also inflammation.

Dose: apply to the affected area 2-3 times a day.
Availability: NHS and private prescription.
Side effects: fluid retention, suppression of adrenal glands, thinning of the skin may occur.
Caution: use for short periods of time only.
Not to be used for: patients suffering from acne or any other skin infections caused by tuberculosis, ringworm, viruses, or fungi, or continuously especially in pregnant women.
Not to be used with:
Contains: MICONAZOLE nitrate, HYDROCORTISONE.
Other preparations: Daktacort Ointment.

Daktarin
(Janssen)

A white, quarter-scored tablet supplied at a strength of 250 mg and used as an anti-fungal treatment for stomach and mouth and throat infections, and as an additional treatment in the prevention of re-infection of the vagina and vulva.

Dose: adults 1 tablet 4 times a day; children use Oral Gel.
Availability: NHS and private prescription.
Side effects: stomach discomfort, phlebitis, itch, fever, diarrhoea, rash, vomiting, flushes.
Caution: in pregnant women.
Not to be used for:
Not to be used with: anti-coagulants, anti-convulsants, anti-diabetic drugs, AMPHOTERICIN B.
Contains: MICONAZOLE.
Other preparations: DAKTARIN ORAL GEL, Daktarin Injection.

Daktarin Cream
(Janssen)

A cream used as an anti-fungal treatment for infections of the skin and nails.

Dose: apply 1-2 times a day until 10 days after the wounds have healed.
Availability: NHS, private prescription, over the counter.
Side effects:
Caution:
Not to be used for:
Not to be used with:
Contains: MICONAZOLE nitrate.
Other preparations: Daktarin Twin Pack, Daktarin Spray Powder, Daktarin Powder.

Daktarin Oral Gel
(Janssen)

A gel supplied at a strength of 25 mg and used as an anti-fungal treatment for fungal infections of the mouth and pharynx.

Dose: adults hold 5-10 ml of gel in the mouth 4 times a day; children under 2 years use 2.5 ml gel twice a day, 2-6 years 5 ml gel twice a day, over 6 years 5 ml gel 4 times a day.
Availability: NHS, private prescription, over the counter.
Side effects: mild stomach upset.
Caution:
Not to be used for:
Not to be used with: WARFARIN.
Contains: MICONAZOLE.
Other preparations:

Dalacin C
(Upjohn)

A lavender capsule or a maroon/lavender capsule according to strengths of 75 mg, 150 mg and used as an antibiotic treatment for serious infections.

Dose: adults 150-450 mg a very 6 hours; children under 12 years use Dalacin C Paediatric.
Availability: NHS and private prescription.
Side effects: stomach disturbances including colitis, jaundice, blood disorders.
Caution: in patients suffering from kidney or liver disease. The treatment should be stopped if diarrhoea and colitis develop.
Not to be used for: patients suffering from sensitivity to lincomycin.
Not to be used with: neuromuscular blocking agents.
Contains: CLINDAMYCIN hydrochloride.
Other preparations: Dalacin C Paediatric, Dalacin C Phosphate.

Dalacin T
(Upjohn)

A solution used as an antibiotic treatment for acne.

Dose: apply to the affected area twice a day for up to 12 weeks.
Availability: NHS and private prescription.
Side effects: dry skin, inflammation, inflammation of the follicles, possible diarrhoea or colitis.
Caution: keep out of the eyes, mouth, and nose.
Not to be used for: patients sensitive to LINCOMYCIN.

Not to be used with: skin-softening agents.
Contains: CLINDAMYCIN phosphate.
Other preparations:

Dalivit Drops
(Paines & Byrne)

Drops used as a multivitamin preparation in the prevention and treatment of vitamin deficiency in children.

Dose: 0-1 year 7 drops a day, over 1 year 14 drops a day.
Availability: NHS, private prescription, over the counter.
Side effects:
Caution:
Not to be used for:
Not to be used with: LEVODOPA.
Contains: VITAMIN A, ERGOCALCIFEROL, THIAMINE, RIBOFLAVINE, PYRIDOXINE, ASCORBIC ACID, NICOTINAMIDE.
Other preparations:

Dalmane
(Roche)

A grey/yellow capsule or a black/grey capsule according to strengths of 15 mg, 30 mg and used as a sleeping capsule for the short-term treatment of sleeplessness where sedation during the day does not cause difficulty.

Dose: elderly 15 mg before going to bed; adults 15-30 mg before going to bed.
Availability: private prescription only.
Side effects:
Caution:
Not to be used for: children.
Not to be used with:
Contains: FLURAZEPAM.
Other preparations:

---

danazol *see* **Danol**

Daneral SA
(Hoechst)

An orange tablet supplied at a strength of 75 mg and used as an anti-histamine treatment for allergies.

Dose: 1-2 tablets at night.
Availability: NHS, private prescription, over the counter.
Side effects: drowsiness, reduced reactions.
Caution: in nursing mothers.
Not to be used for: children.
Not to be used with: sedatives, MAOIS, alcohol.
Contains: PHENIRAMINE MALEATE.
Other preparations:

Danol
(Winthrop)

A white/pink capsule supplied at a strength of 200 mg and used as a gonadotrophin release inhibitor to treat endometriosis (a womb and menstrual disorder), heavy periods, non-malignant breast disorders, premenstrual syndrome.

Dose: 1-4 tablets a day in divided doses.
Availability: NHS and private prescription.
Side effects: nausea, dizziness, rash, backache, flushing, muscle spasm, male hormone effects.
Caution: in patients suffering from severe liver, kidney, or heart disease, epilepsy, migraine, diabetes, or a tendency to gain weight.
Not to be used for: children, pregnant women, nursing mothers, or for patients suffering from porphyria (a rare blood disorder).
Not to be used with: contraceptive pill, anti-coagulants.
Contains: DANAZOL.
Other preparations: Danol-$\frac{1}{2}$

---

danthron *see* Co-Danthrusate, Normax

Dantrium
(Norwich Eaton)

174

An orange/light brown capsule supplied at strengths of 25 mg, 100 mg and used as a muscle relaxant to treat chronic or severe spasticity associated with a stroke, multiple sclerosis, injury to the spinal cord, cerebral palsy.

Dose: 25 mg a day at first increasing as needed to a maximum of 100 mg 4 times a day.
Availability: NHS and private prescription.
Side effects: weakness, tiredness, drowsiness, diarrhoea.
Caution: in pregnant women and in patients suffering from lung or heart disease. Your doctor may advise that your liver should be checked before and 6 weeks after treatment.
Not to be used for: children or for patients suffering from liver disease or where spasticity is useful for movement.
Not to be used with: alcohol, sedatives.
Contains: DANTROLENE SODIUM.
Other preparations:

---

dantrolene sodium *see* **Dantrium**

Daonil
(Hoechst)

A white, oblong, scored tablet supplied at a strength of 5 mg and used as an anti-diabetic drug to treat diabetes.

Dose: 1 tablet a day at breakfast at first increasing if needed by $1/2$ - 1 tablet a day every 7 days to a maximum of 3 tablets a day.
Availability: NHS and private prescription.
Side effects: allergy including skin rash.
Caution: in the elderly and in patients suffering from kidney failure.
Not to be used for: children, pregnant women, nursing mothers, during surgery, or for patients suffering from juvenile diabetes, liver or kidney impairment, hormone disorders, stress, infections.
Not to be used with: ß-BLOCKERS, MAOIS, steroids, DIURETICS, alcohol, anti-coagulants, lipid-lowering agents, ASPIRIN, antibiotics (RIFAMPCIN, sulphonamides, CHLORAMPHENICOL), GLUCAGON, CYCLOPHOSPHAMIDE.
Contains: GLIBENCLAMIDE.
Other preparations: Semi-Daonil, CALABREN (Berk), EUGLUCON (Roussel), LIBANIL (APS), MALIX (Lagap).

dapsone

A tablet supplied at strengths of 50 mg, 100 mg and used as an antileprotic treatment for leprosy.

Dose: 1-2 mg per kg body weight a day.
Availability: NHS and private prescription.
Side effects: liver disease, anorexia, nausea, headache, dizziness, rapid heart rate, sleeplessness, rash, blood changes.
Caution: in patients suffering from heart or lung disease, glucose 6PD deficiency (an inherited disorder). This treatment should only be given under specialist advice.
Not to be used for:
Not to be used with: PARA-AMINOBENZOIC ACID.
Contains: dapsone.
Other preparations:

---

dapsone *see* Maloprim

Daranide
(MSD)

A yellow, scored tablet supplied at a strength of 50 mg used as a fluid balance medication in additonal treatment for glaucoma.

Dose: 2-4 tablets at first then 2 tablets every 12 hours, reducing to $^1/_2$-1 tablet 1-3 times a day.
Availability: NHS and private prescription.
Side effects: stomach upset, loss of weight, constipation, frequent need to urinate, headache, itch, lassitude, prickly sensation.
Caution: in pregnant women. Potassium supplements may be needed.
Not to be used for: children or for patients suffering from liver or kidney disease, adrenocortical weakness, low sodium or potassium levels, severe blockage of the lungs.
Not to be used with: steroids, ACTH, DIGITALIS, anti-diabetic drugs, anti-coagulants, local anaesthetics, SALICYLATES, anti-convulsants, FOLIC ACID ANTAGONISTS.
Contains: DICHLORPHENAMIDE.
Other preparations:

Daraprim
(Wellcome)

A white, scored tablet supplied at a strength of 25 mg and used as an anti-malarial drug for the prevention of malaria.

Dose: adults and children over 10 years 1 tablet a week; children 5-10 years half adult dose.
Availability: NHS, private prescription, over the counter.
Side effects: rash, anaemia.
Caution: in pregnant women, nursing mothers, and in patients suffering from liver or kidney disease.
Not to be used for: children under 5 years.
Not to be used with: CO-TRIMOXAZOLE, LORAZEPAM.
Contains: PYRIMETHAMINE.
Other preparations:

Davenol
(Wyeth)

A linctus used as an antihistamine, SYMPATHOMIMETIC, and opiate preparation to treat cough.

Dose: adults1-2 5 ml teaspoonsful 3-4 times a day; children no more than 1 teaspoonful 3-4 times a day.
Availability: private prescription and over the counter.
Side effects: constipation, drowsiness, reduced reactions, anxiety, hands shaking, irregular or rapid heart rate, dry mouth, excitement, rarely skin eruptions.
Caution: in patients suffering from asthma, kidney disease, diabetes.
Not to be used for: children under 5 years or for patients suffering from liver disease, heart or thyroid isorders.
Not to be used with: MAOIS, alcohol, sedatives, TRICYCLICS.
Contains: CARBINOXAMINE MALEATE, EPHEDRINE HYDROCHLORIDE, PHOLCODINE.
Other preparations:

DDAVP
(Ferring)

Nasal drops supplied in a dropper bottle and used as a hormone to treat diabetes insipidus (a fluid balance disorder).

Dose: adults 0.1-0.2 ml once a day into the nose; children 0.05-0.1 ml once or twice a day.
Availability: NHS and private prescription.
Side effects:
Caution: pregnant women and in patients suffering from high blood pressure.
Not to be used for:
Not to be used with:
Contains: DESMOPRESSIN.
Other preparations:

De-Nol
(Brocades)

A white liquid used as a cell-surface protector to treat gastric and duodenal ulcer.

Dose: adults 10 ml diluted with 15 ml water twice a day 30 minutes before meals.
Availability: NHS and over the counter.
Side effects: black colour to tongue and stools.
Caution:
Not to be used for: children or for patients suffering from kidney failure.
Not to be used with:
Contains: TRI-POTASSIUM DICITRATO BISMUTHATE.
Other preparations: De-Noltab.

De-Noltab *see* De-Nol

Debrisan
(Pharmacia)

A powder used as an absorbant to treat weeping wounds including ulcers.

Dose: wash the wound with a saline solution and, without drying first, coat with 3 mm of powder, and cover with a perforated plastic sheet; repeat before the sheet is saturated.
Availability: NHS, private prescription, over the counter.
Side effects:
Caution:
Not to be used for:
Not to be used with:
Contains: DEXTRANOMER.
Other preparations: Debrisan Paste.

---

debrisoquine sulphate *see* Declinax

Decadron
(MSD)

A white, scored tablet supplied at a strength of 0.5 mg and used as a corticosteroid treatment for rheumatic or inflammatory conditions, allergy.

Dose: as prescribed by your doctor.
Availability: NHS and private prescription.
Side effects: high blood sugar, thin bones, mood changes, ulcers.
Caution: in pregnant women, in patients who have had recent bowel surgery, or who are suffering from inflamed veins, psychiatric disorders, virus infections, some cancers, some kidney diseases, thinning of the bones, ulcers, tuberculosis, other infections, high blood pressure, glaucoma, epilepsy, diabetes, underactive thyroid, liver disease, stress. Withdraw gradually.
Not to be used for: infants under 1 year.
Not to be used with: PHENYTOIN, PHENOBARBITONE, EPHEDRINE, RIFAMPICIN, diuretics, ANTI-CHOLINESTERASES, DIGITALIS, anti-diabetic agents, anti-coagulants, non-steroid anti-inflammatory drugs.
Contains: DEXAMETHASONE.
Other preparations:

Decaserpyl
(Roussel)

A white, scored tablet or a pink, scored tablet according to strengths of 5 mg, 10 mg and used as an anti-hypertensive drug to treat high blood pressure.

Dose: 10 mg 3 times a day at first, increasing by 5-10 mg a day at 7-day intervals if needed.
Availability: NHS and private prescription.
Side effects: lethargy, vertigo, tremor, stomach upset, blocked nose.
Caution: in pregnant women, nursing mothers.
Not to be used for: children or for patients with a history of depression, active peptic ulcer, ulcerative colitis.
Not to be used with: anti-convulsants.
Contains: METHOSERPIDINE.
Other preparations:

Decaserpyl Plus
(Roussel)

A white, scored tablet used as an anti-hypertensive drug to treat high blood pressure.

Dose: 1 tablet 3 times a day increasing by $1/2$-1 tablet a day to a maximum of 5 tablets a day.
Availability: NHS and private prescription.
Side effects: low potassium levels, gout, lethargy, vertigo, tremor, stomach upset, blocked nose.
Caution: in pregnant women, nursing mothers, and in patients suffering from liver disease, gout, diabetes.
Not to be used for: children, for patients with a history of depression, or for patients suffering from active peptic ulcer, ulcerative colitis, severe kidney failure.
Not to be used with: LITHIUM, DIGITALIS, anti-convulsants.
Contains: METHOSERPEDINE, BENTHIAZIDE.
Other preparations:

Declinax
(Roche)

A white tablet scored on one side or a pale-blue tablet scored on one side according to strengths of 10 mg, 20 mg and used as an anti-hypertensive drug to treat high blood pressure.

Dose: 10-20 mg once or twice a day at first, increasing to 120 mg a day if needed.
Availability: NHS and private prescription.
Side effects: low blood pressure when standing up, general feeling of being unwell, headache, failure of ejaculation.
Caution: in patients suffering from kidney disease.
Not to be used for: for children or for patients suffering from phaeochromocytoma (a disease of the adrenal glands) or recent heart attack.
Not to be used with: tricyclic anti-depressants, SYMPATHOMIMETICS.
Contains: DEBRISOQUINE SULPHATE.
Other preparations:

D

Decortisyl
(Roussel)

A white, scored tablet supplied at a strength of 5 mg and used as a corticosteroid treatment for rheumatic conditions, allergies.

Dose: adults 4-8 tablets a day in divided doses reducing by ½-1 tablet every 3-4 days to 1-4 tablets a day; children 1-7 years quarter to half adult dose, 7-12 years half to three-quarters adult dose.
Availability: NHS and private prescription.
Side effects: high blood sugar, thin bones, mood change, ulcers.
Caution: in pregnant women, in patients who have had recent bowel surgery, or who are suffering from inflamed veins, psychiatric disorders, virus infections, some cancers, some kidney diseases, thinning of the bones, ulcers, tuberculosis, other infections, high blood pressure, glaucoma, epilepsy, diabetes, underactive thyroid, liver disease, stress. Withdraw gradually.
Not to be used for: infants under 1 year.
Not to be used with: PHENYTOIN, PHENOBARBITONE, EPHEDRINE, RIFAMPICIN, diuretics, ANTI-CHOLINESTERASES, DIGITALIS, anti-diabetic agents, anti-coagulants, NON-STEROID ANTI-INFLAMMATORY DRUGS.
Contains: PREDNISONE.
Other preparations:

Deltacortril
(Pfizer)

A brown tablet or a red tablet according to strengths of 2.5 mg, 5 mg and used as a corticosteroid treatment for collagen and allergic conditions.

Dose: 5-60 mg a day and then reduce to minimum effective dose.
Availability: NHS and private prescription.
Side effects: high blood sugar, thin bones, mood changes, ulcers.
Caution: in pregnant women, in patients who have had recent bowel surgery, or who are suffering from inflamed veins, psychiatric disorders, virus infections, some cancers, some kidney diseases, thinning of the bones, ulcers, tuberculosis, other infections, high blood pressure, glaucoma, epilepsy, diabetes, underactive thyroid, liver disease, stress. Withdraw gradually.
Not to be used for: infants under 1 year.
Not to be used with: PHENYTOIN, PHENOBARBITONE, EPHEDRINE, RIFAMPICIN, diuretics, ANTI-CHOLINESTERASES, DIGITALIS, anti-diabetic agents, anticoagulants, NON-STEROID ANTI-INFLAMMATORY DRUGS.
Contains: PREDNISOLONE.
Other preparations:

---

demeclocycline *see* Ledermycin

Depixol
(Lundbeck)

A yellow tablet supplied at a strength of 3 mg and used as a sedative to treat schizophrenia and other mental disorders, especially withdrawal or apathy.

Dose: usually 1-3 tablets a day, up to a maximum of 6 tablets a day.
Availability: NHS and private prescription.
Side effects: muscle spasms, restlessness, hands shaking, dry mouth, urine retention, palpitations, low blood pressure, weight gain, changes in libido, low body temperature, breast swelling, menstrual changes, jaundice, blood and skin changes, drowsiness, rarely fits.
Caution: in pregnant women.
Not to be used for: children or for patients suffering from Parkinson's disease, severe hardening of the arteries, senility, advanced kidney,

liver, or heart disease, or for very excitable or overactive patients, or for anyone who is intolerant of these drugs taken by mouth.
Not to be used with: alcohol, tranquillizers, pain killers, anti-hypertensives, anti-depressants, anti-convulsants, anti-diabetic drugs, LEVODOPA.
Contains: FLUPENTHIXOL DIHYDROCHLORIDE.
Other preparations: Depixol Injection, Depixol-Conc.

Deponit
(Schwarz)

D

Self-adhesive patches supplied in strengths of 5 mg, 10 mg and used as a NITRATE preparation for the prevention of angina.

Dose: apply a 5 mg patch at first increasing to 10 mg if required with each subsequent patch applied to a different part of the skin.
Availability: NHS and private prescription.
Side effects: headache, rash, dizziness.
Caution: reduce use of this treatment by replacing with oral nitrates.
Not to be used for: children.
Not to be used with:
Contains: GLYCERYL TRINITRATE.
Other preparations:

---

dequalinium chloride *see* Labosept

Derbac Shampoo
(International)

A shampoo used as a pediculicide to treat head lice.

Dose: use as a shampoo, applying twice and then leaving the second treatment for 5 minutes before rinsing and drying.
Availability: NHS, private prescription, over the counter.
Side effects:
Caution: keep out of the eyes.
Not to be used for:
Not to be used with:
Contains: CARBARYL.

Derbac-M
(International)

A liquid used as a pediculicide and scabicide to treat scabies, lice of the head and pubic areas.

Dose: apply liberally and then shampoo after 24 hours.
Availability: NHS, private prescription, over the counter.
Side effects:
Caution: keep out of the eyes.
Not to be used for:
Not to be used with:
Contains: malathion.
Other preparations:

Dermonistat
(Cilag)

A cream used as an anti-fungal treatment for fungal infections of the skin and nails.

Dose: apply to the affected area twice a day until 10 days after the wounds have healed.
Availability: NHS, private prescription, over the counter.
Side effects:
Caution:
Not to be used for:
Not to be used with:
Contains: MICONAZOLE nitrate.
Other preparations:

Dermovate
(Glaxo)

A cream used as a steroid treatment for psoriasis, eczema, other skin disorders where there is inflammation

Dose: apply a small quantity to the affected area twice a day.

Availability: NHS and private prescription.
Side effects: fluid retention, suppression of adrenal glands, thinning of the skin may occur.
Caution: adults check after 4 weeks; children check after 1 week; use for short periods of time only.
Not to be used for: patients suffering from acne or any other skin infections caused by tuberculosis, ringworm, viruses, or fungi, or continuously especially in pregnant women.
Not to be used with:
Contains: CLOBETASOL PROPIONATE.
Other preparations: Dermovate Ointment, Dermovate Scalp Application, Dermovate-NN.

D

Deseril
(Sandoz)

A white tablet supplied at a strength of 1 mg and used as an anti-spasmodic treatment for diarrhoea associated with carcinoid disease, migraine, severe headache.

Dose: 12-20 tablets a day in divided doses. For migraine 1-2 tablets 3 times a day with food.
Availability: NHS and private prescription.
Side effects: nausea and other stomach disturbances, drowsiness, dizziness, fluid retention, arterial spasm, retroperitonital, pleural, and heart valve fibrosis (membrane thickening).
Caution: patients suffering from or with a history of peptic ulcer.
Not to be used for: children, pregnant mothers, or patients suffering from severe high blood pressure, collagen disorders, coronary, peripheral, or occlusive vascular disease, liver or kidney disease, weight loss, sepsis.
Not to be used with: ergot alkaloids.
Contains: METHYSERGIDE.
Other preparations:

---

desipramine *see* **Pertofran**

---

desmopressin *see* **DDAVP, Desmospray**

Desmospray
(Ferring)

A nasal spray used as a hormone treatment for cranial diabetes insipidus, primary bedwetting, testing kidney function.

Dose: adults diabetes insipidus 1-2 sprays into the nose once or twice a day, kidney testing 2 sprays into each nostril; children diabetes insipidus as adult, kidney testing 1-15 years 1 spray into each nostril. Adults and children over 5 years primary bed wetting 1-2 sprays into each nostril before going to bed for up to 28 days.
Availability: NHS and private prescription.
Side effects:
Caution: in pregnant women or in patients suffering from kidney disease, cardiovascular disease. Patients should not drink excessively after testing.
Not to be used for: children under 5 years.
Not to be used with:
Contains: DESMOPRESSIN.
Other preparations:

---

desogestrel *see* Marvelon, Mercilon

---

desonide *see* Tridesilon

---

desoxymethasone *see* Stiedex

Destolit
(Merrell Dow)

A white, scored tablet supplied at a strength of 150 mg and used as a bile acid to dissolve gallstones.

Dose: 3-4 tablets a day in divided doses after meals with 1 dose always after the evening meal.
Availability: NHS and private prescription.

Side effects:
Caution:
Not to be used for: children, for women who are not taking contraceptive precautions, or for patients with a non-functioning gall bladder, active stomach ulcers, liver or certain diseases of the intestine.
Not to be used with: the contraceptive pill, oestrogens, treatments to reduce cholesterol levels.
Contains: URSODEOXYCHOLIC ACID.
Other preparations: URSOFALK (Thames).

D

Deteclo *see* Tetracycline
(Lederle)

Dexa-Rhinaspray
(Boehringer Ingelheim)

An aerosol used as a corticosteroid, antibiotic, and SYMPATHOMIMETIC treatment for allergic rhinitis.

Dose: adults 1 spray into each nostril no more than 6 times a day; children over 5 years 1 spray into each nostril no more than twice a day.
Availability: NHS and private prescription.
Side effects: itching nose.
Caution: do not use for extended periods.
Not to be used for: children under 5 years.
Not to be used with:
Contains: TRAMAZOLINE HYDROCHLORIDE, DEXAMETHASONE-21 ISONICOTINATE, NEOMYCIN sulphate.
Other preparations:

dexamethasone *see* Decadron, Maxidex, Maxitrol, Oradexon, Sofradex, Sofradex Ointment

dexamethasone-21 isonicotinate *see* Dexa-Rhinaspray

dexamphetamine *see* **Dexedrine**

Dexedrine
(S K B)

A white, scored tablet supplied at a strength of 5 mg and used as a SYMPATHOMIMETIC to stimulate the central nervous system.

Dose: adults 1 tablet twice a day at first increasing every 7 days by 2 tablets a day to a maximum of 12 tablets a day; children 3-5 years ½ tablet a day at first increasing every 7 days by ½ tablet a day, 6-12 years 1-2 tablets a day at first increasing every 7 days by 1 tablet a day to a maximum of 4 tablets a day.
Availability: controlled drug.
Side effects: sleeplessness, restlessness, slowing of growth, euphoria, mood change.
Caution: in pregnant women and in patients suffering from glaucoma.
Not to be used for: infants under 3 years, for patients with a history of drug abuse, or for patients suffering from cardiovascular disease, overactive thyroid gland, hyperexcitability.
Not to be used with: MAOIS, GUANETHIDINE.
Contains: DEXAMPHETAMINE sulphate.
Other preparations:

---

dextran *see* **Tears Naturale**

---

dextranomer *see* **Debrisan**

---

dextrin *see* **Nulacin**

---

dextromethorphan *see* **Actifed Compound, Cosylan, Lotussin**

---

dextromoramide tartrate *see* **Palfium**

---

dextropropoxyphene *see* **Co-proxamol, Doloxene, Doloxene Co.**

DF 118
(Duncan, Flockhart)

A white tablet supplied at a strength of 30 mg and used as an opiate to control pain; for cough use elixir.

Dose: adults 1 tablet every 4-6 hours after meals; children 4-12 years 0.5-1 mg per kg body weight every 4-6 hours.
Availability: NHS (when prescribed as a generic) and private prescription.
Side effects: constipation, nausea, headache, vertigo, vomiting, dizziness.
Caution: in pregnant women, the elderly, and in patients suffering from liver or kidney disease, allergy, underactive thyroid gland.
Not to be used for: children under 4 years, or for patients suffering from respiratory depression or blocked airways.
Not to be used with: alcohol, sedatives, MAOIS.
Contains: DIHYDROCODEINE tartrate.
Other preparations: DF 118 Injection, DF 118 Elixir.

DHC Continus
(Napp)

A white capsule supplied at a strength of 60 mg and used as an opiate to control pain associated with cancer.

Dose: 1 capsule every 12 hours.
Availability: NHS and private prescription.
Side effects: constipation, nausea, headache, vertigo.
Caution: in patients suffering from kidney or liver disease and allergy.
Not to be used for: children or for patients suffering from respiratory depression or blocked airways.
Not to be used with: alcohol, MAOIS, sedatives.

Contains: DIHYDROCODEINE tartrate.
Other preparations:

---

di-methionine *see* Lipotriad

Diabinese
(Pfizer)

A white, scored tablet supplied at strengths of 100 mg, 250 mg and used as an anti-diabetic treatment for diabetes.

Dose: 100-250 mg a day with breakfast, to a maximum of 500 mg a day.
Availability: NHS and private prescription.
Side effects: allergy, including skin rash.
Caution: in the elderly and in patients suffering from kidney failure.
Not to be used for: children, pregnant women, nursing mothers, during surgery, or for patients suffering from juvenile diabetes, liver or kidney disorders, stress, infections.
Not to be used with: ß-BLOCKERS, MAOIS, steroids, diuretics, alcohol, anti-coagulants, lipid-lowering agents, ASPIRIN, some antibiotics (RIFAMPICIN, SULPHONAMIDES, CHLORAMPHENICOL), GLUCAGON, CYCLOPHOSPHAMIDE.
Contains: CHLORPROPAMIDE.
Other preparations:

Diamicron
(Servier)

A white, scored tablet supplied at a strength of 80 mg and used as an anti-diabetic treatment for diabetes.

Dose: $^1/_2$ -1 tablet a day increasing if needed to a maximum of 4 a day in 2 divided doses.
Availability: NHS and private prescription.
Side effects: allergy, including skin rash.
Caution: in the elderly and in patients suffering from kidney failure.
Not to be used for: children, pregnant women, nursing mothers,

during surgery, or for patients suffering from juvenile diabetes, liver or kidney disorders, stress, infections.

Not to be used with: ß-BLOCKERS, MAOIS, steroids, diuretics, alcohol, anti-coagulants, lipid-lowering agents, ASPIRIN, some antibiotics (RIFAMPICIN, SULPHONAMIDES, CHLORAMPHENICOL), GLUCAGON, CYCLOPHOSPHAMIDE.

Contains: GLICLAZIDE.

Other preparations:

Diamox
(Lederle)

A white, scored tablet supplied at a strength of 250 mg and used as a fluid balance drug to treat congestive heart failure, fluid retention, toxaemia of pregnancy, pre-menstrual tension, epilepsy.

Dose: 250-375 mg a day or every other day in the morning at first; for PMT 125-375 mg a day beginning 5-10 days before menstruation. For epilepsy adults 1-4 tablets a day in divided doses; children under 2 years 125 mg a day, 2-12 years 125-750 mg a day individed doses.

Availability: NHS and private prescription.

Side effects: flushing, thirst, headache, drowsiness, increased urination, pins and needles, blood changes, excitement, rash.

Caution: care in pregnant women and for patients suffering from gout or diabetes. Your doctor may advise that potassium supplements may be needed, and that blood, fluids, and electrolytes should be checked regularly.

Not to be used for: patients suffering from a form of glaucoma, some kidney conditions, adrenal insufficiency, low sodium or potassium levels.

Not to be used with: FOLIC ACID ANTAGONISTS, such as TRIMETHOPRIM, anti-diabetics, anti-coagulants taken by mouth.

Contains: ACETAZOLAMIDE.

Other preparations: Diamox Parenteral.

Diamox Sustets *see* Diamox
(Lederle)

Dianette
(Schering)

A beige tablet used as an anti-androgen and oestrogen to treat severe acne in women, hairiness.

Dose: 1 tablet a day for 21 days beginning on day 5 of the cycle, then 7 days without tablets.
Availability: NHS and private prescription.
Side effects: enlarged breasts, bloating and fluid retention, cramps, leg pains, mood change, reduction in sexual desire, headaches, nausea, vaginal erosion, discharge, and bleeding, weight gain, skin changes.
Caution: in patients suffering from high blood pressure, diabetes, vascular disorders, asthma, depression, kidney disease, multiple sclerosis, womb diseases. Your doctor may advise you not to smoke, to have regular examinations. You should stop treatment at the first sign of serious symptoms such as severe headache or jaundice. Treatment should be stopped before surgery.
Not to be used for: children, males, pregnant women, or for patients suffering from sickle-cell anaemia, history of heart disease or thrombosis, liver disorders, some cancers, undiagnosed vaginal bleeding, some ear, skin, and kidney disorders.
Not to be used with: RIFAMPICIN, TETRACYCLINES, GRISEOFULVIN, barbiturates, PHENYTOIN, PRIMIDONE, CARBAMAZEPINE, ETHOSUXIMIDE, CHLORAL HYDRATE, DICHLORALPHENAZONE.
Contains: CYPROTERONE ACETATE, ETHINYLOESTRODIOL.
Other preparations:

Diarrest
(Galen)

A liquid supplied in 200 ml bottles and used as an opiate, antispasmodic, and electrolyte to treat diarrhoea.

Dose: adults 20 ml 4 times a day with water; children under 4 years as advised by manufacturer; children 4-5 years 5 ml 4 times a day; children 6-9 years 10 ml 4 times a day; children 10-13 years 15 ml 4 times a day.
Availability: NHS and private prescription.
Side effects: sedation.
Caution: in patients suffering from thyroid disease, heart failure,

kidney or liver disease, glaucoma, ulcerative colitis.
Not to be used for: patients suffering from pseudomembranous colitis (a bowel disorder), diverticular disease.
Not to be used with: maois.
Contains: CODEINE PHOSPHATE, DICYCLOMINE HYDROCHLORIDE, POTASSIUM CHLORIDE, SODIUM CHLORIDE, SODIUM CITRATE.
Other preparations:

Diatensic
(Gold Cross)

A white tablet supplied at a strength of 50 mg and used as a DIURETIC to treat congestive heart failure, cirrhosis of the liver, malignant fluid retention, some kidney and adrenal gland disorders.

Dose: adults, heart failure100 mg a day increasing if need to 400 mg a day, and then 75-200 mg a day with food; children 3 mg a day per kg of bodyweight. Other conditions as advised by physician.
Availability: NHS and private prescription.
Side effects: breast swelling, stomach upset, rash, drowsiness, headache, confusion.
Caution: in pregnant women, young patients, and for patients suffering from kidney or liver disease.
Not to be used for: nursing mothers or for patients suffering from failure of urination, severe or progressive kidney failure, high potassium levels, Addison's disease.
Not to be used with: potassium supplements, potassium-sparing diuretics, anti-hypertensives, CARBENOXOLONE, ACE INHIBITORS, DIGITALIS.
Contains: SPIRONOLACTONE.
Other preparations:

---

diazepam *see also* Valium

A tablet supplied at strengths of 2 mg, 5 mg, 10 mg and used as a tranquillizer to treat anxiety.

Dose: elderly 3-15 mg a day; adults 6-30 mg a day; children 1-5 mg a day.
Availability: NHS and private prescription.
Side effects: drowsiness, confusion, unsteadiness, low blood pres-

sure, rash, changes in vision, changes in libido, retention of urine. Risk of addiction increases with dose and length of treatment. May impair judgement.

Caution: in the elderly, pregnant women, nursing mothers, in women during labour, and in patients suffering from lung disorders, kidney or liver disorders. Avoid long-term use and withdraw gradually.

Not to be used for: children, or for patients suffering from acute lung diseases, some chronic lung diseases, some obsessional and psychotic diseases.

Not to be used with: alcohol, other tranquillizers, anti-convulsants.

Contains:

Other preparations: ATENSINE (Berk), DIAZEMULS (KabiVitrum), STESOLID (CP Pharmaceuticals), VALIUM (Roche).

---

diazoxide *see* Eudemine

Dibenyline
(S K B)

A red/white capsule supplied at a strength of 10 mg and used as an anti-adrenaline drug to treat high blood pressure associated with phaeochromocytoma (a disease of the adrenal glands).

Dose: adults 1 capsule a day at first increasing by 1 capsule a day as necessary; children 1-2 mg per kg bodyweight per day in divided doses.

Availability: NHS and private prescription.

Side effects: low blood pressure when standing, dizziness, rapid heart rate, failure of ejaculation.

Caution: in patients suffering from congestive heart failure, cardiovascular or kidney disease. The drug has been shown to cause cancer in rodents.

Not to be used for: patients suffering strokes or heart attacks.

Not to be used with:

Contains: PHENOXYBENZAMINE.

Other preparations:

---

dichloralphenazone *see* Welldorm

dichlorphenamide *see* Daranide

---

diclofenac sodium *see* Voltarol

Diconal
(Calmic)

A pink, scored tablet used as an opiate and anti-emetic to control pain.

Dose: 1 tablet at first and then as advised by physician.
Availability: controlled drug.
Side effects: tolerance, dependence, drowsiness, dry mouth, blurred vision.
Caution: in pregnant women and in patients suffering from liver or kidney disease.
Not to be used for: children or for patients suffering from respiratory depression or blocked airways.
Not to be used with: MAOIS, alcohol, sedatives.
Contains: DIPIPANONE HYDROCHLORIDE, CYCLIZINE HYDROCHLORIDE.
Other preparations:

---

dicyclomine *see* Diarrest, Merbentyl, Kolanticon

Dicynene
(Delandale)

A white tablet or an oval, white tablet according to strengths of 250 mg, 500 mg and used as a blood-clotting agent to treat menorrhagia and other bleeding disorders.

Dose: adults 500 mg every 4-6 hours; children half adult dose.
Availability: NHS and private prescription.
Side effects: headache, rash, nausea.
Caution:
Not to be used for: children.
Not to be used with:

Contains: ETHAMSYLATE.
Other preparations: Dicynene Injection.

Didronel
(Norwich Eaton)

A white, rectangular tablet supplied at a strength of 200 mg and used as a calcium-lowering agent to treat Paget's disease, high calcium levels in cancer.

Dose: Paget's disease 5 mg per kg body weight a day as 1 dose 2 hours before food; high calcium levels 20 mg per kg body weight a day for 30-90 days.
Availability: NHS and private prescription.
Side effects: nausea, diarrhoea, metallic or altered taste.
Caution: in pregnant women and in patients suffering from enterocolitis. Kidney function should be checked regularly, and calcium and vitamin D levels should be maintained.
Not to be used for: children or for patients suffering from severe kidney disease.
Not to be used with:
Contains: ETIDRONATE DISODIUM.
Other preparations:

---

dienoesterol *see* **Hormofemin**

---

diethylamine salicylate *see* **Algesal, Aradolene**

---

diethylcarbamazine *see* **Banocide**

---

diethylpropion hydrochloride *see* **Apisate, Tenuate Dospan**

Difflam
(3M Riker)

A cream used as an anti-inflammatory and analgesic rub to relieve muscular and skeletal pain.

Dose: massage gently into the affected area 3-6 times a day.
Availability: NHS, private prescription , over the counter.
Side effects: may be irritant.
Caution:
Not to be used for: areas near the eyes or on broken or inflamed skin, or on membranes (such as the mouth).
Not to be used with:
Contains: BENZYDAMINE HYDROCHLORIDE.
Other preparations:

Difflam Oral Rinse
(3M Riker)

A solution used as an analgesic and anti-inflammatory treatment for painful inflammations of the throat and mouth.

Dose: rinse or gargle with 3 5 ml teaspoonsful every 90 minutes-3 hours.
Availability: NHS, private prescription, over the counter.
Side effects: numb mouth.
Caution:
Not to be used for: children.
Not to be used with:
Contains: BENZYDAMINE HYDROCHLORIDE.
Other preparations: Difflam Spray.

Diflucan
(Pfizer)

A blue/white capsule or a blue capsule according to strengths of 50 mg,150 mg and used as an anti-fungal treatment for vaginal or oral thrush.

Dose: 1 50 mg tablet a day or 150 mg as a single dose for vaginal thrush.

Availability: NHS and private prescription.
Side effects: headache, stomach upset.
Caution: in nursing mothers, or in patients suffering from kidney disease where more than a single dose is prescribed.
Not to be used for: children or pregnant women.
Not to be used with: anti-coagulants, anti-diabetics taken by mouth.
Contains: FLUCONAZOLE.
Other preparations:

D

diflucortolone valerate *see* **Nerisone**

---

diflunisal *see* **Dolobid**

---

digoxin *see* **Lanoxin**

---

dihydrocodeine *see* **co-dydramol, DF 118, DHC Continus, Paramol**

---

dihydrotachysterol *see* **AT 10, Tachyrol**

---

diltiazem *see* **Britiazim, Tildiem**

Dimelor
(Eli Lilly)

A yellow, oval, scored tablet supplied at a strength of 500 mg and used as an anti-diabetic treatment for diabetes.

Dose: $^{1}/_{2}$ -1$^{1}/_{2}$ tablets a day.

Availability: NHS and private prescription.
Side effects: allergy, including skin rash.
Caution: in the elderly and in patients suffering from kidney failure.
Not to be used for: children, pregnant women, nursing mothers, during surgery, or for patients suffering from juvenile diabetes, liver or kidney disorders, stress, infections.
Not to be used with: ß-BLOCKERS, MAOIS, steroids, diuretics, alcohol, anti-coagulants, lipid-lowering agents, ASPIRIN, some antibiotics (RIFAMPICIN, SULPHONAMIDES, CHLORAMPHENICOL), GLUCAGON, CYCLOPHOSPHAMIDE.
Contains: ACETOHEXAMIDE.
Other preparations:

D

---

dimenhydrenate *see* Dramamine

---

dimethicone *see* Actonorm, Altacite Plus, Andursil, Asilone, Conotrane, Diovol, Kolanticon, Loasid, Timodine

---

dimethindene *see* Fenostil Retard, Vibrocil

---

dimethyl sulphoxide *see* Herpid, Virudox

Dimotane Expectorant
(Robins)

A liquid used as an antihistamine, expectorant, and SYMPATHOMIMETIC treatment for cough.

Dose: adults 1-2 5 ml teaspoonsful 3 times a day; children 2-6 years $^1/_2$ teaspoonful 3 times a day, 7-12 years 1 teaspoonful 3 times a day.
Availability: private prescription and over the counter.
Side effects: anxiety, hands shaking, rapid or abnormal heart rate, dry mouth, brain stimulation.

Caution: in patients suffering from diabetes.
Not to be used for: children under 2 years, or for patients suffering from cardiovascular problems, overactive thyroid gland.
Not to be used with: MAOIS, tricyclics, sedatives, alcohol, ANTI-CHOLIN-ERGICS.
Contains: BROMPHENIRAMINE maleate, GUAIPHENESIN, PSEUDOEPHEDRINE hydrochloride.
Other preparations: Dimotane Co, Dimotane Co Paediatric.

Dimotane Plus
(Robins)

A liquid used as an antihistamine and SYMPATHOMIMETIC treatment for allergic rhinitis.

Dose: adults 2 5 ml teaspoonsful 3 times a day; children use paediatric.
Availability: NHS, private prescription, over the counter.
Side effects: drowsiness, reduced reactions, rarely stimulant effects.
Caution: in nursing mothers and in patients suffering from bronchial asthma.
Not to be used for: patients suffering from glaucoma, comatose states, brain damage, epilepsy, retention of urine, cardiovascular problems, overactive thyroid.
Not to be used with: sedatives, MAOIS, TRICYCLICS, ANTI-CHOLINERGICS, alcohol.
Contains: BROMPHENIRAMINE maleate, PSEUDOEPHEDRINE hydrochloride.
Other preparations: Dimotane Plus Paediatric, Dimotane Plus LA, Dimotane LA, Dimotane Tablets, Dimotane Elixir.

Dimotapp LA
(Robins)

A brown tablet used as an antihistamine and SYMPATHOMIMETIC treatment for catarrh, allergic rhinitis, sinusitis.

Dose: adults 1-2 tablets night and morning; children use elixir.
Availability: private prescription and over the counter.
Side effects: drowsiness, reduced reactions, rarely stimulant effects.
Caution: in nursing mothers and in patients suffering from bronchial asthma.

Not to be used for: patients suffering from glaucoma, comatose states, brain damage, epilepsy, retention of urine, cardiovascular problems, overactive thyroid.
Not to be used with: sedatives, MAOIS, TRICYCLICS, ANTI-CHOLINERGICS, alcohol.
Contains: BROMPHENIRAMINE maleate, PHENYLEPHRINE hydrochloride, PHENYLPROPANOLAMINE hydrochloride.
Other preparations: Dimotapp Elixir, Dimotapp Elixir Paediatric.

Dindevan
(Duncan, Flockhart)

A white or a green, scored tablet according to strengths of 10 mg, 25 mg, 50 mg and used as an anti-coagulant to prevent blood from clotting.

Dose: 200 mg a day at first, 100 mg the following day, then 50-150 mg a day.
Availability: NHS and private prescription.
Side effects: rash, fever, white cell count changes, diarrhoea, hepatitis, kidney damage, discoloration of urine.
Caution: in elderly and very ill patients, and for patients suffering from high blood pressure, weight changes, kidney disease, potassium deficiency.
Not to be used for: children, within 24 hours of surgery or labour, for pregnant women, nursing mothers, and for patients suffering from severe liver or kidney disease or haemorrhagic conditions.
Not to be used with: NON-STEROID ANTI-INFLAMMATORY DRUGS, anti-diabetics, sulphonamides, QUINIDINE, antibiotics, PHENFORMIN, CIMETIDINE, drugs affecting the liver chemistry, corticosteroids.
Contains: PHENINDIONE.
Other preparations:

Dioctyl
(Medo)

A yellow tablet supplied at a strength of 100 mg and used as a faecal softener to treat constipation.

Dose: adults up to 500 mg a day in divided doses; children 12.5-25 mg 3 times a day.

Availability: NHS and private prescription.
Side effects:
Caution:
Not to be used for:
Not to be used with:
Contains: DOCUSATE SODIUM.
Other preparations: Dioctyl paediatric syrup, Dioctyl syrup.

Dioctyl Ear Drops
(Medo)

Drops used as a wax softener to remove ear wax.

Dose: 4 drops into the ear twice a day and plug with cotton wool.
Availability: NHS, private prescription, over the counter.
Side effects:
Caution:
Not to be used for: patients suffering from perforated ear drum.
Not to be used with:
Contains: SODIUM DOCUSATE, POLYETHYLENE GLYCOL.
Other preparations:

Dioderm *see* Hydrocortisone
(Dermal)

Dioralyte
(Rorer)

Cherry- or pineapple-flavoured powder supplied as sachets and used as a fluid and electrolyte replacement to treat acute watery diarrhoea including gastroenteritis.

Dose: 1-2 sachets in 200-400 ml water after each occasion of diarrhoea; infants substitute equivalent volume of reconstituted powder to feeds.
Availability: NHS and private prescription.
Side effects:
Caution:

Not to be used for:
Not to be used with:
Contains: SODIUM CHLORIDE, POTASSIUM CHLORIDE, SODIUM BICARBONATE, GLUCOSE.
Other preparations: Dioralyte Effervescent, ELECTROLADE (Nicholas); GLUCO-LYTE (Cupal); REHIDRAT (Searle).

Diovol
(Pharmax)

A white suspension used as an antacid and anti-wind preparation to treat ulcers, hiatus hernias, wind, and acidity.

Dose: adults 10-20 ml as required, children over 6 years half adult dose.
Availability: NHS, private prescription, over the counter.
Side effects: few; occasionally constipation.
Caution:
Not to be used for: infants.
Not to be used with: TETRACYCLINE antibiotics.
Contains: ALUMINIUM HYDROXIDE, MAGNESIUM HYDROXIDE, DIMETHICONE.
Other preparations:

Dipentum
(Pharmacia)

A caramel-coloured capsule supplied at a strength of 250 mg used as a salicylate to treat ulcerative colitis.

Dose: 4-12 capsules a day with food.
Availability: NHS and private prescription.
Side effects: stomach upset, rash, headache, joint pains.
Caution:
Not to be used for: children, pregnant women, or for patients suffering from aspirin allergy or kidney disease.
Not to be used with:
Contains: OLSALAZINE SODIUM.
Other preparations:

diphenhydramine *see* Benylin Expectorant, Guanor, Histalix, Lotussin, Propain, Uniflu and Gregovite C

---

diphenylpyraline *see* Eskornade Spansule, Histryl Spansule, Lergoban

---

dipipanone *see* Diconal

---

dipivefrin *see* Propine

---

dipotassium hydrogen phosphate *see* Glandosane

Diprosalic
(Kirby-Warrick)

An ointment used as a steroid and skin softener to treat hard skin and dry skin disorders.

Dose: apply lightly to the affected area 1-2 times a day.
Availability: NHS and private prescription.
Side effects: fluid retention, suppression of adrenal glands, thinning of the skin may occur.
Caution: use for short periods of time only.
Not to be used for: patients suffering from acne or any other skin infections caused by tuberculosis, ringworm, viruses, or fungi, or continuously especially in pregnant women.
Not to be used with:
Contains: BETAMETHASONE DIPROPIONATE, SALICYLIC ACID.
Other preparations: Diprosalic Scalp Application.

Diprosone *see* Betnovate
(Kirby-Warrick)

dipyridamole *see* **Persantin**

Dirythmin
(Astra)

A white tablet supplied at a strength of 150 mg and used as an anti-arrhythmic drug to treat abnormal heart rhythm.

Dose: 2 tablets every twelve hours but no more than 6 tablets a day.
Availability: NHS and private prescription.
Side effects: ANTI-CHOLINERGIC effects.
Caution: in pregnant women, and in patients suffering from mild heart block, enlarged prostate, glaucoma, retention of urine, low potassium levels, heart failure, kidney or liver failure.
Not to be used for: children or for patients suffering from some types of heart block, heart muscle disease or shock.
Not to be used with: other similar drugs, ß-BLOCKERS, potassium-lowering drugs, ANTI-CHOLINERGICS.
Contains: DISOPYRAMIDE PHOSPHATE.
Other preparations:

Disadine DP
(Stuart)

A powder spray used as an antiseptic for the prevention and treatment of infection in wounds such as burns, bed sores, varicose ulcers.

Dose: spray on to the infected area as needed.
Availability: NHS, private prescription, over the counter.
Side effects:
Caution: care in treating severe burns.
Not to be used for: patients suffering from non-toxic colloid goitre.
Not to be used with:
Contains: POVIDONE-IODINE.
Other preparations:

Disalcid
(3M Riker)

An orange/grey capsule supplied at a strength of 500 mg and used as an analgesic to treat osteoarthritis, rheumatoid arthritis, other joint disorders.

Dose: 4 capsules a day at first in divided doses before or with food, then 2 capsules 2-3 times a day with last dose at bed time if needed.
Availability: NHS and private prescription.
Side effects: stomach upsets, allergy, asthma.
Caution: in the elderly, pregnant women, in patients with a history of allergy to aspirin, asthma, or who are suffering from impaired liver or kidney function, indigestion.
Not to be used for: children, nursing mothers, or for patients suffering from haemophilia, ulcers.
Not to be used with: anti-coagulants (blood-thinning drugs), some anti-diabetic drugs, anti-inflammatory agents, METHOTREXATE, SPIRONOLAC-TONE, steroids, some antacids, some uric acid-lowering drugs.
Contains: SALSALATE.
Other preparations:

Disipal
(Brocades)

A yellow tablet supplied at a strength of 50 mg and used as an ANTI-CHOLINERGIC drug to treat Parkinson's disease.

Dose: 1 tablet 3 times a day at first increasing by 1 tablet a day every 2-3 days usually to 2-6 tablets a day and a maximum of 8 tablets a day.
Availability: NHS and private prescription.
Side effects: euphoria, ANTI-CHOLINERGIC effects, and confusion, agitation, and rash at high dose.
Caution: in patients suffering from heart problems or stomach obstruction. Reduce dose slowly.
Not to be used for: patients suffering from glaucoma, enlarged prostate, some movement disorders.
Not to be used with: PHENOTHIAZINES, antihistamines, anti-depressants.
Contains: ORPHENDRINE hydrochloride.
Other preparations: Disipal Injection.

---

disopyramide *see* **Dirythmin, Rythmodan**

Disprol Paed
(Reckitt & Colman)

A suspension supplied at a strength of 120 mg/ 5 ml teaspoon and used as an analgesic to relieve pain and fever in children.

Dose: 3 months-1 year ¹/₂ -1 5 ml teaspoonful 4 times a day if needed, 1-6 years 1-2 teaspoonsful 4 times a day if needed, 6-12 years 2-4 teaspoonsful 4 times a day if needed.
Availability: NHS, private prescription, over the counter.
Side effects:
Caution: in children suffering from liver or kidney disease..
Not to be used for:
Not to be used with:
Contains: PARACETAMOL.
Other preparations:

D

Distaclor
(Dista)

A violet/white capsule supplied at a strength of 250 mg and used as an antibiotic to treat ear, urinary, respiratory, soft tissue, and skin infections.

Dose: adults and children over 5 years1 capsule every 8 hours to a maximum of 16 capsules a day; children under 5 years half adult dose.
Availability: NHS and private prescription.
Side effects: allergy, stomach disturbances.
Caution: in patients suffering from kidney disease or who are very sensitive to penicillin.
Not to be used for:
Not to be used with: loop DIURETICS.
Contains: CEFACLOR.
Other preparations:

Distalgesic *see* Co-Proxamol
(Dista)

Distamine
(Dista)

A white tablet or a white, scored tablet according to strengths of 50 mg, 125 mg, 250 mg and used as an anti-arthritic drug and binding agent to treat severe active rheumatoid arthritis, cystinuria, Wilson's disease (inherited disorders), heavy metal poisoning, liver disease, cirrhosis.

Dose: adults 125-250 mg a day for 4 weeks increasing by same amount at 4-12 week intervals, usually to 500-750 mg a day or a maximum of 1.5 g a day; elderly 50-125 mg a day at first increasing to a maximum of 1 g a day; children 50 mg a day for 4 weeks, increasing every 4 weeks to a usual dose of 15-20 mg per kg body weight a day. Or as advised.
Availability: NHS and private prescription.
Side effects: nausea, anorexia, fever, rash, loss of taste, blood changes, blood or protein in the urine, kidney changes, muscle disease.
Caution: care in patients suffering from kidney disease, sensitivity to penicillin. Your doctor may advise that your blood and urine should be checked regularly.
Not to be used for: pregnant women, nursing mothers or patients suffering from lupus erythematosus, agranulocytosis, thrombocytopenia (rare blood and multi-system disorders).
Not to be used with: gold salts, anti-malaria or cytotoxic drugs, PHENYLBUTAZONE.
Contains: PENICILLAMINE.
Other preparations:

Distaquaine V-K
(Dista)

A white, scored tablet supplied at strengths of 125 mg, 250 mg and used as a penicillin to treat infections.

Dose: adults 125-250 mg every 4-6 hours; children under 1 year 62.5 mg, 1-5 years 125 mg, over 5 years 125-250 mg, every 6 hours.
Availability: NHS and private prescription.
Side effects: allergy, stomach disturbances.
Caution: in patients suffering from kidney disease.
Not to be used for: patients suffering from penicillin allergy.

Not to be used with:
Contains: PENICILLIN V POTASSIUM.
Other preparations: Distaquaine V-K Syrup.

---

distigmine *see* **Ubretid**

---

disulfiram *see* **Antabuse**

D

---

dithranol *see* **Anthranol, Antraderm, Dithrocream, Dithrolan, Exolan, Psoradrate, Psorin**

---

dithreonine *see* **Cicatrin**

Dithrocream
(Dermal)

A cream used as an anti-psoriatic treatment for psoriasis.

Dose: apply to the affected area once a day and wash off after $^{1}/_{2}$ -1
hour or apply at night and wash off in the morning.
Availability: NHS, private prescription, over the counter.
Side effects: irritation, allergy.
Caution:
Not to be used for: patients suffering from acute psoriasis.
Not to be used with:
Contains: dithranol.
Other preparations: Dithrocream Forte, Dithrocream HP, Dithro-
cream 2%.

Dithrolan
(Dermal)

An ointment used as an anti-psoriatic and skin softener to treat psoriasis.

Dose: before going to bed, bath and then apply the ointment to the affected area.
Availability: NHS, private prescription, over the counter.
Side effects: irritation, allergy.
Caution:
Not to be used for: patients suffering from acute psoriasis.
Not to be used with:
Contains: DITHRANOL, SALICYLIC ACID.
Other preparations:

Diumide-K Continus
(Degussa)

A white/orange tablet supplied at a strength of 600 mg and used as a DIURETIC/ potassium supplement combination to treat fluid retention including that associated with congestive heart failure, kidney and liver disease where a potassium supplement is needed.

Dose: 1 tablet a day in the morning.
Availability: NHS and private prescription.
Side effects: gout.
Caution: pregnant women, nursing mothers, and in patients suffering from kidney or liver disease, diabetes, enlarged prostate, impaired urination, gout.
Not to be used for: children or for patients suffering from liver cirrhosis, raised potassium levels, Addison's disease.
Not to be used with: potassium-sparing DIURETICS, LITHIUM, DIGITALIS, AMINOGLYCOSIDES, NON-STEROID ANTI-INFLAMMATORY DRUGS, cephalosporins, anti-hypertensives.
Contains: FRUSEMIDE, POTASSIUM CHLORIDE.
Other preparations:

Diuresal *see* Lasix
(Lagap)

---

diuretic

a drug which removes salt and water from the body, thus treating fluid retention. Example FRUSEMIDE *see* Lasix.

Diurexan
(Degussa)

A white, scored tablet supplied at a strength of 20 mg and used as a DIURETIC to treat high blood pressure, congestive heart failure, fluid retention.

D

Dose: high blood pressure 1 tablet a day in the morning increasing to 2 tablets a day if needed; fluid retention 2 tablets a day in the morning and then 1-4 tablets a day as needed.
Availability: NHS and private prescription.
Side effects: low potassium levels, dizziness, stomach upset.
Caution: potassium supplements may be needed; care in pregnant women, nursing mothers, and in patients suffering from gout, kidney or liver disease, diabetes, enlarged prostate.
Not to be used for: children or for patients suffering from severe kidney failure or cirrhosis of the liver.
Not to be used with: DIGITALIS, LITHIUM, anti-hypertensives.
Contains: XIPAMIDE.
Other preparations:

Dixarit
(Boehringer Ingelheim)

A blue tablet supplied at a strength of 25 micrograms and used as a blood vessel anti-spasmodic drug to treat migraine, headache, menopausal flushing.

Dose: 2-3 tablets morning and evening.
Availability: NHS and private prescription.
Side effects: sedation, dry mouth, dizziness, sleeplessness.
Caution: in nursing mothers or in patients suffering from depression.
Not to be used for: children.
Not to be used with: anti-hypertensives.
Contains: CLONIDINE hydrochloride.
Other preparations:

docosahexaenoic acid *see* **Maxepa**

---

docusate *see* **Co-Danthrusate, Dioctyl, Dioctyl Ear Drops, Fletcher's Enemette, Normax, Waxsol**

Dolmatil
(Squibb)

A white, scored tablet supplied at a strength of 200 mg and used as a sedative to treat schizophrenia.

Dose: over 14 years 2-4 tablets a day at first in 2 divided doses, the 1-6 tablets a day as needed.
Availability: NHS and private prescription.
Side effects: muscle spasms, restlessness, hands shaking, dry mouth, urine retention, palpitations, low blood pressure, weight gain, changes in libido, low body temperature, breast swelling, menstrual changes, jaundice, blood and skin changes, drowsiness, rarely fits.
Caution: in pregnant women or for patients suffering from hypomania, high blood pressure, kidney disease, or epilepsy.
Not to be used for: for children under 14 years or for patients suffering from phaeochromocytoma (a disease of the adrenal glands).
Not to be used with: alcohol, tranquillizers, pain killers, anti-hypertensives, anti-depressants, anti-coagulants, anti-diabetic drugs, LEVODOPA.
Contains: SULPIRIDE.
Other preparations:

Dolobid
(Morson)

A peach tablet or an orange tablet according to strengths of 250 mg, 500 mg and used as an analgesic to treat pain, rheumatoid arthritis, osteoarthritis.

Dose: 500 mg twice a day at first, then 250-500 mg twice a day. For arthritis 500-1000 mg a day adjusting according to response.
Availability: NHS and private prescription.

Side effects: stomach pain, dyspepsia, diarrhoea, rash, headache, dizziness, tinnitus.
Caution: in patients suffering from kidney disease or with a history of stomach haemorrhage or ulcers.
Not to be used for: children, pregnant women, nursing mothers or for patients suffering from anti-inflammatory-induced allergy, asthma, or peptic ulcer.
Not to be used with: alcohol, INDOMETHACIN, anti-coagulants.
Contains: DIFLUNISAL.
Other preparations:

Doloxene
(Eli Lilly)

An orange capsule supplied at a strength of 60 mg and used as an opiate to control pain.

Dose: 1 capsule 3-4 times a day.
Availability: NHS (when prescribed as a generic), private prescription.
Side effects: tolerance, dependence, drowsiness, constipation, rash, dizziness, nausea.
Caution: in pregnant women and in patients suffering from liver or kidney disease.
Not to be used for: children
Not to be used with: alcohol, sedatives, anti-convulsants, anti-coagulants.
Contains: DEXTROPROPOXYPHENE.
Other preparations:

Doloxene Co.
(Eli Lilly)

A red/grey capsule used as an opiate to control pain.

Dose: 1 capsule 3-4 times a day.
Availability: private prescription only.
Side effects: tolerance, dependence, drowsiness, constipation, dizziness, nausea, rash.
Caution: in pregnant women or in patients suffering from kidney or

liver disease, anti-inflammatory induced allergy, or a history of bron-chospasm.
Not to be used for: children or for patients suffering from peptic ulcer, haemophilia.
Not to be used with: alcohol, sedatives, anti-coagulants, anti-diabetics, uric acid-lowering drugs.
Contains: DEXTROPROPOXYPHENE NAPSYLATE, ASPIRIN, CAFFEINE.
Other preparations:

Dome-Acne
(Lagap)

A cream used as a skin softener to treat acne.

Dose: apply to the affected area night and morning.
Availability: NHS, private prescription, over the counter.
Side effects: irritation, underactive thyroid gland.
Caution: keep out of the eyes, nose, and mouth.
Not to be used for: dark-skinned patients.
Not to be used with:
Contains: SULPHUR, RESORCINOL monoacetate.
Other preparations:

Domical
(Berk)

A blue tablet, orange tablet, or brown tablet according to strengths of 10 mg, 25 mg, 50 mg and used as an anti-depressant to treat depression.

Dose: adults 75 mg a day in divided doses at first increasing to up to 200 mg a day if needed, then usually 50-100 mg at night; elderly 10-50 mg a day at first.
Availability: NHS and private prescription.
Side effects: dry mouth, constipation, urine retention, blurred vision, palpitations, drowsiness, sleeplessness, dizziness, hands shaking, low blood presure, weight change, skin reactions, jaundice or blood changes, loss of libido may occur.
Caution: in nursing mothers or in patients suffering from heart disease, thyroid disease, epilepsy, diabetes, some other psychiatric conditions. Your doctor may advise regular blood tests.

Not to be used for: children, pregnant women, or for patients suffering from heart attacks, heart block, liver disease.
Not to be used with: alcohol, ANTI-CHOLINERGICS, adrenaline, MAOIS, barbiturates, other anti-depressants, anti-hypertensives.
Contains: AMITRYPTILINE hydrochloride.
Other preparations:

---

domiphen *see* **Bradosol**

---

domperidone *see* **Evoxin, Motilium**

Dopamet *see* **Aldomet**
(Berk)

Doralese
(Bridge)

A yellow, triangular tablet supplied at a strength of 20 mg and used as an alpha-blocker to treat urine obstruction due to prostate disease.

Dose: 1-5 tablets a day (low dose in the elderly).
Availability: NHS and private prescription.
Side effects: dry mouth, nose blockage, weight gain, drowsiness, ejaculation failure.
Caution: in patients suffering from poor heart function, kidney or liver disease, Parkinson's disease, epilepsy, depression.
Not to be used for: patients suffering from heart failure.
Not to be used with: MAOIS, anti-hypertensives.
Contains: INDORAMIN.
Other preparations:

Dormonoct
(Roussel)

A yellow, scored tablet supplied at a strength of 1 mg and used as a sleeping tablet for short-term treatment of sleeplessness and nightime waking.

Dose: elderly up to 1 tablet before going to bed; adults 1-2 tablets before going to bed.
Availability: NHS (when prescribed as a generic) and private prescription.
Side effects: drowsiness, confusion, unsteadiness, low blood pressure, rash, changes in vision, changes in libido, retention of urine. Risk of addiction increases with dose and length of treatment. May impair judgement.
Caution: in the elderly, pregnant women, nursing mothers, in women during labour, and in patients suffering from lung disorders, kidney or liver disorders. Avoid long-term use and withdraw gradually.
Not to be used for: children or for patients suffering from acute lung diseases, some chronic lung diseases, some obsessional and psychotic diseases.
Not to be used with: alcohol, other tranquillizers and anti-convulsants.
Contains: LOPRAZOLAM.
Other preparations:

---

dothiepin *see* **Prothiaden**

---

doxazosin *see* **Cardura**

---

doxycycline hydrochloride *see* **Vibramycin, Vibramycin 50**

---

doxylamine succinate *see* **Syndol**

Dozic
(R.P. Drugs)

A liquid used as a sedative to treat schizophrenia, mania, hypomania, organic psychoses, alcohol withdrawal symptoms, delirium tremens, behaviour problems among children.

Dose: elderly psychosis 0.5-2 mg 2-3 times a day at first then increase as needed to a maximum of 200 mg a day then decrease to 5-10 mg a day when control is achieved, anxiety 0.5 mg twice a day; adults 0.5 mg 2-3 times a day at first then as above, anxiety as above; children 0.05 mg per kg body weight a day in 2 divided doses.

Availability: NHS and private prescription.

Side effects: muscle spasms, restlessness, hands shaking, dry mouth, urine retention, palpitations, low blood pressure, weight gain, changes in libido, low body temperature, breast swelling, menstrual changes, jaundice, blood and skin changes, drowsiness, rarely fits.

Caution: in pregnant women or in patients suffering from liver or kidney disease, epilepsy, severe cardiovascular disease, Parkinson's disease, or overactive thyroid gland.

Not to be used for: unconscious patients.

Not to be used with: alcohol, tranquillizers, pain killers, anti-hypertensives, anti-depressants, anti-convulsants, anti-diabetic drugs, LEVODOPA.

Contains: HALOPERIDOL.

Other preparations:

Dramamine
(Searle)

A white, scored tablet supplied at a strength of 50 mg and used as an antihistamine treatment for vertigo, nausea, vomiting, travel sickness.

Dose: adults 1-2 tablets 2-3 times a day; children 1-6 years $1/4$ -$1/2$ tablet, 7-12 years $1/2$ -1 tablet 2-3 times a day.

Availability: NHS and over the counter.

Side effects: drowsiness, reduced reactions, rarely skin eruptions.

Caution: in patients suffering from liver or kidney disease.

Not to be used for: infants under 1 year.

Not to be used with: alcohol, sedatives, some anti-depressants (MAOIS).

Contains: DIMENHYDRENATE.

Other preparations:

Drapolene
(Wellcome)

A cream used as an antiseptic to treat nappy rash.

Dose: apply twice a day or each time the nappy is changed.
Availability: NHS, private prescription, over the counter.
Side effects:
Caution:
Not to be used for:
Not to be used with:
Contains: BENZALKONIUM CHLORIDE, CETRIMIDE.
Other preparations:

---

dried yeast *see* Tonivitan

Droleptan
(Janssen)

A yellow, scored tablet supplied at a strength of 10 mg and used as a sedative to treat manic agitation.

Dose: adults 5-20 mg every 4-8 hours; children 0.2-0.6 mg per kg body weight every 4-8 hours.
Availability: NHS and private prescription.
Side effects: muscle spasms, restlessness, hands shaking, dry mouth, urine retention, palpitations, low blood pressure, weight gain, changes in libido, low body temperature, breast swelling, menstrual changes, jaundice, blood and skin changes, drowsiness, rarely fits.
Caution: in pregnant women, nursing mothers and in patients suffering from severe liver disease, pyramidal or extrapyramidal symptoms (shaking and stiffness).
Not to be used for: patients suffering from severe clinical depression.
Not to be used with: alcohol, tranquillizers, pain killers, anti-hypertensives, anti-depressants, anti-convulsants, anti-diabetic drugs, LEVODOPA.
Contains: DROPERIDOL.
Other preparations: Droleptan Liquid, Droleptan Injection.

Dromoran
(Roche)

A white tablet supplied at a strength of 1.5 mg and used as an opiate to control severe pain.

Dose: 1-3 tablets once or twice a day.
Availability: controlled drug.
Side effects: confusion, nausea, constipation, tolerance, addiction.
Caution: in pregnant women, women in labour, nursing mothers, the elderly, and in patients suffering from kidney or liver damage, head injury, enlarged prostate, or underactive thyroid gland.
Not to be used for: children, unconscious patients or patients suffering from respiratory depression or blocked airways.
Not to be used with: alcohol, MAOIS, sedatives, PHENOTHIAZINES.
Contains: LEVORPHANOL tartrate.
Other preparations:

---

droperidol *see* Droleptan

Droxalin
(Sterling Health)

A white tablet used as an antacid to treat acidity, dyspepsia, hiatus hernia.

Dose: adults 1-3 tablets chewed as required, usually every 4 hours.
Availability: private prescription and over the counter.
Side effects: few; occasionally constipation.
Caution:
Not to be used for: infants.
Not to be used with: TETRACYCLINE antibiotics.
Contains: ALEXITOL SODIUM, MAGNESIUM TRISILICATE.
Other preparations:

Dryptal *see* Lasix
(Berk)

Dubam
(Norma)

An aerosol used as a topical analgesic to relieve muscular pain.

Dose: spray on to the affected area for 2 seconds up to 4 times a day.
Availability: NHS, private prescription, over the counter.
Side effects: may be irritant.
Caution:
Not to be used for: areas near the eyes, or on broken or inflamed skin, or on membranes (such as the mouth).
Not to be used with:
Contains: GLYCOL SALICYLATE, METHYL SALICYLATE, ETHYL SALICYLATE, METHYL NICOTINATE.
Other preparations:

Dulcolax
(Boehringer Ingelheim)

A yellow tablet supplied at a strength of 5 mg and used as a stimulant to treat constipation and for evacuation of the bowels before surgery.

Dose: adults 2 tablets at night; children under 10 years half adult dose.
Availability: NHS (when prescribed as a generic) and private prescription.
Side effects:
Caution:
Not to be used for:
Not to be used with:
Contains: BISACODYL.
Other preparations: Dulcolax suppositories.

Duo-Autohaler
(3M-Riker)

An aerosol used as a broncho-dilator to treat bronchial spasm brought on by chronic bronchitis or bronchial asthma.

Dose: 1-3 sprays and again after 30 minutes if needed up to 24 sprays in 24 hours.
Availability: NHS and private prescription.

Side effects: rapid heart rate, dry mouth, headache, dilation of the blood vessels, abnormal heart rhythms.
Caution: in patients suffering from diabetes.
Not to be used for: patients suffering from heart disease, high blood pressure, cardiac asthma, overactive thyroid gland.
Not to be used with: MAOIS, TRICYCLICS.
Contains: ISOPRENALINE hydrochloride, PHENYLEPHRINE bitartrate.
Other preparations:

Duofilm
(Stiefel)

A liquid used as a skin softener to treat warts.

Dose: apply the liquid to the wart once a day, allow to dry, and cover, rubbing down between applications.
Availability: NHS, private prescription, over the counter.
Side effects:
Caution: do not apply to healthy skin.
Not to be used for: warts on the face or anal and genital areas.
Not to be used with:
Contains: SALICYLIC ACID, LACTIC ACID.
Other preparations:

Duogastrone *see* Biogastrone
(Sterling Research Laboratories)

Duovent
(Boehringer Ingelheim)

An aerosol used as a broncho-dilator to treat blocked airways.

Dose: adults 1-2 sprays 3-4 times a day; children over 6 years 1 spray 3 times a day.
Availability: NHS and private prescription.
Side effects: headache, dry mouth, dilation of the blood vessels.
Caution: in patients suffering from glaucoma, enlarged prostate, high blood pressure, overactive thyroid gland, heart muscle disease, an-

gina, abnormal heart rhythms.

Not to be used for: children under 6 years.
Not to be used with: SYMPATHOMIMETICS.
Contains: FENOTEROL hydrobromide, IPRATROPIUM bromide.
Other preparations:

Duphalac
(Duphar)

A syrup used as a laxative to treat constipation, brain disease due to liver problems.

Dose: children 0-1 year 2.5 ml twice a day; 1-4 years 5 ml twice a day; 5-10 years 10 ml twice a day; adults 15-50 ml 2-3 times a day until 2-3 soft stools are produced each day.
Availability: NHS (when prescribed as a generic) and private prescription.
Side effects:
Caution:
Not to be used for: patients suffering from galactosaemia (an inherited disorder).
Not to be used with:
Contains: LACTULOSE.
Other preparations: LACTULOSE SOLUTION.

Duphaston
(Duphar)

A white, scored tablet supplied at a strength of 10 mg and used as a progestogen to treat period pain, habitual and threatened abortion, endometriosis (a womb disorder), infertility, premenstrual syndrome, and as an additional treatment to oestrogen in hormone replacement.

Dose: period pain 1 tablet twice a day from the fifth to the twenty-fifth day of the cycle; endometriosis 1 tablet 2-3 times a day from the fifth to the twenty-fifth day or continuously; premenstrual syndrome 1 tablet twice a day from the twelfth to the twenty-sixth day; hormone replacement 2 tablets a day for 12 days a month.
Availability: NHS and private prescription.
Side effects: irregular bleeding, breast discomfort, acne, headache.

Caution: in patients suffering from high blood pressure or tendency to thrombosis, migraine, liver abnormalities, ovarian cysts.

Not to be used for: children, pregnant women, women having suffered a previous ectopic pregnancy, or for patients suffering from severe heart or kidney disease, benign liver tumours, undiagnosed vaginal bleeding.

Not to be used with: barbiturates, PHENYTOIN, PYRIDONE, CARBAMAZEPINE, CHLORAL HYDRATE, DICHLORALPHENAZONE, ETHOSUXIMIDE, RIFAMPICIN, CHLOR-PHENESIN, MEPROBAMATE, GRISEOFULVIN.

Contains: DYDROGESTERONE.

Other preparations:

Duromine
(3M Riker)

A grey/green capsule or a grey/maroon capsule according to strengths of 15 mg, 30 mg and used as an appetite suppressant to treat obesity.

Dose: 15-30 mg once a day at breakfast.

Availability: controlled drug.

Side effects: tolerance, addictions, mental disturbances, restlessness, nervousness, agitation, dry mouth, heart palpitations, raised blood pressure.

Caution: do not use for prolonged treatments. Care in patients suffering from high blood pressure, angina, abnormal heart rhythm.

Not to be used for: children, pregnant women, nursing mothers, or for patients suffering from hardening of the arteries, overactive thyroid gland, severe high blood pressure, or with a history of mental illness, alcoholism or drug addiction.

Not to be used with: MAOIS, SYMPATHOMIMETICS, METHYLDOPA, GUANETHIDINE, psychotropics.

Contains: PHENTERMINE.

Other preparations:

Dyazide
(Bridge)

A peach-coloured, scored tablet used as a DIURETIC to treat high blood pressure, fluid retention.

Dose: high blood pressure 1 tablet a day at first; fluid retention 1 tablet twice a day at first after meals and then 1 tablet a day or every other day. No more than 4 tablets a day.

Availability: NHS and private prescription.

Side effects: nausea, diarrhoea, cramps, weakness, headache, dry mouth, rash, blood changes.

Caution: in pregnant women, nursing mothers, and in patients suffering from liver or kidney disease, diabetes, electrolyte changes, and gout.

Not to be used for: patients suffering from severe or progressive kidney failure, or raised potassium levels.

Not to be used with: potassium supplements, potassium-sparing diuretics, LITHIUM, DIGITALIS, anti-hypertensives, INDOMETHACIN, ACE INHIBITORS.

Contains: TRIAMTERENE, HYDROCHLOROTHIAZIDE.

Other preparations: TRIAMCO (Norton).

---

dydrogesterone *see* Duphaston

Dyspamet *see* Tagamet
(Bridge)

Dytac
(S K B)

A maroon capsule supplied at a strength of 50 mg and used as a potassium-sparing DIURETIC to treat fluid retention especially when associated with congestive heart failure, liver or kidney disease.

Dose: 3-5 capsules a day in divided doses for 7 days, and then usually every other day.

Availability: NHS and private prescription.

Side effects: nausea, diarrhoea, cramps, weakness, headache, dry mouth, rash, blood changes.

Caution: in pregnant women, nursing mothers, and in patients suffering from kidney or liver disease, gout, electrolyte changes.

Not to be used for: children or for patients suffering from raised potassium levels, or progressive kidney failure.

Not to be used with: potassium supplements, potassium-sparing DIU-RETICS, anti-hypertensives, INDOMETHACIN, ACE INHIBITORS.
Contains: TRIAMTERENE.
Other preparations:

Dytide
(S K B)

A pale-yellow/maroon capsule used as a potassium-sparing DIURETIC to treat fluid retention.

Dose: 2 capsules after breakfast and 1 capsule after lunch at first, then 1 or 2 capsules every other day.
Availability: NHS and private prescription.
Side effects: nausea, diarrhoea, cramps, weakness, headache, dry mouth, rash, blood changes.
Caution: in pregnant women, nursing mothers, and in patients suffering from liver or kidney disease, diabetes, electrolyte changes, or gout.
Not to be used for: patients suffering from raised potassium levels, or progressive or severe kidney failure.
Not to be used with: potassium supplements, potassium-sparing DIURETICS, LITHIUM, DIGITALIS, anti-hypertensives, INDOMETHACIN, ACE INHIB-ITORS.
Contains: TRIAMTERENE, BENZTHIAZIDE.
Other preparations:

Ebufac *see* Brufen

Econacort
(Squibb)

A cream used as a steroid, anti-fungal, and anti-bacterial treatment for skin infections where there is also inflammation.

Dose: massage into the affected area night and morning.
Availability: NHS and private prescription.
Side effects: fluid retention, suppression of adrenal glands, thinning

of the skin may occur.
Caution: use for short periods of time only.
Not to be used for: patients suffering from acne or any other skin infections caused by tuberculosis, ringworm, viruses, or fungi, or continuously especially in pregnant women.
Not to be used with:
Contains: ECONAZOLE nitrate, HYDROCORTISONE.
Other preparations:

---

econazole see Econacort, Ecostatin, Ecostatin-1, Gyno-Pevaryl 1, Pevaryl

---

Ecostatin
(Squibb)

A cream used as an anti-fungal treatment for fungal infections of the skin.

Dose: apply to the affected area night and morning.
Availability: NHS, private prescription, over the counter.
Side effects:
Caution:
Not to be used for:
Not to be used with:
Contains: ECONAZOLE nitrate.
Other preparations: Ecostatin Lotion, Ecostatin Powder, Ecostatin Spray.

Ecostatin-1
(Squibb)

A pessary plus applicator supplied at a strength of 150 mg and used as an anti-fungal and anti-bacterial treatment for thrush of the vulva or vagina.

Dose: 1 pessary inserted into the vagina at bed time.
Availability: NHS and private prescription.
Side effects: mild burning or irritation.

Caution:
Not to be used for: children.
Not to be used with:
Contains: ECONAZOLE nitrate.
Other preparations: Ecostatin Pessaries, Ecostatin Cream, Ecostatin Twinpack.

ecothiopate iodide *see* Phospholine-Iodide

Edecrin
(MSD)

A white, scored tablet supplied at a strength of 50 mg and used as a DIURETIC to treat fluid retention including that associated with congestive heart failure, or kidney or liver disease.

Dose: adults 1 tablet a day after breakfast at first, increasing by $1/2$ - 1 tablet a day until the minimum effective dose usually of 1-3 tablets a day is found to a maximum of 8 in 2 divided doses; children 2-12 years $1/2$ tablet a day after breakfast, then increasing by $1/2$ tablet a day to the minimum effective dose.
Availability: NHS and private prescription.
Side effects: stomach upset, gout, jaundice, blood changes.
Caution: in pregnant women, and in patients suffering from liver disease, diabetes, enlarged prostate, impaired urination, or gout.
Not to be used for: infants, nursing mothers, or for patients suffering from cirrhosis of the liver, or severe kidney failure.
Not to be used with: LITHIUM, WARFARIN, DIGITALIS, anti-hypertensives, aminoglycosides, cephalosporins.
Contains: ETHACRYNIC ACID.
Other preparations: Edecrin Injection.

Efcortelan *see* Hydrocortisone
(Glaxo)

Effercitrate
(Typharm)

A white, effervescent tablet used as an alkalizing agent to treat cystitis.

Dose: adults and children over 6 years 2 tablets dissolved in water up to 3 times a day with meals; children 1-6 years half adult dose.
Availability: NHS, private prescription, over the counter.
Side effects: raised potassium levels, stomach irritation, mild diuresis.
Caution: in patients suffering from kidney disease.
Not to be used for: infants under 1 year or for patients suffering from ulcerated or blocked small bowel.
Not to be used with: potassium-sparing DIURETICS.
Contains: CITRIC ACID, POTASSIUM BICARBONATE.
Other preparations:

---

eicosapentaenoic acid *see* Maxepa

Elantan
(Schwarz)

A white, scored tablet supplied at strengths of 10 mg, 20 mg, 40 mg and used as a NITRATE treatment for the prevention of angina, and in addition to other treatments for congestive heart failure.

Dose: 10 mg twice a day at first increasing to 40-80 mg a day in 2 or 3 divided doses after meals to a maximum of 120 mg a day.
Availability: NHS and private prescription.
Side effects: headache, flushes, dizziness.
Caution:
Not to be used for: children.
Not to be used with:
Contains: ISOSORBIDE mononitrate.
Other preparations: Elantan LA, IMDUR (Astra).

Elavil *see* Tryptizol
(DDSA)

Eldepryl
(Britannia)

A white, scored tablet supplied at a strength of 5 mg and used as an anti-parkinsonian treatment for Parkinson's disease.

Dose: 2 tablets in the morning or 1 tablet at breakfast and 1 at lunchtime.
Availability: NHS and private prescription.
Side effects: low blood pressure on standing, involuntary movements, nausea, confusion, mental disorders.
Caution:
Not to be used for: children.
Not to be used with:
Contains: SELEGILINE HYDROCHLORIDE.
Other preparations:

E

Electrolade *see* Dioralyte
(Nicholas)

Eltroxin
(Glaxo)

A white, scored tablet or a white tablet according to strengths of

50 micrograms, 100 micrograms and used as a thyroid hormone to treat underactive thyroid gland in adults or children.
Dose: adults 50-100 micrograms a day at first increasing as needed by 50 micrograms a day every 3-4 weeks to a maximum of 150-300 micrograms a day; children 25 micrograms a day at first increasing if needed by 25 micrograms a day every 2-4 weeks and then reduce slightly.
Availability: NHS and private prescription.
Side effects: abnormal rhythms, chest pain, rapid heart rate, muscle cramp, headache, restlessness, excitability, flushing, sweating, diarrhoea, rapid weight loss.
Caution: in nursing mothers and in patients suffering from heart muscle or adrenal weakness.
Not to be used for:
Not to be used with: anti-coagulants, TRICYCLICS, PHENYTOIN, CHOLESTYRAMINE.

Contains: anyhdrous SODIUM THYROXINE.
Other preparations:

Eludril
(Pierre Fabre)

A solution used as an anti-bacterial treatment for throat and mouth infections, gingivitis, ulcers.

Dose: dilute 2 5 ml teaspoonsful with half a glass of warm water and gargle or rinse the mouth 3-4 times a day.
Availability: NHS, private prescription, over the counter.
Side effects:
Caution:
Not to be used for: children under 6 years.
Not to be used with:
Contains: CHLORHEXIDINE DIGLUCONATE, CHLORBUTOL, CHLOROFORM.
Other preparations: Eludril Spray.

Emcor
(Merck)

An orange, heart-shaped tablet supplied at a strength of 10 mg and used as a ß-BLOCKER to treat angina, high blood pressure.

Dose: 10 mg once a day to a maximum of 20 mg a day.
Availability: NHS and private prescription.
Side effects: cold hands and feet, sleep disturbance, slow heart rate, tiredness, wheezing, heart failure, stomach upset.
Caution: in pregnant women, nursing mothers, and in patients suffering from diabetes, kidney or liver disorders, asthma. May need to be withdrawn before surgery. Withdraw gradually. Your doctor may advise additional treatment with DIURETICS or DIGITALIS.
Not to be used for: patients suffering from heart block or failure.
Not to be used with: VERAPAMIL, CLONIDINE withdrawal, some anti-arrhythmic drugs and anaesthetics, some anti-hypertensives, ergot alkoloids, CIMETIDINE, sedatives, SYMPATHOMIMETICS, INDOMETHACIN.
Contains: BISOPROLOL FUMARATE.
Other preparations: Emcor LS.

Emeside
(L.A.B.)

An orange capsule supplied at a strength of 250 mg and used as an anti-convulsant to treat epilepsy.

Dose: adults 4-6 tablets a day; children under 6 years 1 tablet a day, 6-12 years 2 tablets a day.
Availability: NHS and private prescription.
Side effects: stomach and brain disturbances, rash, blood changes, SLE (a multi-system disorder).
Caution: in pregnant women, nursing mothers, and in patients suffering from kidney or liver disease. Dose should be reduced gradually.
Not to be used for:
Not to be used with:
Contains: ETHOSUXIMIDE.
Other preparations:

E

---

enalapril maleate *see* Innovace

Enduron
(Abbott)

A square, pink, scored tablet supplied at a strength of 5 mg and used as a DIURETIC to treat fluid retention, high blood pressure.

Dose: adults $1/2$ -1 tablet a day to a maximum of 2 tablets a day; children in proportion to dose for adult of 70 kg bodyweight.
Availability: NHS and private prescription.
Side effects: low potassium levels, rash, sensitivity to light, blood changes, gout, tiredness.
Caution: in pregnant women, nursing mothers, and in patients suffering from diabetes, gout, or liver or kidney disease. Potassium supplement may be necessary.
Not to be used for: patients suffering from severe kidney failure.
Not to be used with: LITHIUM, DIGITALIS, anti-hypertensives.
Contains: METHYCLOTHIAZIDE.
Other preparations:

Enteromide
(Consolidated)

A white tablet supplied at a strength of 500 mg and used as a sulpho-namide to treat dysentery, enteritis, ileitis, colitis, food poisoning, and for sterilization of the colon.

Dose: adults 2 tablets 3 times a day; infants quarter adult dose, other children half adult dose.
Availability: NHS and private prescription.
Side effects: anaemia, stomach disturbances, inflammation of the tongue, rash, blood changes if used for a long period.
Caution: in patients suffering from blood changes, kidney and liver disease. Blood should be checked if long-term treatment is used.
Not to be used for: new-born babies, or mothers in the late stages of pregnancy.
Not to be used with: FOLATE ANTAGONISTS (such as TRIMETHOPRIM), anti-diabetics.
Contains: CALCIUM SULPHALOXATE.
Other preparations:

Epanutin
(Parke-Davis)

A white/purple capsule, a white/pink capsule, or a white/orange capsule according to strengths of 25 mg, 50 mg, 100 mg and used as an anti-convulsant to treat epilepsy, migraine, neuralgia.

Dose: adults and children over 7 years 100 mg 2-4 times a day before food to a maximum of 600 mg a day; children under 3 years up to 50 mg 2-3 times a day, 4-6 years 5-10 mg per kg body weight.
Availability: NHS and private prescription.
Side effects: stomach upset, sleeplessness, unsteadiness, allergies, gum swelling, hairiness and motor activity in young people, blood changes, lymph gland swelling, nystagmus (abnormal eye move-ments).
Caution: in pregnant women, nursing mothers, and in patients suffering from liver disease. Dose should be reduced gradually.
Not to be used for:
Not to be used with: COUMARIN anti-coagulants, ISONIAZID, CHLORAM-PHENICOL, SULTHIAME, the contraceptive pill.
Contains: PHENYTOIN sodium.

Other preparations: Epanutin Suspension, Epanutin Infatabs, Epanutin Parenteral.

---

ephedrine *see* **Auralgicin, CAM, Davenol, Expurhin, Franol, Haymine, Phensedyl**

Ephynal
(Roche)

A white tablet or a white, scored tablet according to strengths of 10 mg, 50 mg, 200 mg and used as a source of vitamin E to treat vitamin E deficiency, tropical vitamin E deficiency.

Dose: adults 10-15 mg a day; children 1-10 mg per kg body weight a day.
Availability: NHS, private prescription, over the counter.
Side effects:
Caution:
Not to be used for:
Not to be used with:
Contains: TOCOPHERYL ACETATE.
Other preparations:

Epifoam
(Stafford-Miller)

A foam supplied in an aerosol and used as a corticosteroid, local anaesthetic treatment for damage to the external genital area, skin disorders.

Dose: apply foam 3-4 times a day (2-3 times a day for skin disorders) with a sterile, non-absorbent pad.
Availability: NHS and private prescription.
Side effects:
Caution:
Not to be used for: patients suffering from infected wounds.
Not to be used with:
Contains: HYDROCORTISONE acetate, PRAMOXINE hydrochloride.
Other preparations:

Epifrin
(Allergan)

Drops used as a SYMPATHOMIMETIC to treat glaucoma.

Dose: 1 drop into the eye 1-2 times a day.
Availability: NHS and private prescription.
Side effects: pain in the eye, deposits during extended use, head-ache, reddening of the eye.
Caution:
Not to be used for: patients suffering from narrow angle glaucoma or who wear soft contact lenses.
Not to be used with:
Contains: ADRENALINE.
Other preparations:

Epilim
(Sanofi)

A lilac tablet supplied at strengths of 200 mg, 500 mg and used as an anti-convulsant to treat epilepsy.

Dose: adults 600 mg a day at first in 2 divided doses then increase by 200 mg every 3 days usually to 1-2 g a day and a maximum of 2.5 g a day; children under 20 kg body weight 20 mg per kg a day at first, over 20 kg 400 mg a day at first, increasing gradually to 40 mg per kg a day if needed.
Availability: NHS and private prescription.
Side effects: gain in weight, loss of hair, fluid retention, pancreatitis, liver failure, blood changes, neurological effects.
Caution: in pregnant women, in patients suffering from mental retardation, or who are undergoing major surgery.
Not to be used for: patients suffering from liver disease.
Not to be used with: anti-depressants, other anti-convulsants.
Contains: SODIUM VALPROATE.
Other preparations: Epilim Crushable, Epilim Syrup, Epilim Liquid, Epilim Intravenous.

Epinal
(Alcon)

Drops used as a SYMPATHOMIMETIC and lubricant. to treat glaucoma.

Dose: 1 drop into the eye 1-2 times a day.
Availability: NHS, private prescription, over the counter.
Side effects: pain in the eye, headache, skin reactions, reddening of the eye, melanosis, rarely systemic effects.
Caution:
Not to be used for: patients suffering from narrow angle glaucoma or who wear soft contact lenses
Not to be used with:
Contains: ADRENALINE, HYPROMELLOSE.
Other preparations:

Eppy
(SNP)

Drops used as a SYMPATHOMIMETIC to treat glaucoma.

Dose: 1 drop into the eye 1-2 times a day.
Availability: NHS, private prescription, over the counter.
Side effects: pain in the eye, headache, skin reactions, melanosis, red eye, rarely systemic effects.
Caution:
Not to be used for: patients suffering from absence of the lens, narrow angle glaucoma.
Not to be used with:
Contains: ADRENALINE.
Other preparations:

Equagesic
(Wyeth)

A pink/white/yellow tablet used as an opiate, analgesic, and muscle relaxant to control pain in muscles or bones.

Dose: 2 tablets 3-4 times a day.
Availability: controlled drug.
Side effects: drowsiness, dizziness, nausea, unsteadiness, rash, blood changes.
Caution: in the elderly in patients with a history of epilepsy, or

suffering from depression or suicidal behaviour.

Not to be used for: pregnant women, or for patients suffering from porphyria (a rare blood disorder), alcoholism, peptic ulcer, haemophilia, kidney disease, allergy to anti-inflammatory drugs.

Not to be used with: alcohol, sedatives, anti-coagulants, antidiabetics, uric acid-lowering agents.

Contains: ETHOHEPTAZINE, MEPROBAMATE, ASPIRIN.

Other preparations:

Equanil
(Wyeth)

A white tablet or a white, scored tablet according to strengths of 200 mg, 400 mg and used as a tranquillizer for short-term treatment of anxiety, muscular tension.

Dose: elderly 200 mg 3 times a day; adults 400 mg 3 times a day and before going to bed.

Availability: NHS and private prescription.

Side effects: brain and stomach disturbances disturbances, low blood pressure, pins and needles, allergy, excitement, blood disorders.

Caution: in pregnant women, nursing mothers, and in patients with a history of epilepsy or depression, or patients suffering from liver or kidney disease. Patients should be warned that the drug is addictive

Not to be used for: alcoholics or for patients suffering from acute intermittent porphyria (a rare blood disorder).

Not to be used with: alcohol, sedatives, anti-coagulants, PHENYTOIN, GRISEOFULVIN, RIFAMPICIN, systemic steroids, contraceptive pill.

Contains: MEPROBAMATE.

Other preparations:

Eradacin
(Sterling Research Laboratories)

A red/yellow capsule supplied at a strength of 150 mg and used as an antibiotic to treat acute gonorrhoea.

Dose: 2 capsules as a single dose.

Availability: NHS and private prescription.

Side effects: stomach upset, headache, dizziness, drowsiness.
Caution: in pregant women and in patients suffering from liver or kidney disease.
Not to be used for: children.
Not to be used with:
Contains: ACROSOXACIN.
Other preparations:

---

ergotamine tartrate *see* **Cafergot, Lingraine, Medihaler-Ergotamine, Migril**

Erycen *see* **Erythrocin**
(Berk)

E

Erymax *see* **Erythrocin**
(Park-Davis)

Erythrocin
(Abbott)
A white, oblong tablet supplied at strengths of 250 mg, 500 mg and used as an antibiotic to treat infections.
Dose: 1-2 g a day.
Availability: NHS and private prescription.
Side effects: stomach disturbances, allergies.
Caution: in patients suffering from liver disease.
Not to be used for: children.
Not to be used with: THEOPHYLLINE, anti-coagulants taken by mouth, CARBAMAZEPINE.
Contains: ERYTHROMYCIN stearate.
Other preparations: Erythrocin IV Lactobionate, ARPIMYCIN (RP Drugs), ERYCEN (Berk), ERYMAX (Parke-Davis), ERYTHROMID (Abbott), ERYTHROPED A (Abbott), ILOSONE (Dista), LOTYCIN (Eli Lilly), RECTIN (DDSA).

Erythromid *see* **Erythrocin**
(Abbott)

---

erythromycin *see* **Erythrocin, Stromba**

Erythroped A *see* **Erythrocin**

Esbatal
(Calmic)

A peach, scored tablet supplied at strengths of 10 mg, 50 mg and used as an anti-hypertensive to treat high blood pressure.

Dose: adults 10 mg 3 times a day at first to a maximum of 200 mg a day; children as advised by physician.
Availability: NHS and private prescription.
Side effects: low blood pressure on standing, failure of ejaculation, blocked nose.
Caution: in patients suffering from weak kidneys.
Not to be used for: for patients suffering from phaeochromocytoma (a disease of the adrenal glands).
Not to be used with: SYMPATHOMIMETICS, TRICYCLIC anti-depressants, MAOIS.
Contains: BETHANIDINE sulphate.
Other preparations: BENDOGEN (Lagap).

Esidrex K
(Ciba)

A white tablet used as a DIURETIC with potassium supplement to treat fluid retention, high blood pressure where a potassium supplement is needed.

Dose: adults 2-8 tablets a day as a single dose after breakfast at first, then 2-4 tablets every other day; children as advised by the physician.
Availability: NHS and private prescription.

Side effects: rash, sensitivity to light, blood changes, gout, tiredness.
Caution: in pregnant women, nursing mothers, and in patients suffering from diabetes, gout, liver or kidney disease.
Not to be used for: patients suffering from a severe kidney failure, Addison's disease, or raised potassium levels.
Not to be used with: potassium-sparing diuretics, LITHIUM, DIGITALIS, anti-hypertensives.
Contains: HYDROCHLOROTHIAZIDE, POTASSIUM CHLORIDE.
Other preparations:

Eskamel
(S K B)

E

A cream used as a skin softener to treat acne.

Dose: apply a little to the affected area once a day.
Availability: NHS, private prescription, over the counter.
Side effects: irritation.
Caution: in patients suffering from acute local infection; keep out of the eyes, nose, and mouth.
Not to be used for:
Not to be used with:
Contains: RESORCINOL, SULPHUR.
Other preparations:

Eskornade Spansule
(S K B)

A grey/clear capsule used as an antihistamine and SYMPATHOMIMETIC to treat congestion, running nose, and phlegm brought on by common cold, rhinitis, flu, sinusitis.

Dose: adults 1 capsule every 12 hours; children use syrup.
Availability: private prescription and over the counter.
Side effects: drowsiness.
Caution: in patients suffering from diabetes.
Not to be used for: patients suffering from cardiovascular problems, overactive thyroid gland.
Not to be used with: MAOIS, TRICYCLICS, alcohol.
Contains: PHENYLPROPANOLAMINE HYDROCHLORIDE, DIPHENYLPYRALINE HYDRO-CHLORIDE.

Other preparations: Eskornade Syrup.

Estraderm
(Ciba)

A patch supplied at strengths of 25 micrograms, 50 micrograms, 100 micrograms and used as an oestrogen in oestrogen replacement.

Dose: apply a 50 microgram patch at first to a clean, hairless area of skin below the waist and replace with a new patch every 3-4 days on a different place. Increase the dose as needed after 1 month to a maximum of 100 micrograms a day.
Availability: NHS and private prescription.
Side effects: headache, nausea, tender breasts, redness at the site of the patch.
Caution: in patients with breast disease or a family history of breast cancer. Your doctor may advise that your blood pressure, breasts, pelvic organs should be checked regularly.
Not to be used for: patients suffering from severe liver, kidney, or heart disease, breast, genital tract, or other oestrogen-dependent cancers, genital bleeding, some ear disorders, or a history of or tendency towards thrombophlebitis, thromoboembolic diseases, or cerebrovascular disease.
Not to be used with: liver enzyme-inducing drugs.
Contains: OESTRADIOL.
Other preparations:

Estrapak
(Ciba)

A patch plus a red tablet supplied at strengths of 50 microgram and 1 mg respectively and used as oestrogen and progestogen in hormone replacement.

Dose: place patch on a clean, hairless are of skin below the waist and replace with a new patch every 3-4 days on a different area. 1 tablet a day from the fifteenth to the twenty-sixth days of each 28 days of oestrogen replacement. Start the treatment on the fifth day of the period if present.
Availability: NHS and private prescription.

Side effects: headache, nausea, tender breasts, redness at site of patch.
Caution: in patients with breast disease or a family history of breast cancer, high blood pressure, cholelithiasis (gallstones). Your doctor may advise that your blood pressure, breasts, pelvic organs should be checked regularly.
Not to be used for: children or for patients suffering from severe liver, kidney, or heart disease, breast, genital tract, or other oestrogen-dependent cancers, genital bleeding, some ear disorders, or a history of or tendency towards thrombophlebitis, thromboembolic disorders, or cerebrovascular disease.
Not to be used with: liver enzyme-inducing drugs.
Contains: OESTRADIOL, NORETHISTERONE.
Other preparations:

E

ethacrynic acid *see* **Edecrin**

ethambutol *see* **Myambutol, Mynah**

ethamsylate *see* **Dicynene**

ethinyloestradiol *see* **BiNovum, Brevinor, Conova 30, Controvlar, Dianette, Eugynon 30, Femodene, Loestrin 20, Logynon, Logynon ED, Marvelon, Mercilon, Microgynon 30, Minilyn, Minulet, Neocon 1/35, Norimin, Ovran, Ovranette, Ovysmen, PC4, Synphase, Trinordiol, Trinovum**

ethoheptazine *see* **Equagesic**

ethosuximide *see* **Emeside, Zarontin**

ethyl nicotinate *see* **Transvasin**

---

ethyl salicylate *see* **Dubam**

---

ethynodiol diacetate *see* **Conova 30**

---

etidronate disodium *see* **Didronel**

E

etodolac *see* **Lodine**

---

etretinate *see* **Tigason**

Eudemine
(A & H)

A white tablet supplied at a strength of 50 mg and used as a vasodilator and blood sugar elevator to treat severe high blood pressure especially when associated with kidney disease, low blood sugar.

Dose: high blood pressure 8-20 tablets a day in divided doses; low blood sugar 5 mg per kg body weight a day in 2-3 divided doses as needed.
Availability: NHS and private prescription.
Side effects: raised blood sugar, nausea, tremor, blood changes, anorexia, vomiting, low blood pressure, fluid retention, rapid heart rate, abnormal heart rhythm.
Caution: in pregnant women and in patients suffering from severe kidney disease. Your doctor may advise that your blood glucose levels should be checked.
Not to be used for: children.
Not to be used with: DIURETICS, anti-hypertensives, anti-coagulants

(blood-thinning drugs).
Contains: DIAZOXIDE.
Other preparations: Eudemine Injection.

Euglucon *see* **Daonil**
(Roussel)

Eugynon 30
(Schering)

A white tablet used as an oestrogen, progestogen contraceptive.

Dose: 1 tablet a day for 21 days starting on day 5 of the period.
Availability: NHS and private prescription.
Side effects: enlarged breasts, bloating and fluid retention, cramps, leg pains, mood change, reduction in sexual desire, headaches, nausea, vaginal erosion, discharge, and bleeding, weight gain, skin changes.
Caution: in patients suffering from high blood pressure, diabetes, vascular disorders, asthma, depression, kidney disease, multiple sclerosis, womb diseases. Your doctor may advise you not to smoke, to have regular examinations. You should stop treatment at the first sign of serious symptoms such as severe headache or jaundice. Treatment should be stopped before surgery.
Not to be used for: pregnant women, or for patients suffering from sickle-cell anaemia, history of heart disease or thrombosis, liver disorders, some cancers, undiagnosed vaginal bleeding, some ear, skin, and kidney disorders.
Not to be used with: RIFAMPICIN, TETRACYCLINES, GRISEOFULVIN, barbiturates, PHENYTOIN, PRIMIDONE, CARBAMAZEPINE, ETHOSUXIMIDE, CHLORAL HYDRATE, DICHLORALPHENAZONE.
Contains: ETHINYLOESTRADIOL, LEVONORGESTEROL.
Other preparations:

Eumovate
(Glaxo)

Drops used as a corticosteroid treatment for inflammation of the eyes where there is no infection present.

Dose: 1-2 drops into the eye 4 times a day or every 1-2 hours for severe inflammation.
Availability: NHS and private prescription.
Side effects: rise in eye pressure, sensitization, resistance to neomycin, fungal infection, cataract, thinning cornea.
Caution: in pregnant women and infants — do not use for extended periods. Avoid using unnecessarily for any patients.
Not to be used for: patients suffering from glaucoma, dendritic ulcer, viral, fungal, tubercular, or weeping infections, or for patients who wear soft contact lenses.
Not to be used with:
Contains: CLOBETASONE BUTYRATE.
Other preparations:

Eumovate Cream
(Glaxo)

A cream used as a steroid treatment for mild eczema and other skin disorders.

Dose: apply to the affected area 1-4 times a day.
Availability: NHS and private prescription.
Side effects: fluid retention, suppression of adrenal glands, thinning of the skin may occur.
Caution: use for short periods of time only.
Not to be used for: patients suffering from acne or any other skin infections caused by tuberculosis, ringworm, viruses, or fungi, or continuously especially in pregnant women.
Not to be used with:
Contains: CLOBETASONE BUTYRATE.
Other preparations: Eumovate Ointment.

Eurax
(Geigy)

A lotion used as a scabicide to treat scabies.

Dose: apply to the body apart from the head and face after a hot bath.

Availability: NHS, private prescription, over the counter.
Side effects:
Caution: keep out of the eyes.
Not to be used for: patients suffering from acute exudative derma-
titis.
Not to be used with:
Contains: CROTAMITON.
Other preparations: Eurax Cream.

Eurax-Hydrocortisone
(Zyma)

A cream used as a steroid and anti-itch treatment for itching skin disorders.

Dose: apply to the affected area 2-3 times a day.
Availability: NHS and private prescription.
Side effects: fluid retention, suppression of adrenal glands, thinning
of the skin may occur.
Caution: use for short periods of time only.
Not to be used for: patients suffering from acne or any other skin
infections caused by tuberculosis, ringworm, viruses, or fungi, or con-
tinuously especially in pregnant women.
Not to be used with:
Contains: CROTAMITON, HYDROCORTISONE.
Other preparations:

Evadyne
(Wyeth)

An orange tablet or a pink tablet according to strengths of 25 mg, 50
mg and used as an anti-depressant to treat depression.

Dose: 25 mg 3 times a day at first increasing if needed by 25 mg a day
or avery other day to a maximum of 100-150 mg a day, then 25 mg 3
times a day.
Availability: NHS and private prescription.
Side effects: dry mouth, constipation, urine retention, blurred vision,
palpitations, drowsiness, sleeplessness, dizziness, hands shaking,
low blood presure, weight change, skin reactions, jaundice or blood
changes, loss of libido may occur.

Caution: in nursing mothers or in patients suffering from heart disease, thyroid disease, epilepsy, diabetes, some other psychiatric conditions. Your doctor may advise regular blood tests.

Not to be used for: children, pregnant women , or patients suffering from heart attacks, liver disease, heart block.

Not to be used with: alcohol, ANTI-CHOLINERGICS, ADRENALINE, MAOIS, barbiturates, other anti-depressants, anti-hypertensives.

Contains: BUTRYPTILINE HYDROCHLORIDE.

Other preparations:

Evoxin
(Sterling Research Laboratories)

A white tablet supplied at a strength of 10 mg and used as an anti-nauseant to treat acute nausea and vomiting.

Dose: 1-2 tablets every 4-8 hours.

Availability: NHS and private prescription.

Side effects: raised serum prolactin (a hormone).

Caution:

Not to be used for: children or for pregnant women.

Not to be used with:

Contains: DOMPERIDONE maleate.

Other preparations: Evoxin Suppositories.

Exelderm
(ICI)

A cream used as an anti-fungal treatment for fungal infections of the skin.

Dose: rub into the affected area twice a day for 2-3 weeks after the wounds have healed.

Availability: NHS, private prescription, over the counter.

Side effects:

Caution: keep out of the eyes; if the area becomes irritated, the treatment should be stopped.

Not to be used for:

Not to be used with:

Contains: SULCONAZOLE nitrate.

Other preparations:

Exirel
(Pfizer)

An olive green/turquoise-blue capsule or a beige/turquoise-blue capsule according to strengths of 10 mg, 15 mg and used as a broncho-dilator to treat bronchial spasm brought on by bronchial asthma, bronchitis, emphysema.

Dose: adults 10-15 mg 3-4 times a day up to a maximum of 60 mg a day; children 6-12 years use syrup.
Availability: NHS and private prescription.
Side effects: shaking of the hands, nervous tension, headache, dilation of the blood vessels.
Caution: in pregnant women and in patients suffering from high blood pressure, abnormal heart rhythms, angina, heart muscle disease, overactive thyroid.
Not to be used for: children under 6 years.
Not to be used with: SYMPATHOMIMETICS.
Contains: PIRBUTEROL hydrochloride.
Other preparations: Exirel Syrup, Exirel Inhaler.

Exolan
(Dermal)

A cream used as an anti-psoriatic treatment for psoriasis.

Dose: apply to the affected area 1-2 times a day.
Availability: NHS, private prescription, over the counter.
Side effects: irritation, allergy.
Caution:
Not to be used for: patients suffering from acute psoriasis.
Not to be used with:
Contains: DITHRANOL triacetate.
Other preparations:

Expulin
(Galen)

A linctus used as an antihistamine, opiate, and SYMPATHOMIMETIC treatment for cough and congestion.

Dose: adults 2 5 ml teaspoonsful 4 times a day; children 2-6 years
$^1/_2$ -1 teaspoonful 4 times a day; 7-12 years 1-2 teaspoonsful 4 times
a day.
Availability: private prescription and over the counter.
Side effects: constipation, drowsiness, reduced reactions, anxiety,
hands shaking, irregular or rapid heart rate, dry mouth, excitement,
rarely skin eruptions.
Caution: in patients suffering from asthma, kidney disease, diabetes.
Not to be used for: children under 5 years or for patients suffering
from liver disease, heart or thyroid isorders.
Not to be used with: MAOIS, alcohol, sedatives, TRICYCLICS.
Contains: PHOLCODINE, PSEUDOEPHEDRINE HYDROCHLORIDE, CHLORPHENIRAM-
INE HYDROCHLORIDE, CHLORPHENIRAMINE MALEATE.
Other preparations: Expulin Paediatric.

Expurhin
(Galen)

A linctus used as an antihistamine and SYMPATHOMIMETIC treatment for
congestion, phlegm, and running nose in children.

Dose: 3 months-1 year $^1/_2$ -1 5 ml teaspoonful twice a day, 1-5 years1-
2 teaspoonsful 3 times a day, 6-12 years 2-3 teaspoonsful 3 times a
day.
Availability: private prescription and over the counter.
Side effects: drowsiness, reduced reactions, anxiety, hands shaking,
irregular or rapid heart rate, dry mouth, excitement, rarely skin erup-
tions.
Caution: patients suffering from liver or kidney disease, diabetes.
Not to be used for: infants under 3 months, or for patients suffering
from heart or thyroid disorders.
Not to be used with: alcohol, sedatives, some anti-depressants
(MAOIS), TRICYCLICS.
Contains: EPHEDRINE HYDROCHLORIDE, CHLORPHENIRAMINE MALEATE, MEN-
THOL.
Other preparations:

Exterol
(Dermal)

Drops used as a wax softener to remove ear wax.

Dose: hold 5-10 drops in the ear 1-2 times a day for 3-4 days.
Availability: NHS, private prescription, over the counter.
Side effects: slight fizzing.
Caution:
Not to be used for: patients suffering from perforated ear drum.
Not to be used with:
Contains: UREA HYDROGEN PEROXIDE, GLYCERIN.
Other preparations:

Fabahistin
(Bayer)

An orange tablet supplied at a strength of 50 mg and used as an anti-histamine to treat rhinitis, hay fever, other allergies.

Dose: adults 1-2 tablet 3 times a day; children use suspension.
Availability: NHS and private prescription.
Side effects: drowsiness, reduced reactions, excitement in children, rarely white cell depression.
Caution:
Not to be used for:
Not to be used with: sedatives, MAOIS, alcohol.
Contains: MEBHYDROLIN.
Other preparations: Fabahistin Suspension.

Fabrol
(Zyma)

A sachet of granules of 200 mg and used as a protein to treat bronchitis, infections of the respiratory tract where phlegm is produced, complications in the abdomen associated with cystic fibrosis.

Dose: up to 6 sachets a day.
Availability: NHS in some circumstances (when prescribed as a generic), private prescription.
Side effects: nausea, heartburn, vomiting, headache, tinnitus, allergy, rarely bronchial spasm.
Caution: in patients suffering from diabetes.

Not to be used for:
Not to be used with:
Contains: ACETYLCYSTEINE.
Other preparations:

---

famotidine *see* Pepcid PM

Fansidar
(Roche)

A white, quarter-scored tablet used as a sulphonamide for the prevention and treatment of malaria.

Dose: prevention adults and children over 14 years 1 tablet a week, treatment 2-3 tablets as one dose or as advised by the physician; prevention children under 4 years quarter adult dose, treatment $1/2$ tablet as one dose; prevention children 4-8 years half adult dose, treatment 1 tablet as one dose; prevention children 9-14 years three-quarters adult dose, treatment 2 tablets as one dose.
Availability: NHS and private prescription.
Side effects: rash, inflammation of the pharynx, itch, stomach upset, rare skin and blood changes.
Caution: patients should keep out of the sun. Your doctor may advise regular blood tests if the treatment is prolonged.
Not to be used for: new-born infants, pregnant women, nursing mothers or for patients suffering from severe kidney or liver disease, or sensitivity to sulphonamides.
Not to be used with: FOLATE INHIBITORS such as TRIMETHOPRIM.
Contains: SULFADOXINE, PYRIMETHAMINE.
Other preparations:

Fasigyn
(Pfizer)

A white tablet supplied at a strength of 500 mg and used as an antibiotic for the treament and prevention of infection.

Dose: prevention 4 tablets as a single dose, treatment 4 tablets at first

then 2 tablets a day for at least 5-6 days.
Availability: NHS and private prescription.
Side effects: stomach upset, furred tongue, unpleasant taste, swelling and brain disturbances, dark-coloured urine.
Caution: in pregnant women and nursing mothers.
Not to be used for: children or for patients suffering from nervous disorders, blood changes. Your doctor may advise regular blood tests
Not to be used with: alcohol.
Contains: TINIDAZOLE.
Other preparations:

Faverin
(Duphar)

A yellow tablet supplied at a strength of 50 mg and used as an anti-depressant to treat depression.

Dose: 2 tablets in the evening at first then usually 2-4 tablets a day in divided doses, up to a maximum of 6 tablets a day if needed.
Availability: NHS and private prescription.
Side effects: nausea, vomiting, sleepiness, diarrhoea, agitation, anorexia, tremor, convulsions
Caution: in patients suffering from liver or kidney disease.
Not to be used for: children, pregnant women, nursing mothers, or for patients with a history of epilepsy.
Not to be used with: PROPANOLOL, THEOPHYLLINE, PHENYTOIN, WARFARIN, MAOIS, alcohol.
Contains: FLUVOXAMINE MALEATE.
Other preparations:

Fectrim Forte *see* Septrin
(DDSA)

Fefol Spansule
(S K B)

A clear/green capsule used for the prevention of iron and folic acid deficiency in pregnancy.

Dose: 1 capsule a day.
Availability: NHS, private prescription, over the counter.
Side effects: mild stomach upset.
Caution:
Not to be used for: children.
Not to be used with: TETRACYCLINES.
Contains: FERROUS SULPHATE, FOLIC ACID.
Other preparations:

Fefol Z Spansule
(S K B)

A clear/blue capsule used for the prevention of iron and folic acid deficiency in pregnancy where zinc supplement is also needed.

Dose: 1 capsule a day.
Availability: NHS, private prescription, over the counter.
Side effects: mild stomach upset.
Caution: in patients suffering from kidney disease.
Not to be used for: children.
Not to be used with: TETRACYCLINES.
Contains: FERROUS SULPHATE, FOLIC ACID, ZINC SULPHATE MONOHYDRATE.
Other preparations:

Fefol-Vit Spansule
(S K B)

A white/clear capsule used for the prevention of iron, folic acid, and vitamin deficiency in pregnancy.

Dose: 1 capsule a day.
Availability: private prescription and over the counter.
Side effects: mild stomach upset.
Caution:
Not to be used for: children.
Not to be used with: TETRACYCLINES.
Contains: FERROUS SULPHATE, FOLIC ACID, THIAMINE mononitrate, RIBOFLAVINE, PYRIDOXINE hydrochloride, NICOTINAMIDE, ASCORBIC ACID.
Other preparations:

---

felbinac *see* **Traxam**

Feldene
(Pfizer)

A maroon/blue capsule or a maroon capsule according to strengths of 10 mg, 20 mg and used as a NON-STEROID ANTI-INFLAMMATORY DRUG to treat rheumatoid arthritis, osteoarthritis, ankylosing spondylitis, acute muscle or bone problems, acute gout, juvenile chronic arthritis.

Dose: adults 20 mg a day; for muscle or bone problems 40 mg a day for 2 days at first then 20 mg a day for 7-14 days; for gout 40 mg a day for 4-6 days. Children over 6 years and under 15 kg body weight 5 mg, 16-25 kg 10 mg, 26-45 kg 15 mg, over 46 kg 20 mg.
Availability: NHS and private prescription.
Side effects: stomach disturbances, swelling, brain disturbances, feeling of being unwell, tinnitus.
Caution: in pregnant women, nursing mothers, and in patients suffering from kidney or liver disease.
Not to be used for: patients suffering from anti-inflammatory or aspirin induced allergy, peptic ulcer, history of recurring ulcers, recent anal inflammation.
Not to be used with: anti-coagulants, other non-steroid anti-inflammatory drugs, anti-diabetics, LITHIUM.
Contains: PIROXICAM.
Other preparations: Feldene Dispersible, Feldene Suppositories, LARAPAM (Lagap).

Femerital
(MCP)

A white, scored tablet used as an anti-spasmodic and analgesic drug for the relief of period pain.

Dose: 1-2 tablets 2-3 times a day beginning 2 days before the start of the period.
Availability: private prescription and over the counter.
Side effects:
Caution: in patients suffering from liver or kidney disease.
Not to be used for: children.

Not to be used with:
Contains: AMBUCETAMIDE, PARACETAMOL.
Other preparations:

Femodene
(Schering)

A white tablet used as an oestrogen, progestogen contraceptive.

Dose: 1 tablet a day for 21 days starting on day 1 of the period.
Availability: NHS and private prescription.
Side effects: enlarged breasts, bloating and fluid retention, cramps, leg pains, mood change, reduction in sexual desire, headaches, nausea, vaginal erosion, discharge, and bleeding, weight gain, skin changes.
Caution: in patients suffering from high blood pressure, diabetes, vascular disorders, asthma, depression, kidney disease, multiple sclerosis, womb diseases. Your doctor may advise you not to smoke, to have regular examinations. You should stop treatment at the first sign of serious symptoms such as severe headache or jaundice. Treatment should be stopped before surgery.
Not to be used for: pregnant women, or for patients suffering from sickle-cell anaemia, history of heart disease or thrombosis, liver disorders, some cancers, undiagnosed vaginal bleeding, some ear, skin, and kidney disorders.
Not to be used with: RIFAMPICIN, TETRACYCLINES, GRISEOFULVIN, barbiturates, PHENYTOIN, PRIMIDONE, CARBAMAZEPINE, ETHOSUXIMIDE, CHLORAL HYDRATE, DICHLORALPHENAZONE.
Contains: ETHINYLOESTRADIOL, GESTODENE.
Other preparations:

Femulen
(Gold Cross)

A white tablet used as a progesterone contraceptive.

Dose: 1 tablet at the same time every day starting on day 1 of the period.
Availability: NHS and private prescription.
Side effects: irregular bleeding, breast discomfort, acne, headache.
Caution: in patients suffering from high blood pressure, tendency to

thrombosis, migraine, liver abnormalities, ovarian cysts. Your doctor
may advise regular check-ups.
Not to be used for: pregnant women, or for patients suffering from
severe heart or artery disease, benign liver tumours, vaginal bleeding,
previous ectopic pregnancy.
Not to be used with: barbiturates, PHENYTOIN, PRIMIDONE, CARBAMAZEP-
INE, CHLORAL HYDRATE, DICHLORALPHENAZONE, ETHOSUXIMIDE, RIFAMPICIN,
GLUTETHIMIDE, CHLORPROMAZINE, MEPROBAMATE, GRISEOFULVIN.
Contains: ETHYNODIOL DIACETATE.
Other preparations:

Fenbid Spansule
(S K B)

A pink/maroon capsule supplied at a strength of 300 mg and used as
a NON-STEROID ANTI-INFLAMMATORY DRUG to treat pain, rheumatoid arthritis, osteoarthritis, ankylosing spondylitis, other joint diorders.

F

Dose: 2 capsules twice a day at first, then 3 capsules twice a day if
needed, usually 1-2 capsules twice a day.
Availability: NHS and private prescription.
Side effects: dyspepsia, gastro-intestinal bleeding, rash, blood
changes.
Caution: in pregnant women, in patients allergic to anti-inflammatory
drugs, and in patients suffering from asthma.
Not to be used for: children or patients suffering from peptic ulcer.
Not to be used with:
Contains: IBUPROFEN.
Other preparations: APSIFEN (APS), BRUFEN (Boots), EBUFAC (DDSA),
LIDIFEN (Berk), MOTRIN (Upjohn), PAXOFEN (Steinhard).

---

fenbufen *see* **Lederfen**

---

fenchone *see* **Rowatinex**

---

fenfluramine *see* **Ponderax Pacaps**

fenofibrate *see* **Lipantil**

---

fenoprofen *see* **Fenopron**

Fenopron
(Dista)

An orange, oval tablet or orange, oblong, scored tablet according to strengths of 300 mg, 600 mg and used as a NON-STEROID ANTI-INFLAMMATORY DRUG to treat pain, rheumatoid arthritis, osteoarthritis, ankylosing spondylitis.

Dose: 300-600 mg 3-4 times a day to a maximum of 3 g a day.
Availability: NHS and private prescription.
Side effects: stomach intolerance, allergy, kidney and liver disorders, blood changes.
Caution: in pregnant women, nursing mothers, and in patients with a history of peptic ulcer or stomach bleeding, or suffering from asthma or liver disease.
Not to be used for: children or for patients suffering from peptic ulcer, kidney disease, or allergy to ASPIRIN or anti-inflammatory drugs.
Not to be used with: anti-coagulants, aspirin, hypoglycaemics, hydantoins.
Contains: FENOPROFEN.
Other preparations: PROGESIC (Eli Lilly).

Fenostil Retard
(Zyma)

A white tablet supplied at a strength of 2.5 mg and used as an antihistamine treatment for rhinitis, urticaria, hay fever, other allergies.

Dose: 1 tablet night and morning.
Availability: NHS, private prescription, over the counter.
Side effects: drowsiness, reduced reactions.
Caution: in nursing mothers.
Not to be used for: children.
Not to be used with: sedatives, MAOIS, alcohol.
Contains: DIMETHINDENE maleate.

Other preparations:

---

fenoterol *see* **Berotec**

---

fenoterol *see* **Duovent**

Fentazin
(A & H)

A white tablet supplied at strengths of 2 mg, 4 mg and used as a sedative to treat anxiety, tension, chronic mental disorders, schizophrenia, vomiting, nausea, and other psychiatric problems.

F

Dose: usually 12 mg day in divided doses to a maximum of 24 mg day.
Availability: NHS and private prescription.
Side effects: muscle spasms, restlessness, hands shaking, dry mouth, urine retention, palpitations, low blood pressure, weight gain, changes in libido, low body temperature, breast swelling, menstrual changes, jaundice, blood and skin changes, drowsiness, rarely fits.
Caution: in pregnant women, nursing mothers, and in patients suffering from Parkinson's disease, liver disease, or cardiovascular disease.
Not to be used for: children, unconscious patients, or those suffering from bone marrow depression.
Not to be used with: alcohol, tranquillizers, pain killers, anti-hypertensives, anti-depressants, anti-convulsants, anti-diabetic drugs, LEVODOPA.
Contains: PERPHENAZINE.
Other preparations: Fentazin Injection.

Feospan Spansule
(S K B)

A red/clear capsule supplied at a strength of 150 mg and used as a iron supplement to treat iron deficiency, anaemia

Dose: adults 1-2 capsules a day; children 1-12 years 1 capsule a day.
Availability: NHS, private prescription, over the counter.
Side effects: mild stomach upset.
Caution:
Not to be used for: infants under 1 year.
Not to be used with: TETRACYCLINES.
Contains: FERROUS SULPHATE.
Other preparations:

Ferfolic SV
(Sinclair)

A pink tablet used as an iron supplement to treat iron and folic acid deficiencies.

Dose: 1 tablet 3 times a day.
Availability: NHS and private prescription.
Side effects: nausea, constipation
Caution:
Not to be used for: patients suffering from megaloblastic anaemia.
Not to be used with: TETRACYCLINES.
Contains: FOLIC ACID, FERROUS GLUCONATE.
Other preparations:

Fergon
(Winthrop)

A red tablet supplied at a strength of 300 mg and used as an iron supplement to treat iron deficiency, anaemia.

Dose: adults treatment 4-8 tablets in divided doses 1 hour before food, prevention 2 tablets a day; children 6-12 years 1-3 tablets a day.
Availability: NHS, private prescription, over the counter.
Side effects: nausea, constipation.
Caution:
Not to be used for: children under 6 years.
Not to be used with: TETRACYCLINES.
Contains: FERROUS GLUCONATE.
Other preparations:

---

ferric ammonium citrate *see* Tonivitan A & D

Ferrocap *see* Fersamal
(Consolidated)

Ferrocontin Continus
(Degussa)

A red tablet supplied at a strength of 100 mg and used as an iron supplement to treat iron deficiency, anaemia.

Dose: 1 tablet a day.
Availability: NHS, private prescription, over the counter.
Side effects:
Caution:
Not to be used for: children.
Not to be used with: TETRACYCLINES.
Contains: FERROUS GLYCINE SULPHATE.
Other preparations: Ferrocontin Folic Continus.

Ferrograd
(Abbott)

A red tablet supplied at a strength of 325 mg and used as an iron supplement to treat iron deficiency anaemia.

Dose: 1 tablet a day before food.
Availability: NHS, private prescription, and over the counter.
Side effects:
Caution: in patients suffering from slow bowel actions.
Not to be used for: children or for patients suffering from diverticular disease, blocked intestine.
Not to be used with: TETRACYCLINES.
Contains: FERROUS SULPHATE.
Other preparations:

Ferrograd C
(Abbott)

A red, oblong tablet used as an iron supplement to treat iron deficiency anaemia where absorption is difficult.

Dose: 1 tablet a day before food.
Availability: private prescription and over the counter.
Side effects:
Caution: in patients suffering from slow bowel action.
Not to be used for: children or for patients suffering from diverticular disease, blocked intestine.
Not to be used with: TETRACYCLINE, Clinistix urine test.
Contains: FERROUS SULPHATE, ASCORBIC ACID.
Other preparations:

Ferrograd Folic
(Abbott)

A yellow/red tablet used as an iron supplement to treat anaemia in pregnancy.

Dose: 1 tablet a day before food.
Availability: NHS, private prescription, over the counter.
Side effects:
Caution: in patients suffering from slow bowel movements.
Not to be used for: children or for patients suffering from diverticular disease, intestinal blockage, vitamin B12 deficiency.
Not to be used with: TETRACYCLINES.
Contains: FERROUS SULPHATE, FOLIC ACID.
Other preparations:

Ferromyn
(Calmic)

An elixir used as an iron supplement to treat iron deficiency anaemia.

Dose: adults and children over 10 years1 5 ml teaspoonful 3 times a day; children up to 2 years 1 ml twice a day, 2-5 years $1/2$ teaspoonful 3 times a day, 5-10 years 1 teaspoonful twice a day.
Availability: NHS, private prescription, over the counter.

Side effects: stomach upset.
Caution:
Not to be used for:
Not to be used with: TETRACYCLINES, antacids.
Contains: FERROUS SUCCINATE.
Other preparations:

---

ferrous fumarate *see* BC 500 with Iron, Fersaday, Fersamal, Folex-350, Galfer, Galfervit, Givitol, Meterfolic, Pregaday

---

ferrous gluconate *see* Ferfolic SV, Fergon

---

ferrous glycine sulphate *see* Ferrocontin Continus, Plesmet

---

ferrous perchloride *see* Glykola

---

ferrous succinate *see* Ferromyn

---

ferrous sulphate *see* Fefol Spansule, Fefol Z Spansule, Fefol-Vit Spansule, Feospan Spansule, Ferrograd, Ferrograd C, Ferrograd Folic, Fesovit Spansule, Fesovit Z Spansule, Folicin, Irofol C, Octovit, Pregnavite Forte F, Slow-Fe, Slow-Fe Folic

---

Fersaday
(Duncan, Flockhart)

A brown tablet supplied at a strength of 100 mg and used as an iron supplement to treat iron deficiency.

Dose: 1 tablet 1-2 times a day.
Availability: NHS, private prescription, over the counter.
Side effects: stomach upset.
Caution: in patients with a history of peptic ulcer.
Not to be used for: children.
Not to be used with: TETRACYCLINES, antacids.
Contains: FERROUS FUMARATE.
Other preparations:

Fersamal
(Duncan, Flockhart)

A brown tablet supplied at a strength of 65 mg and used as an iron
supplement to treat iron deficiency.

Dose: adults 1 tablet 3 times a day; children use Fersamal Syrup.
Availability: NHS, private prescription, over the counter.
Side effects: stomach upset.
Caution: in patients with a history of peptic ulcer.
Not to be used for:
Not to be used with: TETRACYCLINES, antacids.
Contains: FERROUS FUMARATE.
Other preparations: Fersamal Syrup, FERROCAP (Consolidated).

Fesovit Spansule
(S K B)

A yellow/clear capsule used as an iron and vitamin supplement to treat
iron deficiency anaemia needing vitamins B and C.

Dose: adults 1 capsule 1-2 times a day; children 1-12 years 1 capsule
a day.
Availability: private prescription and over the counter.
Side effects: mild stomach upset.
Caution:
Not to be used for: infants under 1 year.
Not to be used with: TETRACYCLINES.
Contains: FERROUS SULPHATE, ASCORBIC ACID, THIAMINE mononitrate,
RIBOFLAVINE, PYRIDOXINE hydrochloride, NICOTINAMIDE.

Fesovit Z Spansule
(S K B)

An orange/clear capsule used as an iron, zinc, and vitamin supplement to treat iron defficiency anaemia where vitamins B and C and zinc are needed.

Dose: adults 1-2 capsules a day; children 1-12 years 1 capsule a day.
Availability: private prescription, over the counter.
Side effects: mild stomach upset.
Caution: in patients suffering from kidney disease.
Not to be used for: infants under 1 year.
Not to be used with: TETRACYCLINES.
Contains: FERROUS SULPHATE, ZINC SULPHATE MONOHYDRATE, ASCORBIC ACID, THIAMINE mononitrate, RIBOFLAVINE, PYRIDOXINE hydrochloride, NICOTINAMIDE.
Other preparations:

F

Finalgon
(Boehringer Ingelheim)

An ointment supplied with an applicator. and used as an analgesic rub to relieve muscular and skeletal pain.

Dose: massage gently into the affected area as needed.
Availability: NHS, private prescription, over the counter.
Side effects: may be irritant.
Caution:
Not to be used for: areas near the eyes, or on broken or inflamed skin, or on membranes (such as the mouth).
Not to be used with:
Contains: NONIVAMIDE, BUTOXYETHYL NICOTINATE.
Other preparations:

Flagyl
(M & B)

An off-white tablet or an off-white, capsule-shaped tablet according to strengths of 200 mg, 400 mg and used as an anti-bacterial treatment for trichomoniasis, non-specific vaginitis, other infections, dysentery, abscess of the liver, ulcerative gingivitis (gum disease).

Dose: adults up to 400 mg 2-3 times a day; children 7.5 mg per kg body weight 3 times a day.
Availability: NHS and private prescription.
Side effects: stomach upset, furred tongue, unpleasant taste, allergy, swelling, brain disturbances, dark-coloured urine, nerve changes, seizures, white cell changes.
Caution: short-term high-dose treatment should not be used for pregnant women or nursing mothers.
Not to be used for: children under 10 years.
Not to be used with: alcohol, phenobarbitones, anti-coagulants (blood-thinning drugs) taken by mouth.
Contains: METRONIDAZOLE.
Other preparations: Flagyl-S Suspension, Flagyl Suppositories, Flagyl Injection, Flagyl Compak, METROLYL (Lagap), ZADSTAT (Lederle).

F

Flamazine
(SNP)

A cream used as an anti-bacterial treatment for wounds, burns, infected ulcers of the leg, bed sores, and where skin has been removed for grafting.

Dose: apply a layer up to 0.5 cm thick to the affected area; change dressing 3 times a week.
Availability: NHS and private prescription.
Side effects:
Caution: in patients suffering from kidney or liver disease.
Not to be used for: infants under 3 months or for pregnant women.
Not to be used with:
Contains: SILVER SULPHADIAZINE.
Other preparations:

---

flavoxate hydrochloride *see* Urispas

---

flecainide *see* **Tambocor**

Fletchers' Arachis Oil
(Pharmax)

A 130 ml, single-dose enema used as a faecal softener to treat faecal impactation.

Dose: 1 enema as required; children in proportion according to age and body weight.
Availability: NHS and private prescription.
Side effects:
Caution: warm before use.
Not to be used for:
Not to be used with:
Contains: ARACHIS OIL.
Other preparations:

Fletchers' Enemette
(Pharmax)

A 5 ml, single-dose micro-enema supplied at a strength of 90 mg and used as a faecal softener to treat constipation, and for evacuation of bowels before surgery etc.

Dose: adults 1 as required; children over 3 years in proportion to age.
Availability: NHS and private prescription.
Side effects:
Caution:
Not to be used for: children under 3 years.
Not to be used with:
Contains: DOCUSATE SODIUM.
Other preparations:

Fletchers' Phosphate
(Pharmax)

A 128 ml, single-dose enema used as a bowel evacuator to treat constipation, and for evacuation of the bowels before surgery etc.

Dose: adults 1 enema as required; children over 3 years in proportion to age.
Availability: NHS and private prescription.
Side effects:
Caution: in patients with restricted sodium intake.
Not to be used for: patients where the absorptive capacity of the colon is increased.
Not to be used with:
Contains: SODIUM ACID PHOSPHATE, SODIUM PHOSPHATE.
Other preparations:

Flexin Continus
(Napp)

A yellow, scored tablet supplied at a strength of 75 mg and used as a NON-STEROID ANTI-INFLAMMATORY DRUG to treat acute rheumatoid arthritis, osteoarthritis, ankylosing spondylitis, degenerative joint disease of the hip, acute muscle or bone problems, lower back pain, other joint disorders, painful periods.

Dose: 1 tablet 1-2 times a day with food, milk, or an antacid.
Availability: NHS and private prescription.
Side effects: stomach bleeding, headache, corneal deposits, disturbances of the retina, stomach intolerance, dizziness, brain effects, blood changes.
Caution: in patients suffering from liver or kidney disease, brain disorders.
Not to be used for: children, pregnant women, nursing mothers, or for patients suffering from peptic ulcer, a history of stomach lesions, or allergy to aspirin or anti-inflammatory drugs.
Not to be used with: salicylates, anti-coagulants, LITHIUM, corticosteroids, DIURETICS, ß-BLOCKERS, PROBENECID.
Contains: INDOMETHACIN.
Other preparations:

Florinef
(Squibb)

A pink, scored tablet supplied at a strength of 0.1 mg and used as a corticosteroid replacement treatment in Addison's disease, salt-losing adrenogenital syndrome (adrenal disorders).

Dose: adults $^1/_2$-3 tablets a day; children in proportion to adult dose according to age, body weight, and severity of illness.
Availability: NHS and private prescription.
Side effects: high blood sugar, thin bones, mood change, ulcers.
Caution: in pregnant women, in patients who have had recent bowel surgery, or who are suffering from inflamed veins, psychiatric disorders, virus infections, some cancers, some kidney diseases, thinning of the bones, ulcers, tuberculosis, other infections, high blood pressure, glaucoma, epilepsy, diabetes, underactive thyroid, liver disease, stress. Withdraw gradually.
Not to be used for: infants under 1 year.
Not to be used with: PHENYTOIN, PHENOBARBITONE, EPHEDRINE, RIFAMPICIN, DIURETICS, anti-cholinesterases, DIGITALIS, anti-diabetic agents, anti-coagulants, NON-STEROID ANTI-INFLAMMATORY DRUGS.
Contains: FLUDROCORTISONE acetate.
Other preparations:

Floxapen
(S K B)

A black/caramel-coloured capsule supplied at strengths of 250 mg, 500 mg and used as a penicillin treatment for skin, soft tissue, ear, nose, and throat, and other infections.

Dose: adults and children over 10 years 1 capsule 4 times a day; children under 2 years quarter adult dose, 2-10 years half adult dose.
Availability: NHS and private prescription.
Side effects: allergy, stomach disturbances.
Caution:
Not to be used for: patients suffering from penicillin allergy.
Not to be used with:
Contains: FLUCLOXACILLIN sodium.
Other preparations: Floxapen Syrup, Floxapen Syrup Forte, Floxapen Injection.

---

fluandrenolone *see* **Haelan**

Fluanxol
(Lundbeck)

A red tablet supplied at strengths of 0.5 mg, 1 mg and used as a sedative for the short-term treatment of depression and anxiety.

Dose: adults 1-2 mg in the morning to a maximum of 3 mg a day in divided doses; elderly 0.5 mg in the morning to a maximum of 2 mg a day in divided doses.
Availability: NHS and private prescription.
Side effects: muscle spasms, restlessness, hands shaking, dry mouth, urine retention, palpitations, low blood pressure, weight gain, changes in libido, low body temperature, breast swelling, menstrual changes, jaundice, blood and skin changes, drowsiness, rarely fits.
Caution: in patients suffering from Parkinson's disease, severe hardening of the arteries, confusion in the elderly, severe kidney, liver, or heart disease.
Not to be used for: children or for excitable, overactive, or severely clinically depressed patients.
Not to be used with: alcohol, tranquillizers, pain killers, anti-hypertensives, anti-depressants, anti-convulsants, anti-diabetic drugs, LEVODOPA.
Contains: FLUPENTHIXOL DIHYDROCHLORIDE.
Other preparations:

---

fluclorolone acetonide *see* **Topilar**

---

flucloxacillin *see* **Floxapen, Magnapen, Stafoxil, Staphlipen**

---

fluconazole *see* **Diflucan**

---

fludrocortisone *see* **Florinef**

---

flumethasone *see* **Lorocorten-Vioform**

flunisolide *see* **Syntaris**

flunitrazepam *see* **Rohypnol**

fluocinolone *see* **Synalar**

fluocinonide *see* **Metosyn**

fluocortolone hexanoate *see* **Ultradil, Ultralanum Plain Cream, Ultraproct**

fluocortolone pivalate *see* **Ultradil, Ultralanum Plain Cream, Ultraproct**

Fluorescein
(SNP)

Drops used as a dye for staining purposes to enable abrasions or foreign bodies in the eye to be found.

Dose: 1 or more drops into the eye as needed.
Availability: NHS, private prescription, over the counter.
Side effects:
Caution:
Not to be used for:
Not to be used with:
Contains: sodium FLUORESCEIN.
Other preparations:

fluorescein *see* Fluorescein

---

fluorometholone *see* FML

---

fluoxetine *see* Prozac

---

flupenthixol *see* Depixol, Fluanxol

---

fluphenazine *see* Moditen, Motipress, Motival

---

flurazepam *see* Dalmane

---

flurbiprofen *see* Froben

---

fluvoxamine *see* Faverine

FML
(Allergan)

Drops used as a corticosteroid treatment for inflammation of the eye where no infection is present.

Dose: 1-2 drops into the eye 2-4 times a day.
Availability: NHS and private prescription.
Side effects: rise in eye pressure, thinning cornea, fungal infection, cataract.
Caution: in pregnant women and infants — do not use for extended

periods — or for patients suffering from glaucoma.
Not to be used for: infants under 2 years, or for patients suffering from viral, fungal, tubercular, or weeping infections, or who wear soft contact lenses.
Not to be used with:
Contains: FLUOROMETHOLONE.
Other preparations:

Folex-350
(Rybar)

A pink tablet used as an iron supplement for the prevention of iron and folic acid deficiency in pregnancy.

Dose: 1 tablet a day.
Availability: NHS, private prescription, over the counter.
Side effects: nausea, constipation.
Caution:
Not to be used for: children or for patients suffering from megaloblastic anaemia.
Not to be used with: TETRACYCLINES.
Contains: FERROUS FUMARATE, FOLIC ACID.
Other preparations:

F

---

folic acid *see* **Fefol Spansule, Fefol Z Spansule, Fefol-Vit Spansule, Ferfolic SV, Ferrograd Folic, Folex-350, Folicin, Givitol, Irofol C, Ketovite, Lexpec, Meterfolic, Pregaday, Pregnavite Forte F, Slow-Fe Folic**

Folicin
(Paines & Byrne)

A white tablet used as an iron and mineral supplement for the prevention and treatment of anaemia in pregnancy.

Dose: 1-2 tablets a day.
Availability: NHS and private prescription.
Side effects: nausea, constipation.

Caution:
Not to be used for: children or patients suffering from megaloblastic anaemia.
Not to be used with: TETRACYCLINES.
Contains: FOLIC ACID, COPPER SULPHATE, MANGANESE SULPHATE, FERROUS SULPHATE.
Other preparations:

Forceval
(Unigreg)

A brown/red capsule used as a source of multivitamins and minerals to treat vitamin and mineral deficiencies.

Dose: adults 1 capsule a day; children over 5 years use Forceval Junior.
Availability: private prescription and over the counter.
Side effects:
Caution:
Not to be used for: children under 5 years.
Not to be used with: LEVODOPA.
Contains: multivitamins and minerals.
Other preparations: Forceval Junior.

formaldehyde *see* Veracur

Fortagesic
(Sterling Research Laboratories)

A white tablet used as an analgesic to relieve pain in the bones and muscles.

Dose: 2 tablets up to 4 times a day.
Availability: controlled drug.
Side effects: sedation, dizziness, nausea, psychological effects.
Caution: in pregnant women and in patients suffering from kidney, liver, or respiratory disease.
Not to be used for: children or for patients with respiratory depres-

sion, raised intracranial pressure, head injuries, or certain brain conditions, or for patients who depend on narcotics.
Not to be used with: MAOIS, narcotics, alcohol.
Contains: PENTAZOCINE HYDROCHLORIDE, PARACETAMOL.
Other preparations:

Fortral
(Sterling Research Laboratories)

A white tablet supplied at a strength of 25 mg and used as an analgesic to relieve pain.

Dose: adults 1-4 tablets every 3-4 hours after meals; children 1-6 years by injection; children 6-12 years 1 tablet every 3-4 hours.
Availability: controlled drug.
Side effects: sedation, dizziness, nausea, psychological effects.
Caution: in pregnant women and in patients suffering from kidney, liver, or respiratory disease.
Not to be used for: children under 1 year or for patients suffering from respiratory depression, raised intracranial pressure, head injury, certain brain conditions, or dependence on narcotics.
Not to be used with: MAOIS, narcotics, alcohol.
Contains: PENTAZOCINE HYDROCHLORIDE.
Other preparations: Fortral Capsules, Fortral Injection, Fortral Suppositories.

Fortunan *see* Dozic
(Steinhard)

Fosfor
(Chancellor)

A syrup used as a food supplement.

Dose: adults 4 5 ml teaspoonsful 3 times a day; children half adult dose.
Availability: private prescription and over the counter.
Side effects:

Caution:
Not to be used for:
Not to be used with:
Contains: PHOSPHORYLCOLAMINE.
Other preparations:

---

framycetin *see* Framycort, Framycort Ointment, Framygen, Framygen Ointment, Sofradex, Sofradex Ointment, Soframycin, Soframycin Cream, Soframycin Drops

---

Framycort
(Fisons)

Drops used as an antibiotic, corticosteroid treatment for inflammation of the outer ear, bacterial eye infections, conjunctivitis, eyelid inflammation, ulceration of the cornea.

Dose: 1-4 drops into the ear or eye 3-4 times a day.
Availability: NHS and private prescription.
Side effects: sensitization, hearing damage, rise in eye pressure, thinning cornea, cataract, fungal infection.
Caution: in pregnant women, in infants — avoid using for extended periods — and in patients suffering from perforated ear drum.
Not to be used for: patients suffering from viral infections, or viral, tubercular, fungal, or weeping infections of the eye, glaucoma, or for patients who wear soft contact lenses.
Not to be used with:
Contains: FRAMYCETIN sulphate, HYDROCORTISONE acetate.
Other preparations: Framycort Ointment.

Framycort Ointment
(Fisons)

An ointment used as an anti-bacterial, steroid treatment for infected eczema, seborrhoeic dermatitis, itch of the anal and genital areas.

Dose: apply to the affected area 2-3 times a day and cover.
Availability: NHS and private prescription.

Side effects: sensitization, hearing damage, fluid retention, suppression of adrenal glands, thinning of the skin may occur.
Caution: use for short periods of time only.
Not to be used for: patients suffering from acne or any other skin infections caused by tuberculosis, ringworm, viruses, or fungi, or continuously especially in pregnant women.
Not to be used with:
Contains: FRAMYCETIN sulphate.
Other preparations:

Framygen
(Fisons)

Drops used as an antibiotic treatment for inflammation of the outer ear.

Dose: 1-4 drops into the ear 3-4 times a day.
Availability: NHS and private prescription.
Side effects: hearing damage, sensitization.
Caution: in patients suffering from perforated ear drum.
Not to be used for:
Not to be used with:
Contains: FRAMYCETIN sulphate.
Other preparations:

Framygen Ointment
(Fisons)

An ointment used as an antibiotic treatment for inflammation of the eyelid, styes, infected conjunctivitis.

Dose: apply into the eye 4-6 times a day.
Availability: NHS and private prescription.
Side effects:
Caution:
Not to be used for:
Not to be used with:
Contains: FRAMYCETIN sulphate.
Other preparations: Framygen Eye Drops.

frangula *see* **Roter**

Franol
(Winthrop)

A white tablet used as a broncho-dilator to treat blocked airway brought on by chronic bronchitis or bronchial asthma.

Dose: 1 tablets 3 times a day and 1 tablet before going to bed if needed.
Availability: NHS and private prescription.
Side effects: nausea, stomach upset, headache, sleeplessness, rapid or abnormal heart rate.
Caution: in pregnant women, nursing mothers, and in patients suffering from heart or liver disease, diabetes, peptic ulcer.
Not to be used for: children or for patients suffering from heart disease, high blood pressure, cardiac asthma, overactive thyroid gland.
Not to be used with: CIMETIDINE, ERYTHROMYCIN, CIPROFLOXACIN, MAOIS, TRICYCLICS, SYMPATHOMIMETICS, INTERFERON, the contraceptive pill.
Contains: EPHEDRINE hydrochloride, THEOPHYLLINE.
Other preparations: Franol Plus.

Frisium
(Hoechst/Albert)

A blue capsule supplied at a strength of 10 mg and used as a sedative to treat anxiety, tension, agitation, and as an additional treatment for epilepsy.

Dose: elderly 1 tablet twice a day or 2 tablets at night; adults 1 tablet 2-3 times a day or 2-3 tablets at night. Maximum dose 6 tablets a day.
Availability: NHS (for epilepsy when prescribed as a generic) and private prescription.
Side effects: drowsiness, confusion, unsteadiness, low blood pressure, rash, changes in vision, changes in libido, retention of urine. Risk of addiction increases with dose and length of treatment. May impair judgement.
Caution: in the elderly, pregnant women, nursing mothers, in women during labour, and in patients suffering from lung disorders, kidney

or liver disorders. Avoid long-term use and withdraw gradually.
Not to be used for: children or for patients suffering from acute lung disorders, some chronic lung disorders, some obsessional and psychotic diseases.
Not to be used with: alcohol, other tranquillizers and anti-convulsants.
Contains: CLOBAZAM.
Other preparations:

Froben
(Boots)

A yellow tablet supplied at strengths of 50 mg, 100 mg and used as a NON-STEROID ANTI-INFLAMMATORY DRUG to treat rheumatoid disease, osteoarthritis, ankylosing spondylitis.

Dose: 150-200 mg a day in divided doses to a maximum of 300 mg a day.
Availability: NHS and private prescription.
Side effects: stomach intolerance, rash, rarely jaundice, blood changes, fluid retention.
Caution: in pregnant women, nursing mothers, and in patients suffering from asthma, kidney disease, allergy to ASPIRIN or anti-inflammatory drugs.
Not to be used for: children or for patients suffering from peptic ulcer or stomach bleeding.
Not to be used with: FRUSEMIDE, anti-coagulants.
Contains: FLURBIPROFEN.
Other preparations: Froben Suppositories, Froben SR.

Frumil
(Rorer)

An orange, scored tablet used as a potassium-sparing DIURETIC to treat fluid retention associated with heart failure, liver and kidney disease.

Dose: 1-2 tablets a day in the morning.
Availability: NHS and private prescription.
Side effects: feeling of being unwell, stomach upset, rash, blood changes.

Caution: in pregnant women, nursing mothers, and in patients suffering from liver or kidney disease, diabetes, electrolyte changes, enlarged prostate, gout, or impaired urination.

Not to be used for: children or for patients suffering from liver cirrhosis, progressive kidney failure, raised potassium levels.

Not to be used with: potassium supplements, potassium-sparing diuretics, LITHIUM, DIGITALIS, aminoglycosides, cephalosporins, anti-hypertensives, NON-STEROID ANTI-INFLAMMATORY DRUGS, ACE INHIBITORS.

Contains: FRUSEMIDE, AMILORIDE hydrochloride.

Other preparations:

---

frusemide *see* **Diumide-K Continus, Frumil, Frusene, Lasikal, Lasilactone, Lasipressin, Lasix, Lasix + K, Lasoride**

Frusene
(Fisons)

A yellow, scored tablet used as a potassium-sparing DIURETIC to treat fluid retention caused by heart or liver problems.

Dose: 1-2 tablets a day.

Availability: NHS and private prescription.

Side effects: stomach upset, feeling of being unwell.

Caution: in pregnant women, nursing mothers, and in patients suffering from kidney or liver disease, diabetes, electrolyte changes, enlarged prostate, impaired urination, gout.

Not to be used for: children or for patients suffering from cirrhosis of the liver, progressive kidney failure, or raised potassium levels.

Not to be used with: potassium supplements, potassium-sparing diuretics, LITHIUM, DIGITALIS, anti-hypertensives, aminoglycosides, cephalosporin antibiotics, NON-STEROID ANTI-INFLAMMATORY DRUGS, ACE INHIBITORS.

Contains: FRUSEMIDE, TRIAMTERENE.

Other preparations:

Fucibet
(Leo)

A cream used as an anti-bacterial and steroid treatment for eczema where there is also infection.

Dose: apply to the affected area 2-3 times a day at first and then reduce if possible.
Availability: NHS and private prescription.
Side effects: fluid retention, suppression of the adrenal glands, thinning of the skin may occur.
Caution: use for short periods of time only.
Not to be used for: patients suffering from acne or any other skin infections caused by tuberculosis, ringworm, viruses, or fungi, or continuously especially in pregnant women.
Not to be used with:
Contains: BETAMETHASONE valerate, FUSIDIC ACID.
Other preparations:

F

Fucidin
(Leo)

A white, oval tablet supplied at a strength of 250 mg and used as an antibiotic to treat infections.

Dose: 2 tablets 3 times a day; children use Fucidin Suspension.
Availability: NHS and private prescription.
Side effects: jaundice, stomach disturbances.
Caution: the liver should be checked regularly.
Not to be used for:
Not to be used with:
Contains: SODIUM FUSIDATE.
Other preparations: Fucidin Suspension, Fucidin IV Infusion.

Fucidin Cream
(Leo)

A cream used as an anti-bacterial treatment for skin infections.

Dose: apply to the affected area 3-4 times a day.
Availability: NHS and private prescription.

Side effects:
Caution:
Not to be used for:
Not to be used with:
Contains: FUSIDIC ACID.
Other preparations: Fucidin Gel, Fucidin Ointment, Ficidin Caviject.

Fucidin H
(Leo)

An ointment used as a steroid and anti-bacterial treatment for skin disorders where there is inflammation and infection.

Dose: apply to the affected area 3-4 times a day.
Availability: NHS and private prescription.
Side effects: fluid retention, suppression of the adrenal glands, thinning of the skin may occur.
Caution: use for short periods of time only.
Not to be used for: patients suffering from acne or any other skin infections caused by tuberculosis, ringworm, viruses, or fungi, or continuously especially in pregnant women.
Not to be used with:
Contains: SODIUM FUSIDATE, HYDROCORTISONE acetate.
Other preparations: Fucidin H Cream, Fucidin H Gel.

Fucithalmic
(Leo)

Drops used as an antibacterial treatment for conjunctivitis.

Dose: 1 drop into the eye twice a day.
Availability: NHS and private prescription.
Side effects: temporary irritation, allergy.
Caution:
Not to be used for:
Not to be used with:
Contains: FUSIDIC ACID.
Other preparations:

Fulcin
(ICI)

A white, scored tablet or a white tablet according to strengths of 125 mg, 500 mg and used as an anti-fungal treatment for scalp, skin, and nail infections.

Dose: adults 125 mg 4 times a day or 500 mg once a day; children 10 mg per kg body weight in one or divided doses.
Availability: NHS and private prescription.
Side effects: drowsiness, thirst, stomach upset, headache, allergy, sensitivity to light, rarely a collagen disease.
Caution:
Not to be used for: pregnant women or for patients suffering from porphyria (a rare blood disorder), severe liver disease.
Not to be used with: COUMARIN, anti-coagulants, barbiturates, the contraceptive pill, alcohol.
Contains: GRISEOFULVIN.
Other preparations: Fulcin Suspension.

Fungilin
(Squibb)

A light-brown, scored tablet supplied at a strength of 100 mg and used as an antibiotic to treat intestinal thrush, and for the prevention of vaginal or skin thrush.

Dose: adults 1-2 tablets 4 times a day; children use Suspension.
Availability: NHS and private prescription.
Side effects: stomach upset.
Caution:
Not to be used for:
Not to be used with:
Contains: AMPHOTERICIN.
Other preparations: Fungilin Suspension.

Fungilin Cream
(Squibb)

A cream used as an anti-fungal treatment for skin and mucous membrane thrush.

Dose: apply to the affected area 2-4 times a day.
Availability: NHS and private prescription.
Side effects:
Caution:
Not to be used for:
Not to be used with:
Contains: AMPHOTERICIN.
Other preparations: Fungilin Ointment.

Fungilin Lozenges
(Squibb)

A yellow lozenge supplied at a strength of 10 mg and used as an anti-fungal treatment for thrush.

Dose: 1 lozenge allowed to dissolve slowly in the mouth 4-8 times a day.
Availability: NHS and private prescription.
Side effects:
Caution:
Not to be used for:
Not to be used with:
Contains: AMPHOTERICIN.
Other preparations: fungilin, Fungilin Suspension

Furacin
(Norwich Eaton)

An ointment used as an anti-bacterial treatment for infected wounds, burns, ulcers, or where skin has been removed for grafting.

Dose: apply to the affected area as needed.
Availability: NHS and private prescription.
Side effects:
Caution:
Not to be used for:
Not to be used with:
Contains: NITROFURAZONE.
Other preparations:

Furadantin
(Norwich Eaton)

A yellow, pentagonal, scored tablet supplied at strengths of 50 mg, 100 mg and used as an antiseptic to treat infection of the urinary tract.

Dose: adults treatment 100 mg 4 times a day with food or milk, prevention 100-200 mg a day; children 3 months-$2\frac{1}{2}$ years eighth adult dose, $2\frac{1}{2}$-6 years quarter adult dose, 6-11 years half adult dose, 11-14 years three-quarters adult dose.
Availability: NHS, private prescription, over the counter.
Side effects: stomach upset, allergy, jaundice, nerve inflammation, blood changes, possible liver damage.
Caution:
Not to be used for: infants under 1 month or for patients suffering from kidney problems resulting in reduced urine output.
Not to be used with:
Contains: NITROFURANTOIN.
Other preparations: Furadantin Suspension.

---

fusafungine *see* Locabiotal

---

fusidic acid *see* Fucibet, Fucidin Cream, Fucithalmic

Fybogel
(Reckiit & Colman)

Plain or orange-flavoured, effervescent granules supplied in sachets of 3.5 g and used as a bulking agent in the treatment of diverticular disease, spastic and irritable colon.

Dose: adults 1 sachet in water evening and morning; children 2.5-5 ml in water evening and morning.
Availability: NHS and private prescription.
Side effects:
Caution:
Not to be used for: patients suffering from intestinal obstruction.
Not to be used with:

Contains: ISPAGHULA husk.
Other preparations:

Fybranta
(Norgine)

A mottled, pale-brown, chewable, 2 g tablet used as a bulking agent in the treatment of diverticular disease, irritable colon syndrome, constipation through a diet lacking in fibre.

Dose: adults 1-3 tablets with liquid 3-4 times a day; children in proportion.
Availability: private prescription andover the counter.
Side effects:
Caution:
Not to be used for:
Not to be used with:
Contains: BRAN.
Other preparations:

Galcodine
(Galen)

A linctus supplied at a strength of 15 mg and used as an opiate to treat dry cough.

Dose: adults 1 5 ml teaspoonful 4 times a day; children 1-5 years $\frac{1}{2}$ -1 teaspoonful 3-4 times a day, 6-12 years 1 teaspoonful 3-4 times a day.
Availability: NHS, private prescription, over the counter.
Side effects: constipation.
Caution: in patients suffering from asthma.
Not to be used for: infants under 1 year, or for patients suffering from liver disease.
Not to be used with: MAOIS.
Contains: CODEINE phosphate.
Other preparations: Galcodine Paediatric.

Galenphol
(Galen)

A liquid supplied at a strength of 5 mg and used as an opiate to treat dry cough.

Dose: adults 1-2 5 ml teaspoonsful 3-4 times a day; children 1-5 years $^1/_2$-1 teaspoonful 3-4 times a day, 6-12 years 1 teaspoonful 3-4 times a day.
Availability: NHS, private prescription, over the counter.
Side effects: constipation.
Caution: in patients suffering from asthma.
Not to be used for: infants under 1 year, or for patients suffering from liver disease.
Not to be used with: MAOIS.
Contains: PHOLCODINE.
Other preparations: Galenphol Linctus Strong, Galenphol Linctus Paediatric.

Galfer
(Galen)

G

A green/red capsule supplied at a strength of 290 mg and used as an iron supplement to treat iron-deficiency anaemia.

Dose: adults 1 capsule 1-2 times a day before food; children as advised by the physician.
Availability: private prescription and over the counter.
Side effects: nausea, constipation.
Caution:
Not to be used for:
Not to be used with: TETRACYCLINES.
Contains: FERROUS FUMARATE.
Other preparations: Galfer FA.

Galfervit
(Galen)

An orange/maroon capsule used as an iron and vitamin supplement to treat iron deficiency anaemia where a vitamin supplement is also needed.

Dose: adults 1 capsule 1-2 times a day; children as advised by the physician.
Availability: private prescription and over the counter.
Side effects: nausea, constipation.
Caution:
Not to be used for:
Not to be used with: TETRACYCLINES, LEVODOPA.
Contains: FERROUS FUMARATE, ASCORBIC ACID, RIBOFLAVINE, NICOTINAMIDE, PYRIDOXINE hydrochloride, THIAMINE mononitrate.
Other preparations:

Galpseud
(Galen)

A white tablet supplied at a strength of 60 mg and used as a SYMPATH-OMIMETIC to treat congestion of the nose, sinuses, and upper respiratory tract.

Dose: adults 1 tablet 3 times a day; children use linctus.
Availability: NHS, private prescription, and over the counter.
Side effects: anxiety, hands shaking, irregular or rapid heart rate, dry mouth, excitement.
Caution: in patients suffering from diabetes.
Not to be used for: children under 2 years, or for patients suffering from heart or thyroid disorders.
Not to be used with: MAOIS, TRICYCLICS.
Contains: PSEUDOEPHEDRINE hydrochloride.
Other preparations: Galpseud Linctus.

Gamanil
(Merck)

A maroon, scored tablet supplied at a strength of 70 mg and used as an anti-depressant to treat depression.

Dose: 1 tablet in the morning and 1-2 tablets at night.
Availability: NHS and private prescription.
Side effects: dry mouth, constipation, urine retention, blurred vision, palpitations, drowsiness, sleeplessness, dizziness, hands shaking, low blood presure, weight change, skin reactions, jaundice or blood

changes, loss of libido may occur.

Caution: in nursing mothers or in patients suffering from heart disease, thyroid disease, epilepsy, diabetes, some other psychiatric conditions. Your doctor may advise regular blood tests.

Not to be used for: children, pregnant women, or for patients suffering from heart attacks, heart block, liver disease.

Not to be used with: alcohol, ANTI-CHOLINERGICS, ADRENALINE, MAOIS, barbiturates, other anti-depressants, anti-hypertensives.

Contains: LOFEPRAMINE hydrochloride.

Other preparations:

Ganda
(SNP)

Drops used as a fluid channel drug to treat glaucoma.

Dose: 1 drop into the eye 1-2 times a day.

Availability: NHS and private prescription.

Side effects: pain in the eye, headache, redness, skin reactions, melanosis, rarely systemic effects, increase in eye pressure.

Caution: your doctor may advise that the conjucntiva and cornea should be checked every 6 months if you are undergoing prolonged treatment.

Not to be used for: patients suffering from narrow-angle glaucoma, absence of the lens.

Not to be used with: MAOIS.

Contains: GUANETHIDINE monosulphate, ADRENALINE.

Other preparations:

Garamycin *see* Cidomycin Drops
(Kirby-Warrick)

Gastrobid Continus *see* Maxolon
(Napp)

Gastrocote
(MCP)

A white tablet used as an antacid and reflux suppressant to treat dyspepsia, hiatus hernia, oesophagitis

Dose: adults 1-2 tablets 4 times a day, children over 6 years as adult.
Availability: NHS and over the counter.
Side effects: few; occasionally constipation.
Caution:
Not to be used for: infants.
Not to be used with: TETRACYCLINE antibiotics.
Contains: ALGINIC ACID, ALUMINIUM HYDROXIDE, MAGNESIUM TRISILICATE, SODIUM BICARBONATE.
Other preparations: Gastrocote liquid.

Gastromax *see* Maxolon
(Farmitalia CE)

Gastron
(Sterling Research Laboratories)

A white tablet used as an antacid and reflux suppressant to treat reflux symptoms.

Dose: adults 1-2 tablets 3 times a day and 2 at bedtime.
Availability: NHS and over the counter.
Side effects: few; occasionally constipation.
Caution: in pregnant women, and in patients suffering from high blood pressure, heart or kidney failure.
Not to be used for: infants.
Not to be used with: TETRACYCLINE antibiotics.
Contains: ALGINIC ACID, ALUMINIUM HYDROXIDE, SODIUM BICARBONATE, MAGNESIUM TRISILICATE.
Other preparations:

Gastrozepin
(Boots)

A white tablet used as an anti-spasm, ANTI-CHOLINERGIC treatment for gastric and duodenal ulcers.

Dose: adults 1 tablet twice a day before meals.
Availability: NHS and private prescription.
Side effects: blurred vision, confusion, dry mouth.
Caution:
Not to be used for: patients with glaucoma, inflammatory bowel disease, intestinal obstruction, or enlarged prostate.
Not to be used with:
Contains: PIRENZEPINE.
Other preparations:

Gaviscon
(Reckitt & Colman)

A white tablet used as an antacid and reflux suppressant to treat reflux symptoms.

Dose: children $^1/_2$ infant sachet after meals, adults 1-2 tablets or 10-20 ml after meals and at night.
Availability: NHS, private prescription, over the counter.
Side effects: few; occasionally constipation.
Caution: in pregnant women, and in patients suffering from high blood pressure, heart or kidney failure.
Not to be used for: infants.
Not to be used with: TETRACYCLINE antibiotics.
Contains: SODIUM ALGINATE, SODIUM BICARBONATE, CALCIUM CARBONATE.
Other preparations: Gaviscon liquid, Gaviscon Infant.

G

---

gelatin *see* Orabase

Gelcosal
(Quinoderm)

A gel used as an anti-psoriatic and skin softener to treat psoriasis, dermatitis, when the condition is scaling.

Dose: massage into the affected area twice a day.

Availability: NHS, private prescription, over the counter.
Side effects:
Caution:
Not to be used for:
Not to be used with:
Contains: COAL TAR SOLUTION, TAR, SALICYLIC ACID.
Other preparations:

Gelcotar
(Quinoderm)

A gel used as an anti-psoriatic treatment for psoriasis, dermatitis.

Dose: massage into the affected area twice a day.
Availability: NHS, private prescription, over the counter.
Side effects: irritation, sensitivity to light.
Caution:
Not to be used for: patients suffering from acute psoriasis.
Not to be used with:
Contains: COAL TAR SOLUTION, TAR.
Other preparations: Gelcotar Liquid.

gemfibrozil *see* Lopid

Genisol
(Fisons)

A liquid used as an anti-psoriatic and anti-dandruff treatment for psoriasis, dandruff, seborrhoeic inflammation of the scalp.

Dose: shampoo once a week or as needed.
Availability: NHS, private prescription, over the counter.
Side effects: irritation, sensitivity to light.
Caution:
Not to be used for: patients suffering from acute psoriasis.
Not to be used with:
Contains: COAL TAR, SODIUM SULPHOSUCCINATED UNDECYLENIC MONOAL-KYOLAMIDE.
Other preparations:

Gentamicin

(SNP)

Drops used as an aminoglycoside antibiotic to treat bacterial infections of the eye.

Dose: 1 drop into the eye as needed.
Availability: NHS and private prescription.
Side effects:
Caution:
Not to be used for:
Not to be used with:
Contains: GENTAMICIN sulphate.
Other preparations:

---

gentamicin *see* Cidomycin Cream, Cidomycin Drops, Gentamicin, Genticin Cream, Genticin HC, Gentisone HC

---

gentian mixture, acid

A tonic used to to improve appetite.

Dose: 2-4 5 ml teaspoonsful ½ hour before a meal.
Availability: NHS, private prescription, over the counter.
Side effects:
Caution:
Not to be used for: children.
Not to be used with:
Contains:
Other preparations: gentian mixture, alkaline.

Genticin Cream

(Nicholas)

A cream used as an aminoglycoside antibiotic to treat skin infections such as ulcers, burns, wounds, impetigo, inflammation of the follicles.

Dose: apply to the affected area 3-4 times a day.
Availability: NHS and private prescription.

Side effects: sensitization.
Caution: in patients with large areas of affected skin.
Not to be used for:
Not to be used with:
Contains: GENTAMICIN.
Other preparations: Genticin Ointment.

Genticin HC
(Nicholas)

A cream used as a steroid and anti-bacterial treatment for allergic or other skin disorders where there is also infection and inflammation.

Dose: apply to the affected area 3-4 times a day.
Availability: NHS and private prescription.
Side effects: fluid retention, suppression of adrenal glands, thinning of the skin.
Caution: use for short periods of time only.
Not to be used for: continuously especially for pregnant women, or for patients suffering from tubercular, fungal, viral, or ringworm infections.
Not to be used with:
Contains: GENTAMICIN sulphate, HYDROCORTISONE acetate.
Other preparations: Genticin HC Ointment.

Genticin *see* Cidomycin Drops
(Nicholas)

Gentisone HC
(Nicholas)

Drops used as an antibiotic, corticosteroid treatment for inflammation of the outer ear, acute weeping inflammation of the middle ear.

Dose: 2-4 drops into the ear 3-4 times a day and at night.
Availability: NHS and private prescription.
Side effects: additional infection, fluid retention, suppression of adrenal glands, thinning of the skin may occur.

Caution: in pregnant women, infants, and in patients suffering from perforated ear drum. Use for short periods of time only.
Not to be used for: continuously especially for pregnant women, or for patients suffering from acne or any other viral, fungal, tubercular, or ringworm infections.
Not to be used with:
Contains: GENTAMICIN sulphate, HYDROCORTISONE acetate.
Other preparations:

Genusil
(Warner-Lambert)

A white tablet used as an antacid to treat dyspepsia, heartburn.

Dose: adults 1-2 tablets after meals, children over 6 years half adult dose.
Availability: private prescription and over the counter.
Side effects: few; occasionally constipation.
Caution:
Not to be used for: infants.
Not to be used with: TETRACYCLINE antibiotics.
Contains: MAGNESIUM TRISILICATE, ALUMINIUM HYDROXIDE.
Other preparations:

G

Gestanin
(Organon)

A white tablet supplied at a strength of 5 mg and used as a progestogen treatment for threatened or habitual abortion, failure of implantation of fertilized eggs.

Dose: 1-4 tablets a day.
Availability: NHS and private prescription.
Side effects: nausea.
Caution: in patients suffering from diabetes, migraine, epilepsy.
Not to be used for: children or for patients with a history of thromboembolic disorders, breast or genital cancer, liver disease, abnormal vaginal bleeding.
Not to be used with:
Contains: ALLYLOESTRENOL.
Other preparations:

gestodene *see* **Femodene, Minulet**

Gevral
(Lederle)

A brown capsule used as a source of multivitamins and minerals to treat vitamin and mineral deficiencies.

Dose: 1 capsule a day.
Availability: private prescription and over the counter.
Side effects:
Caution:
Not to be used for:
Not to be used with: LEVODOPA.
Contains: multivitamins and minerals.
Other preparations:

Givitol
(Galen)

A maroon/red capsule used as an iron, folic acid, and vitamin supplement to treat iron and folic acid deficiencies in pregnancy where vitamin supplements are also needed.

Dose: 1 capsule a day before food.
Availability: private prescription and over the counter.
Side effects: nausea, constipation.
Caution:
Not to be used for: children.
Not to be used with: TETRACYCLINES, LEVADOPA.
Contains: FERROUS FUMARATE, ASCORBIC ACID, RIBOFLAVINE, PYRIDOXINE hydrochloride, NICOTINAMIDE, FOLIC ACID.
Other preparations:

Glandosane
(Fresenius)

An aerosol used to provide artificial saliva for dry mouth and throat.

Dose: spray into the mouth and throat for 1-2 seconds as needed.
Availability: NHS, private prescription, over the counter.
Side effects:
Caution:
Not to be used for:
Not to be used with:
Contains: CARBOXYMETHYLCELLULOSE SODIUM, SORBITOL, POTASSIUM CHLO-
RIDE, SODIUM CHLORIDE, MAGNESIUM CHLORIDE, CALCIUM CHLORIDE, DIPOTASSIUM
HYDROGEN PHOSPHATE.
Other preparations:

Glauline
(SNP)

Drops used as a ß-BLOCKER to treat glaucoma.

Dose: 1 drop into the eye twice a day.
Availability: NHS and private prescription.
Side effects: slight smarting, temporary headache.
Caution: in patients suffering from heart block.
Not to be used for: pregnant women, for patients who wear soft
contact lenses, or for patients suffering from heart failure, blocked
airways disease.
Not to be used with: VERAPAMIL, other ß-blockers.
Contains: METIPRANOLOL.
Other preparations:

G

---

glibenclamide *see* Daonil

Glibenese
(Pfizer)

A white, oblong, scored tablet supplied at a strength of 5 mg and used
as a sulphonylurea to treat diabetes.

Dose: $^1/_2$-1 tablet a day with breakfast or lunch at first increasing if
needed by $^1/_2$-1 tablet a day every 3-5 days to a maximum of 6 tablets
a day in divided doses.

Availability: NHS and private prescription.
Side effects: allergy including skin rash.
Caution: in the elderly and in patients suffering from kidney failure.
Not to be used for: children, pregnant women, nursing mothers, during surgery, or for patients suffering from juvenile diabetes, liver or kidney impairment, hormone disorders, stress, infections.
Not to be used with: ß-BLOCKERS, MAOIS, steroids, DIURETICS, alcohol, anti-coagulants, lipid-lowering agents, ASPIRIN, some antibiotics (RIFAMPICIN, sulphonamides, CHLORAMPHENICOL), GLUCAGON, CYCLOPHOSPHAMIDE.
Contains: GLIPIZIDE.
Other preparations:

---

gliclazide *see* Diamicron

---

glipizide *see* Glibenese, Minodiab

Gluco-lyte *see* Dioralyte
(Cupal)

Glucophage
(Lipha)

A white tablet supplied at strengths of 500 mg, 850 mg and used as an anti-diabetic to treat diabetes.

Dose: 500-850 mg twice a day with meals at first increasing gradually if needed to a maximum of 3 g a day, and then reduce to 2 x 850 mg or 3 x 500 mg a day in divided doses.
Availability: NHS and private prescription.
Side effects: allergy including skin rash, rarely acidosis (a metabolic disorder).
Caution: in the elderly and in patients suffering from kidney failure.
Not to be used for: children, pregnant women, nursing mothers, during pregnancy, or for patients suffering from juvenile diabetes, liver

or kidney impairment, hormone disorders, stress, infections.
Not to be used with: ß-BLOCKERS, MAOIS, steroids, DIURETICS, alcohol, anti-coagulants, lipid-lowering agents, ASPIRIN, some antibiotics (RIFAMPICIN, sulphonamides, CHLORAMPHENICOL), GLUCAGON, CYCLOPHOSPHAMIDE.
Contains: METFORMIN HYDROCHLORIDE.
Other preparations: ORABET (Lagap).

---

glucose *see* Dioralyte, Rehidrat

Glucotard
(MCP)

Mini-tablets in 5 g sachets used as a bulking agent to treat diabetes.

Dose: 1 sachet 1-3 times a day before main meals taken with water.
Availability: NHS, private prescription, over the counter.
Side effects: wind, swollen abdomen.
Caution: glucose levels should be checked initially.
Not to be used for: children or patients suffering from blocked intestine, oesophageal disease.
Not to be used with:
Contains: GUAR GUM.
Other preparations:

Glurenorm
(Sterling Research Laboratories)

A white, scored tablet supplied at a strength of 30 mg and used as an anti-diabetic to treat diabetes.

Dose: 1½-2 tablets a day in divided doses before food to a maximum of 6 tablets a day.
Availability: NHS and private prescription.
Side effects: allergy including skin rash.
Caution: in the elderly and in patients suffering from kidney failure.
Not to be used for: children, pregnant women, nursing mothers, during surgery, or for patients suffering from juvenile diabetes, liver or

kidney impairment, hormone disorders, stress, infections.
Not to be used with: ß-BLOCKERS, MAOIS, steroids, DIURETICS, alcohol, anti-coagulants, lipid-lowering agents, ASPIRIN, some antibiotics (RIFAMPICIN, sulphonamides, CHLORAMPHENICOL), glucagon, CYCLOPHOSPHAMIDE.
Contains: GLIQUIDONE.
Other preparations:

---

glutamic acid hydrochloride *see* Muripsin

---

glutaraldehyde *see* Glutarol, Verucasep

Glutarol
(Dermal)

A solution used as a virucidal, skin-drying agent to treat warts.

Dose: apply the solution to the wart twice a day and rub down hard skin.
Availability: NHS, private prescription, over the counter.
Side effects: staining of the skin.
Caution: do not apply to healthy skin.
Not to be used for: warts on the face or anal and genital areas.
Not to be used with:
Contains: GLUTARALDEHYDE.
Other preparations:

---

glycerin *see* Auralgicin, Exterol

---

glycerol *see* Micolette, Relaxit

---

glycerol suppositories

Suppositories supplied at strengths of 1 g, 2 g, 4 g and used as a lubricant to treat constipation.

Dose: adults 4 g suppository as necessary; children 1 g suppository.
Availability: NHS and private prescription.
Side effects:
Caution:
Not to be used for:
Not to be used with:
Contains:
Other preparations:

---

glyceryl trinitrate *see* Coro-Nitro, Deponit, Nitrocontin Continus, Nitrolingual, Percutol, Suscard Buccal. Sustac, Transiderm-Nitro

---

glycine *see* Cicatrin, Paynocil, Titralac

---

glycol salicylate *see* Bayolin, Cremalgin, Dubam, Salonair

Glykola
(Sinclair)

A liquid used as a tonic.

Dose: 1-2 5 ml teaspoonsful 3 times a day.
Availability: private prescription and over the counter.
Side effects:
Caution: in patients with a history of peptic ulcer.
Not to be used for: children.
Not to be used with:
Contains: CAFFEINE, CALCIUM GLYCEROPHOSPHATE, KOLA LIQUID EXTRACT, CHLOROFORM suspension, alcohol, FERROUS PERCHLORIDE LIQUID.
Other preparations:

grain fibre *see* **Proctofibe**

---

gramicidin *see* Graneodin, Neosporin, Sofradex, Sofradex
Ointment, Tri-Adcortyl, Tri-Adcortyl Otic,

Graneodin
(Squibb)

An ointment used as an aminoglycoside and protein to treat infections
of the cornea, eyelid, and conjunctiva; skin infections such as impetigo
and beard infections.

Dose: apply 1 cm length of the ointment inside the eyelid as needed;
for skin infections apply 2-4 times a day.
Availability: NHS and private prescription.
Side effects: hearing damage, sensitization.
Caution: in patients with large areas of affected skin; do not use with
dressings.
Not to be used for: fungal, viral, or deep infections.
Not to be used with:
Contains: NEOMYCIN sulphate, GRAMICIDIN.
Other preparations:

Gregoderm
(Unigreg)

An ointment used as a steroid, anti-bacterial treatment for psoriasis,
itch of the anal and genital area, and other skin disorders where there
is also inflammation and infection.

Dose: apply to the affected area 2-3 times a day.
Availability: NHS and private prescription.
Side effects: fluid retention, suppression of the adrenal glands,
thinning of the skin may occur.
Caution: use for short periods of time only.
Not to be used for: continuously especially for pregnant women, or
for patients suffering from acne or any other tubercular, fungal, viral,
or ringworm infections.
Not to be used with:

Contains: NEOMYCIN sulphate, NYSTATIN, POLYMYXIN B SULPHATE.
Other preparations:

---

griseofulvin *see* **Fulcin, Grisovin**

Grisovin
(Glaxo)

A white tablet supplied at strengths of 125 mg, 500 mg and used as an anti-fungal treatment for infections of the nails, skin, and scalp.

Dose: adults 500 mg-1 g a day in divided doses after meals; children 10 mg per kg body weight a day in divided doses.
Availability: NHS and private prescription.
Side effects: drowsiness, gastric upset, headache, allergies, sensitivity to light, rarely precipitation of SLE (a rare collagen disease).
Caution: in pregnant women and in patients on prolonged treatment.
Not to be used for: patients suffering from porphyria (a rare blood disease), liver disease, SLE (a rare collagen disease).
Not to be used with: barbiturates, COUMARIN anti-coagulants.
Contains: GRISEOFULVIN.
Other preparations:

G

---

guaiphenesin *see* **Bricanyl Expectorant, Dimotane, Expectorant, Noradran**

---

guanethidine *see* **Ganda, Ismelin (Ciba), Ismelin (Zyma)**

Guanor
(R P Drugs)

A liquid used as an expectorant, antihistamine, mucus softener to treat cough, bronchial congestion.

Dose: adults 1-2 5 ml teaspoonsful every 2-3 hours; children 1-5 years

¹/₂ teaspoonful every 3-4 hours, 6-12 years 1 teaspoonful every 3-4 hours.
Availability: private prescription and over the counter.
Side effects: drowsiness, reduced reactions, rarely skin eruptions.
Caution: in patients suffering from liver or kidney disease.
Not to be used for: infants under 1 year.
Not to be used with: sedatives, alcohol, some anti-depressants (MAOIS).
Contains: AMMONIUM CHLORIDE, DIPHENHYDRAMINE hydrochloride, SODIUM CITRATE, MENTHOL.
Other preparations:

---

guar gum *see* Glucotard, Guarem

Guarem
(Rybar)

Dispersible granules in a 5 g sachet used as a bulking agent to treat diabetes.

Dose: 1 sachet dispersed in 200 ml of liquid immediately before each meal or stirred into food and eaten with 200 ml liquid.
Availability: NHS, private prescription, over the counter.
Side effects: wind, swollen abdomen.
Caution: glucose levels should be checked.
Not to be used for: children or for patients suffering from a blocked intestine or oesophageal disease.
Not to be used with:
Contains: GUAR GUM.
Other preparations: GUARINA (Norgine)

Guarina *see* Guarem
(Norgine)

Gyno-Daktarin 1
(Janssen)

A white vaginal capsule supplied at a strength of 120 mg and used as an anti-fungal treatment for thrush of the vulva or vagina.

Dose: 1 capsule inserted high into the vagina as a single dose.
Availability: NHS and private prescription.
Side effects: mild burning or irritation.
Caution:
Not to be used for: children.
Not to be used with:
Contains: MICONAZOLE nitrate.
Other preparations: Gyno-Daktarin Pessaries, Gyno-Daktarin CombiPack, Gyno-Daktarin Tampons, GynoDaktarin Cream.

Gyno-Pevaryl 1
(Cilag)

A pessary supplied at a strength of 150 mg and used as an anti-fungal treatment for vaginal thrush.

Dose: 1 pessary inserted into the vagina at night as a single dose.
Availability: NHS and private prescription.
Side effects: mild burning or irritation.
Caution:
Not to be used for: children.
Not to be used with:
Contains: ECONAZOLE nitrate.
Other preparations: Gyno-Pevaryl 1 CP, Gyno-Pevaryl Cream, Gyno-Pevaryl Pessaries, Gyno-Pevaryl Combipack.

H_2 antagonist

a drug which works on the stomach to reduce acid production by blocking the histamine pathway. Example RANITIDINE *see* Zantac.

Haelan
(Dista)

A cream used as a steroid treatment for skin disorders.

H

Dose: apply to the affected area 2-3 times a day.
Availability: NHS and private prescription.
Side effects: fluid retention, suppression of the adrenal glands, thinning of the skin may occur.
Caution: use for short periods of time only.
Not to be used for: continuously especially for pregnant women, or for patients suffering from acne, or any other tubercular, viral, fungal, or ringworm skin infections.
Not to be used with:
Contains: FLURANDRENOLONE.
Other preparations: Haelan Ointment, Haelan-X, Haelan Tape.

Halciderm
(Squibb)

A cream used as a steroid treatment for acute skin disorders.

Dose: apply to the affected area 2-3 times a day.
Availability: NHS and private prescription.
Side effects: fluid retention, suppression of the adrenal glands, thinning of the skin may occur.
Caution: do not dilute the cream. Use for short periods of time only.
Not to be used for: continuously especially for pregnant women, or for patients suffering from other tubercular, fungal, viral, or ringworm infections.
Not to be used with:
Contains: HALCINONIDE.
Other preparations:

---

halcinonide *see* Halciderm

Halcion
(Upjohn)

A lavender, oval, scored tablet or a blue, oval, scored tablet according to strengths of 0.125 mg, 0.25 mg and used as a sleeping tablet for the short-term and occasional treatment of sleeplessness.

Dose: elderly 0.125 mg before going to bed; adults 0.25 mg before going to bed.
Availability: NHS (when prescribed as a generic) and private prescription.
Side effects: drowsiness, confusion, unsteadiness, low blood pressure, rash, changes in vision, changes in libido, retention of urine. Risk of addiction increases with dose and length of treatment. May impair judgement.
Caution: in the elderly, pregnant women, nursing mothers, in women during labour, and in patients suffering from lung disorders, kidney or liver disorders. Avoid long-term use and withdraw gradually.
Not to be used for: children, or for patients suffering from acute lung diseases, some chronic lung diseases, some obsessional and psychotic diseases.
Not to be used with: alcohol, other tranquillizers and anti-convulsants.
Contains: TRIAZOLAM.
Other preparations:

Haldol
(Janssen)

A blue tablet or a yellow tablet according to strengths of 5 mg, 10 mg and used as a sedative to treat schizophrenia, mental or behavioural disorders, mania, hypomania, alcohol withdrawal symptoms, delirium tremens, behavioural disorders in children, nausea, vomiting, medication before an anaesthetic.

Dose: adults 0.5-5 mg 2-3 times a day at first increasing gradually to a maximum of 200 mg a day if needed; children 0.05 mg per kg body weight a day in 2 divided doses.
Availability: NHS and private prescription.
Side effects: muscle spasms, restlessness, hands shaking, dry mouth, urine retention, palpitations, low blood pressure, weight gain, changes in libido, low body temperature, breast swelling, menstrual changes, jaundice, blood and skin changes, drowsiness, rarely fits.
Caution: in pregnant women, nursing mothers, and in patients suffering from liver or kidney failure, severe cardiovascular disease, Parkinson's disease, overactive thyroid gland.
Not to be used for: children, unconscious patients.
Not to be used with: alcohol, tranquillizers, pain killers, anti-hy-

pertensives, anti-depressants, anti-convulsants, anti-diabetics, LEVODOPA.
Contains: HALOPERIDOL DECANOATE.
Other preparations: Haldol Decanoate, Haldol Oral Liquid, Haldol Injection.

---

haloperidol decanoate *see* Haldol

---

haloperidol *see* Dozic, Serenace

Halycitrol
(LAB)

An emulsion used as a multivitamin preparation to treat vitamin A and vitamin D deficiencies.

Dose: adults and children over 6 months 1 5 ml teaspoonful a day; infants under 6 months $1/2$ teaspoonful a day.
Availability: private prescription and over the counter.
Side effects: vitamin poisoning.
Caution: in patients suffering from kidney disease, sarcoidosis (a chest disease that affects calcium levels).
Not to be used for:
Not to be used with:
Contains: VITAMIN A, VITAMIN D.
Other preparations:

Hamarin *see* Zyloric
(Nicholas)

Harmogen
(Abbott)

An orange, oval, scored tablet supplied at a strength of 1.5 mg and used as an oestrogen to treat menopausal oestrogen deficiency.

Dose: 1-3 tablets a day for 3-4 weeks then 7 days without tablets.
Availability: NHS and private prescription.
Side effects: enlarged breasts, bloating and fluid retention, cramps, leg pains, mood change, reduction in sexual desire, headaches, nausea, vaginal erosion, discharge, and bleeding, weight gain, skin changes.
Caution: in patients suffering from high blood pressure, diabetes, vascular disorders, asthma, depression, kidney disease, multiple sclerosis, womb diseases. Your doctor may advise you not to smoke, to have regular examinations. You should stop treatment at the first sign of serious symptoms such as severe headache or jaundice. Treatment should be stopped before surgery.
Not to be used for: pregnant women, or for patients suffering from sickle-cell anaemia, history of heart disease or thrombosis, liver disorders, some cancers, undiagnosed vaginal bleeding, some ear, skin, and kidney disorders.
Not to be used with: RIFAMPICIN, TETRACYCLINES, GRISEOFULVIN, barbiturates, PHENYTOIN, PRIMIDONE, CARBAMAZEPINE, ETHOSUXIMIDE, CHLORAL HYDRATE, DICHLORALPHENAZONE.
Contains: PIPERAZINE OESTRONE SULPHATE.
Other preparations:

Haymine
(Pharmax)

A yellow tablet used as an antihistamine and SYMPATHOMIMETIC treatment for allergies.

Dose: 1 tablet in the morning and 1 tablet at night if needed.
Availability: NHS, private prescription, over the counter.
Side effects: drowsiness, reduced reactions, dizziness.
Caution:
Not to be used for: children or for patients suffering from overactive thyroid gland, high blood pressure, coronary thrombosis.
Not to be used with: sedatives, MAOIS, alcohol.
Contains: CHLORPHENIRAMINE maleate, EPHEDRINE hydrochloride.
Other preparations:

Heminevrin
(Astra)

A syrup used as a sedative for the short-term treatment of sleeplessness in the elderly, agitated states, tension and anxiety, daytime sedation in senile mental disorder, confusion, alcohol withdrawal symptoms, pre-eclamptic toxaemia, severe epilepsy.

Dose: 10 ml in water or fruit juice before going to bed. For sedation 5-10 ml 3 times a day.
Availability: NHS and private prescription.
Side effects: blocked and irritating nose, irritating eyes, stomach disturbances, severe allergy, sedation, excitement, confusion.
Caution: in patients suffering from long-term lung weakness, kidney or liver disease. Patients should be warned of impaired ability.
Not to be used for: children, nursing mothers, or patients suffering from acute lung weakness.
Not to be used with: alcohol and sedatives.
Contains: CHLORMETHIAZOLE EDISYLATE.
Other preparations: Heminevrin Capsules, Heminevrin IV.

---

heparinoid *see* **Anacal, Bayolin, Lasonil, Movelat**

Herpid
(Boehringer Ingelheim)

A solution used as an anti-viral treatment for herpes-type skin infections.

Dose: apply locally.
Availability: NHS and private prescription.
Side effects:
Caution:
Not to be used for: children, pregnant women, nursing mothers.
Not to be used with:
Contains: IDOXURIDINE, DIMETHYL SULPHOXIDE.
Other preparations:

hexachlorophane *see* Anacal, Ster-Zac DC, Ster-Zac Powder, Torbetol

---

hexamine hippurate *see* Hiprex

---

hexetidine *see* Oraldene

Hexopal
(Winthrop)

A white, scored tablet supplied at a strength of 500 mg and used as a vasodilator to treat Raynaud's phenomenon (a condition caused by spasm of the blood vessels), intermittent claudication (difficulty walking caused by circulation disorders).

Dose: 2 tablets 3-4 times a day.
Availability: NHS and private prescription.
Side effects:
Caution: in pregnant women.
Not to be used for: children.
Not to be used with:
Contains: INOSITOL NICOTINATE.
Other preparations: Hexopal Forte, Hexopal Suspension.

Hibiscrub
(ICI)

A solution used as a disinfectant for cleansing and disinfecting skin and hands.

Dose: use as a liquid soap.
Availability: NHS, private prescription, over the counter.
Side effects:
Caution:
Not to be used for:
Not to be used with:

Contains: CHLORHEXIDINE gluconate.
Other preparations:

Hibisol
(ICI)

A solution used as a disinfectant for cleansing and disinfecting skin and hands.

Dose: rub vigorously on to the skin until dry.
Availability: NHS, private prescription, over the counter.
Side effects:
Caution:
Not to be used for:
Not to be used with:
Contains: CHLORHEXIDINE gluconate, ISOPROPYL ALCOHOL.
Other preparations:

Hibitane
(ICI)

A cream used as a disinfectant for cleansing and disinfecting hands and skin before surgery, and for prevention of infections in wounds and after surgery.

Dose: apply freely to the affected area as needed.
Availability: NHS, private prescription, over the counter.
Side effects:
Caution:
Not to be used for:
Not to be used with:
Contains: CHLORHEXIDINE gluconate.
Other preparations: Hibitane Obstetric Cream, Hibitane Concentrate, Hibitane 20% Gluconate.

Hioxyl
(Quinoderm)

A cream used as a disinfectant to treat minor wounds, infections, bed sores, leg ulcers.

Dose: apply freely as needed and cover with a dressing.
Availability: NHS, private prescription, over the counter.
Side effects:
Caution:
Not to be used for:
Not to be used with:
Contains: HYDROGEN PEROXIDE.
Other preparations:

Hiprex
(3M Riker)

A white, oblong, scored tablet supplied at a strength of 1 g and used as an anti-bacterial treatment for infections of the urinary tract.

Dose: adults 1 g twice a day; children 6-12 years half adult dose.
Availability: NHS, private prescription, over the counter.
Side effects: stomach upset, rash, bladder irritation.
Caution:
Not to be used for: in patients suffering from severe dehydration, severe kidney failure, or electrolyte changes.
Not to be used with: sulphonamides, alkalizing agents.
Contains: HEXAMINE HIPPURATE.
Other preparations:

H

Hismanal
(Janssen)

A white, scored tablet supplied at a strength of 10 mg and used as an antihistamine treatment for hay fever, allergic rhinitis, skin allergies.

Dose: adults 1 tablet a day 1 hour before food; children 6-12 years half adult dose.
Availability: NHS and private prescription.
Side effects: rarely drowsiness or gain in weight.
Caution: women of child-bearing age should take steps to avoid conception during and for some weeks after the treatment.

Not to be used for: pregnant women.
Not to be used with:
Contains: ASTEMIZOLE.
Other preparations: Hismanal Suspension.

Histalix
(Wallace)

A syrup used as an antihistamine, expectorant, and sputum softener to treat bronchial and nasal congestion.

Dose: adults 1-2 5 ml teaspoonsful every 3 hours; children half adult dose.
Availability: private prescription and over the counter.
Side effects: drowsiness, reduced reactions, rarely skin eruptions.
Caution: patients suffering from liver or kidney disease.
Not to be used for:
Not to be used with: alcohol, sedatives, MAOIS.
Contains: DIPHENHYDRAMINE HYDROCHLORIDE, AMMONIUM CHLORIDE, SODIUM CITRATE, MENTHOL.
Other preparations:

Histryl Spansule
(S K B)

A pink/clear capsule supplied at a strength of 5 mg and used as an antihistamine treatment for rhinitis, severe allergic conditions, insect bites and stings, allergies to food or other drugs.

Dose: 1-2 capsules night and morning.
Availability: NHS, private prescription, over the counter.
Side effects: drowsiness, reduced reactions, dry mouth, blurred vision, dizziness.
Caution: in nursing mothers.
Not to be used for: children.
Not to be used with: sedatives, MAOIS, alcohol.
Contains: DIPHENYL PYRALINE HYDROCHLORIDE.
Other preparations: Histryl Paediatric.

Homatropine
(SNP)

Drops used as an ANTI-CHOLINERGIC treatment for glaucoma.

Dose: 1 or more drops into the eye as needed.
Availability: NHS and private prescription.
Side effects:
Caution:
Not to be used for: patients suffering from narrow-angle glaucoma.
Not to be used with:
Contains: HOMATROPINE HYDROBROMIDE.
Other preparations:

---

homatropine hydrobromide *see* Homatropine

---

homatropine *see* APP

Hormofemin
(Medo)

H

A cream with applicator used as an oestrogen for the short-term treatment of senile or atrophic inflammation of the vagina, vulval itch.

Dose: $^1/_2$ -1 application into the vagina once a day for 1-2 weeks then reducing to half that dose.
Availability: NHS and private prescription.
Side effects: enlarged breasts, bloating and fluid retention, cramps, leg pains, mood change, reduction in sexual desire, headaches, nausea, vaginal erosion, discharge, and bleeding, weight gain, skin changes.
Caution: in patients suffering from high blood pressure, diabetes, vascular disorders, asthma, depression, kidney disease, multiple sclerosis, womb diseases. Your doctor may advise you not to smoke, to have regular examinations. You should stop treatment at the first sign of serious symptoms such as severe headache or jaundice. Treatment should be stopped before surgery.
Not to be used for: children, pregnant women, or for patients

suffering from sickle-cell anaemia, history of heart disease or thrombosis, liver disorders, some cancers, undiagnosed vaginal bleeding, some ear, skin, and kidney disorders.

Not to be used with: RIFAMPICIN, TETRACYCLINES, GRISEOFULVIN, barbiturates, PHENYTOIN, PRIMIDONE, CARBAMAZEPINE, ETHOSUXIMIDE, CHLORAL HYDRATE, DICHLORALPHENAZONE.

Contains: DIENOESTEROL.
Other preparations:

Hormonin
(Carnrick)

A pink, scored tablet used as an oestrogen treatment for symptoms associate with the menopause.

Dose: $1/2$ -2 tablets a day.
Availability: NHS and private prescription.
Side effects: enlarged breasts, bloating and fluid retention, cramps, leg pains, mood change, reduction in sexual desire, headaches, nausea, vaginal erosion, discharge, and bleeding, weight gain, skin changes.
Caution: in patients suffering from high blood pressure, diabetes, vascular disorders, asthma, depression, kidney disease, multiple sclerosis, womb diseases. Your doctor may advise you not to smoke, to have regular examinations. You should stop treatment at the first sign of serious symptoms such as severe headache or jaundice. Treatment should be stopped before surgery.
Not to be used for: pregnant women, or for patients suffering from sickle-cell anaemia, history of heart disease or thrombosis, liver disorders, some cancers, undiagnosed vaginal bleeding, some ear, skin, and kidney disorders.
Not to be used with: RIFAMPICIN, TETRACYCLINES, GRISEOFULVIN, barbiturates, PHENYTOIN, PRIMIDONE, CARBAMAZEPINE, ETHOSUXIMIDE, CHLORAL HYDRATE, DICHLORALPHENAZONE.
Contains: OESTRIOL, OESTRONE, OESTRADIOL.
Other preparations:

Hydergine
(Sandoz)

A white tablet supplied at strengths of 1.5 mg, 4.5 mg and used as a vasodilator as an additional treatment for elderly patients suffering from dementia.

Dose: 4.5 mg a day.
Availability: NHS and private prescription.
Side effects: stomach upset, flushes, rash, blocked nose, cramps, headache, dizziness.
Caution: in patients suffering from slow heart rate.
Not to be used for: children
Not to be used with:
Contains: CODERGOCRINE MESYLATE.
Other preparations:

---

hydralazine *see* **Apresoline**

Hydrenox
(Boots)

A white, scored tablet supplied at a strength of 50 mg and used as a DIURETIC to treat fluid retention, high blood pressure.

Dose: adults fluid retention 1-4 tablets a day as a single dose in the morning, then $^1/_2$-1 tablet a day every other day, high blood pressure $^1/_2$-1 tablet a day; children 1 mg per kg bodyweight a day.
Availability: NHS and private prescription.
Side effects: low potassium levels, rash, sensitivity to light, blood changes, gout, tiredness.
Caution: in the elderly, in pregnant women, nursing mothers, and in patients suffering from diabetes, liver or kidney disease, or gout; your doctor may advise that a potassium supplement is needed.
Not to be used for: patients suffering from severe kidney failure.
Not to be used with: LITHIUM, DIGITALIS, anti-hypertensives.
Contains: HYDROFLUMETHIAZIDE.
Other preparations:

---

hydrochlorothiazide *see* **Capozide, Co-Betaloc, Dyazide, Esidrex K, Hydromet, Hydrosaluric, Hypertane, Kalten,**

H

Moducren, Moduret 25, Moduretic, Normetic, Secadrex, Serpasil Esidrex, Sotazide, Tolerzide

---

Hydrocortisone
(Roussel)

A cream used as a steroid treatment for eczema, itch, and other skin disorders.

Dose: apply to the affected area 1-4 times a day.
Availability: NHS and private prescription.
Side effects: fluid retention, suppression of adrenal glands, thinning of the skin may occur.
Caution: use for short periods of time only.
Not to be used for: continuously especially for pregnant women, or for patients suffering from acne or any other tubercular, viral, fungal, or ringworm skin infections.
Not to be used with:
Contains: HYDROCORTISONE.
Other preparations: Hydrocortisone Ointment, HYDROCORTISTAB (Boots), DIODERM (Dermal), EFCORTELAN (Glaxo), LOCOID (Brocades).

H

hydrocortisone *see* Actinac, Alphaderm, Alphosyl HC, Anugesic-HC, Anusol HC, Barquinol HC, Calmurid HC, Canesten-HC, Carbo-Cort, Chloromycetin Hydrocortisone, Cobadex, Colifoam, Corlan, Cortenema, Cortucid, Daktacort, Econacort, Epifoam, Eurax-Hydrocortisone, Framycort, Fucidin H, Genticin HC, Gentisone HC, Gregoderm, Hydrocortistab, Hydroderm, Mildison Lipocream, Neo-Cortef, Nystaform-HC, Otosporin, Proctofoam HC, Proctosedyl, Quinocort, Sential, Tarcortin, Terra-Cortril, Timodine, Tri-Cicatrin, Uniroid, Vioform-Hydrocortisone, Xyloproct

---

Hydrocortistab
(Boots)

A white, scored tablet supplied at a strength of 20 mg and used as a corticosteroid for replacement treatment in adrenocortical deficiency, inflammation in allergies, and rheumatic and collagen diseases.

Dose: adults $^1/_2$ -3 tablets a day; children as advised by the physician.
Availability: NHS and private prescription.
Side effects: high blood sugar, thin bones, mood changes, ulcers.
Caution: in pregnant women, in patients who have had recent bowel surgery, or who are suffering from inflamed veins, psychiatric disorders, virus infections, some cancers, some kidney diseases, thinning of the bones, ulcers, tuberculosis, other infections, high blood pressure, glaucoma, epilepsy, diabetes, underactive thyroid, liver disease, stress. Withdraw gradually.
Not to be used for: infants under 1 year.
Not to be used with: PHENYTOIN, PHENOBARBITONE, EPHEDRINE, RIFAMPICIN, DIURETICS, ANTI-CHOLINESTERASES, DIGITALIS, anti-diabetic agents, anti-coagulants, NON-STEROID ANTI-INFLAMMATORY DRUGS.
Contains: HYDROCORTISONE.
Other preparations: Hydrocortistab Injection.

Hydrocortone
(MSD)

A white, quarter-scored tablet or a white, scored, oval tablet according to strengths of 10 mg, 20 mg and used as a corticosteroid replacement treatment in adrenocortical deficiency.

H

Dose: as advised by the physician.
Availability: NHS and private prescription.
Side effects: high blood sugar, thin bones, mood changes, ulcers.
Caution: in pregnant women, in patients who have had recent bowel surgery, or who are suffering from inflamed veins, psychiatric disorders, virus infections, some cancers, some kidney diseases, thinning of the bones, ulcers, tuberculosis, other infections, high blood pressure, glaucoma, epilepsy, diabetes, underactive thyroid, liver disease, stress. Withdraw gradually.
Not to be used for: infants under 1 year.
Not to be used with: PHENYTOIN, PHENOBARBITONE, EPHEDRINE, RIFAMPICIN, DIURETICS, ANTI-CHOLINESTERASES, DIGITALIS, anti-diabetic agents, anti-coagulants, NON-STEROID ANTI-INFLAMMATORY DRUGS.
Contains: HYDROCORTISONE.
Other preparations:

Hydroderm
(MSD)

An ointment used as an anti-bacterial and steroid treatment for eczema, itch, and other skin disorders where there is also infection.

Dose: apply to the affected area 2-3 times a day.
Availability: NHS and private prescription.
Side effects: fluid retention, suppression of the adrenal glands, thinning of the skin may occur.
Caution: use for short periods of time only.
Not to be used for: continuously especially in pregnant women, or for patients suffering from acne or any other tubercular, viral, fungal, or ringworm skin infections.
Not to be used with:
Contains: HYDROCORTISONE, NEOMYCIN sulphate, ZINC BACITRACIN.
Other preparations:

---

hydroflumethiazide *see* Hydrenox

---

hydrogen peroxide *see* Hioxyl

Hydromet
(MSD)

A pink tablet used as an anti-hypertensive treatment for high blood pressure.

Dose: adults 1 tablet twice a day at first increasing at 2-day intervals to a maximum of 12 tablets a day; children as advised by physician.
Availability: NHS and private prescription.
Side effects: sedation, headache, weakness, depression, slow heart rate, blocked nose, dry mouth, stomach upset, blood changes.
Caution: in pregnant women, nursing mothers, and in patients with a history of liver disease, or in patients suffering from some blood disorders, gout, diabetes, liver or kidney disease. Your doctor may advise that potassium supplements may be needed.
Not to be used for: patients suffering from depression, liver disease,

severe kidney failure, phaeochromocytoma (a disease of the adrenal glands).
Not to be used with: TRICYCLICS, MAOIS, RESERPINE-like anti-hypertensives, HYDRALAZINE, DIGITALIS, LITHIUM, or other anti-hypertensives.
Contains: METHYLDOPA, HYDROCHLOROTHIAZIDE.
Other preparations:

Hydrosaluric
(MSD)

A white, scored tablet supplied at strengths of 25 mg, 50 mg and used as a DIURETIC to treat fluid retention, high blood pressure.

Dose: adults as a diuretic 50-100 mg once or twice a day, high blood pressure 50-100 mg a day at first, then up to not more than 200 mg a day; infants under 6 months up to 3.5 mg per kg bodyweight a day, 6 months-2 years 12.5-37.5 mg a day, 2-12 years 37.5-100 mg a day all in 2 divided doses.
Availability: NHS and private prescription.
Side effects: low potassium levels, rash, sensitivity to light, blood changes, gout, tiredness.
Caution: in pregnant women and in patients suffering from diabetes, liver or kidney disease, or gout. Your doctor may advise that a potassium supplement is needed.
Not to be used for: nursing mothers or for patients suffering from severe kidney failure.
Not to be used with: LITHIUM, DIGITALIS, anti-hypertensives.
Contains: HYDROCHLOROTHIAZIDE.
Other preparations:

H

---

hydrotalcite *see* Altacite Plus

---

hydroxocobalamin *see* Lipoflavonoid, Lipotriad

---

hydroxyapatite compound *see* **Ossopan**

---

hydroxychloroquine *see* **Plaquenil**

---

hydroxyzine *see* **Atarax**

Hygroton
(Geigy)

A pale-yellow, scored tablet or a white, scored tablet according to strengths of 50 mg, 100 mg and used as a DIURETIC to treat high blood pressure, fluid retention, toxaemia of pregnancy.

Dose: adults fluid retention 50 mg a day or 100-200 mg every other day at first, then 100 mg twice a week as a single dose after breakfast, high blood pressure 25-50 mg a day as a single dose after breakfast; children up to 10 kg body weight 5 mg per kg every other day, up to 5 years 50 mg every other day, 5-12 years 50-100 mg every other day.
Availability: NHS and private prescription.
Side effects: abnormal heart rhythm, stomach disturbances, low potassium levels, rash, sensitivity to light, blood changes, gout, tiredness.
Caution: in the elderly, pregnant women, nursing mothers, and in patients suffering from diabetes, kidney or liver disease, or gout. Your doctor may advise that a potassium supplement is needed.
Not to be used for: patients suffering from severe kidney failure.
Not to be used with: LITHIUM, DIGITALIS, antihypertensives.
Contains: CHLORTHALIDONE.
Other preparations:

Hygroton K
(Geigy)

A pink tablet used as a DIURETIC with potassium supplement to treat high blood pressure, fluid retention, toxaemia of pregnancy.

Dose: high blood pressure 1-2 tablets at breakfast, fluid retention 1-2 tablets once or twice a day.
Availability: NHS and private prescription.
Side effects: abnormal heart rhythm, stomach disturbances, rash, sensitivity to light, blood changes, gout, tiredness.
Caution: in the elderly, pregnant women, nursing mothers, and in patients suffering from diabetes, gout, liver or kidney disease.
Not to be used for: patients suffering from severe kidney failure, Addison's disease, raised potassium levels.
Not to be used with: LITHIUM, DIGITALIS, anti-hypertensives.
Contains: CHLORTHALIDONE, POTASSIUM CHLORIDE.
Other preparations:

---

hyoscine *see* Buscopan, Scopoderm

---

hyoscyamine sulphate *see* Peptard

Hypertane
(Schwarz)

A white, scored tablet used as a DIURETIC and potassium-sparing diuretic to treat congestive heart failure, high blood pressure, cirrhosis of the liver with ascites especially where the potassium balance must be controlled.

Dose: adults usually 1-2 tablets a day up to a maximum of 4 tablets; elderly according to kidney function and response.
Availability: NHS and private prescription.
Side effects: rash, sensitivity to light, blood changes, gout.
Caution: in patients suffering from diabetes, electrolyte changes, gout, kidney or liver disease.
Not to be used for: children, pregnant women, nursing mothers, or for patients suffering from raised potassium levels, progressive or severe kidney failure.
Not to be used with: potassium supplements and potassium-sparing diuretics, DIGITALIS, LITIUM, anti-hypertensives, ACE INHIBITORS.
Contains: HYDROCHLOROTHIAZIDE, AMILORIDE hydrochloride.
Other preparations:

Hypon
(Calmic)

A yellow tablet used as an analgesic for the relief of headache, rheumatism, neuralgia, period pain, colds.

Dose: 1-2 tablets every 4 hours.
Availability: private prescription only.
Side effects: stomach upset, allergy, asthma.
Caution: in the elderly, pregnant women, and in patients with a history of allergy to aspirin or asthma, impaired liver or kidney function, indigestion.
Not to be used for: children, nursing mothers, or for patients suffering from haemophilia, ulcers.
Not to be used with: anti-coagulants (blood-thinning drugs), some anti-diabetic drugs, anti-inflammatory agents, METHOTREXATE, SPIRONOLACTONE, steroids, some antacids, some uric acid-lowering drugs.
Contains: ASPIRIN, CAFFEINE, CODEINE phosphate
Other preparations:

Hypotears
(Iolab)

Drops used to moisten dry eyes.

Dose: 1-2 drops every 3-4 hours or as needed.
Availability: NHS, private prescription, over the counter.
Side effects:
Caution:
Not to be used for: patients who wear soft contact lenses.
Not to be used with:
Contains: POLYETHYLENE GLYCOL, POLYVINYL ALCOHOL.
Other preparations:

Hypovase
(Pfizer)

A white tablet, orange, scored tablet, or white, scored tablet according to strengths of 500 micrograms, 1 mg, 2 mg, 5 mg and used as a vasodilator to treat congestive heart failure, high blood pressure,

Raynaud's phenomenon, additional treatment in urinary obstruction caused by prostate enlargement.

Dose: 500 micrograms 3-4 times a day at first, increasing to 1 mg 3-4 times a day, followed by 4-20 mg a day in divided doses to maintain treatment. For high blood pressure 500 micrograms on first evening, then 500 micrograms 2-3 times a day for 3-7 days increasing as needed to a maximum of 20 mg a day. For Raynaud's phenomenon or prostate enlargement 500 micrograms twice a day at first then 1-2 mg twice a day.
Availability: NHS and private prescription.
Side effects: loss of consciousness, dizziness, lassitude, dry mouth, blurred vision, rash.
Caution: in patients suffering from fainting when they urinate.
Not to be used for: children.
Not to be used with: anti-hypertensive drugs.
Contains: PRAZOSIN HYDROCHLORIDE.
Other preparations:

---

hypromellose *see* **Carbachol, Carpine, Epinal, Ilube, Isopto Alkaline, Isopto Plain, Maxidex, Maxitrol, Tears Naturale**

H

Hytrin
(Abbott)

A white, yellow, brown, or blue tablet according to strengths of 1 mg, 2 mg, 5 mg, 10 mg and used as an anti-hypertensive to treat high blood pressure.

Dose: 1 mg at bed time at first, then increase dose at weekly intervals to a usual dose of 2-10 mg once a day.
Availability: NHS and private prescription.
Side effects: fainting with first dose, dizziness, lowered blood pressure on standing, lassitude, swelling of the limbs.
Caution: in patients with a history of liver disease or suffering from fainting.
Not to be used for: children.
Not to be used with:
Contains: TERAZOSIN HYDROCHLORIDE.
Other preparations:

ibuprofen *see* **Brufen**

Idoxene
(Spodefell)

An ointment used as an anti-viral treatment for herpetic keratitis (viral infection of the cornea).

Dose: Apply 4 times a day and at night for 3-5 days after symptoms have gone but for no more than 3 weeks.
Availability: NHS and private prescription.
Side effects: local irritation, swelling, pain.
Caution: in pregnant women.
Not to be used for:
Not to be used with: corticosteroids, boric acid.
Contains: IDOXURIDINE.
Other preparations:

---

idoxuridine *see* **Herpid, Idoxene, Kerecid, Virudox**

Ilosone *see* **Erythrocin**
(Dista)

Ilube
(Duncan, Flockhart)

Drops used to moisten dry eyes.

Dose: 1-2 drops into the eye 3-4 times a day.
Availability: NHS and private prescription.
Side effects:
Caution:
Not to be used for: patients who wear soft contact lenses.
Not to be used with:
Contains: ACETYLCYSTEINE, HYPROMELLOSE.
Other preparations:

Imbrilon *see* **Indocid**
(Berk)

Imdur *see* **Elantan**
(Astra)

---

imipramine *see* **Tofranil**

Imperacin *see* **Tetracycline**
(ICI)

---

indapamide hemihydrate *see* **Natrilix**

Inderal
(ICI)

A pink tablet supplied at strengths of 10 mg, 40 mg, 80 mg and used as a ß-ʙʟᴏᴄᴋᴇʀ to treat angina, migraine, high blood pressure, and as an additional treatment for thyrotoxicosis.

Dose: adults high blood pressure 80 mg twice a day at first, then adjust each weak according to response, thyrotoxicosis 10-40 mg 3-4 times a day, migraine 40 mg 2-3 times a day, angina 40 mg 2-3 times a day up to 480 mg a day; children thyrotoxicosis 0.25-0.5 mg per kg bodyweight 3-4 times a day, migraine half adult dose.
Availability: NHS and private prescription.
Side effects: cold hands and feet, sleep disturbance, slow heart rate, tiredness, wheezing, heart failure, stomach upset.
Caution: in pregnant women, nursing mothers, and in patients suffering from diabetes, kidney or liver disorders, asthma. May need to be withdrawn before surgery. Withdraw gradually. Your doctor may advise additional treatment with ᴅɪᴜʀᴇᴛɪᴄs or ᴅɪɢɪᴛᴀʟɪs.
Not to be used for: patients suffering from heart block or failure.

Not to be used with: VERAPAMIL, CLONIDINE withdrawal, some anti-arrhythmic drugs and anaesthetics, RESERPINE, some anti-hypertensives, ergot alkaloids, CIMETIDINE, sedatives, SYMPATHOMIMETICS, INDOMETHACIN.
Contains: PROPANOLOL HYDROCHLORIDE.
Other preparations: berkolol (Berk), Inderal Injection, Inderal LA, Half-Inderal LA, ANGILOL (DDSA).

Inderal LA
(ICI)

A lavender/pink capsule supplied at a strength of 160 mg and used as ß-BLOCKER to treat angina, high blood pressure, and as an additional treatment for thyrotxicosis.

Dose: 80 or 160 mg a day to a maximum of 240 mg a day. High blood pressure 160 mg a day at first increasing by 80 mg at a time until there is an effective response. Thyrotoxicosis 80 or 160 mg a day to a maximum of 240 mg a day.
Availability: NHS and private prescription.
Side effects: cold hands and feet, sleep disturbance, slow heart rate, tiredness, wheezing, heart failure, stomach upset.
Caution: in pregnant women, nursing mothers, and in patients suffering from diabetes, kidney or liver disorders, asthma. May need to be withdrawn before surgery. Withdraw gradually. Your doctor may advise additional treatment with DIURETICS or DIGITALIS.
Not to be used for: for children or patients suffering from heart block or failure.
Not to be used with: VERAPAMIL, CLONIDINE withdrawal, some anti-arrhythmic drugs and anaesthetics, RESERPINE, some anti-hypertensives, ergot alkaloids, CIMETIDINE, sedatives, SYMPATHOMIMETICS, INDOMETHACIN.
Contains: PROPANOLOL HYDROCHLORIDE.
Other preparations: Half-Inderal-LA, Inderal Tablets

Inderetic
(ICI)

A white capsule used as a ß-BLOCKER to treat high blood pressure.

Dose: 1 capsule twice a day.
Availability: NHS and private prescription.
Side effects: cold hands and feet, sleep disturbance, slow heart rate, tiredness, wheezing, heart failure, stomach upset, low blood potassium, rash, sensitivity to light, blood changes, gout, tiredness.
Caution: in pregnant women, nursing mothers, and in patients suffering from diabetes, kidney or liver disorders, asthma, gout. May need to be withdrawn before surgery. Withdraw gradually. Your doctor may advise additional treatment with DIURETICS or DIGITALIS, blood tests. Potassium supplements may be needed.
Not to be used for: for children or patients suffering from heart block or failure, severe kidney failure.
Not to be used with: VERAPAMIL, CLONIDINE withdrawal, some anti-arrhythmic drugs and anaesthetics, RESERPINE, some anti-hypertensives, ergot alkaloids, CIMETIDINE, sedatives, SYMPATHOMIMETICS, INDOMETHACIN, LITHIUM, DIGITALIS, other diuretics.
Contains: propanolol hydrochloride, bendrofluazide
Other preparations: Inderex (double strength).

Indocid
(Morson)

An ivory capsule supplied at strengths of 25 mg, 50 mg and used as a NON-STEROID ANTI-INFLAMMATORY DRUG to treat rheumatoid arthritis, osteoarthritis, degenerative disease of the hip joint, ankylosing spondylitis, acute gout, lumbago, acute joint disorders, orthopaedic procedures, period pain.

Dose: 50-200 mg a day in divided doses.
Availability: NHS and private prescription.
Side effects: gastro-intestinal bleeding, headache, corneal deposits, disturbances of the retina, gastro-intestinal intolerance, dizziness, brain disturbances, blood changes.
Caution: in patients suffering from kidney or liver disease, brain disorders.
Not to be used for: children, pregnant women, nursing mothers, or for patients suffering from peptic ulcer, history of stomach lesions, aspirin/anti-inflammatory drug allergy, recent proctitis, severe allergic swelling.
Not to be used with: SALICYLATES, anti-coagulants, LITHIUM, corticosteroids, DIURETICS, ß-BLOCKERS, PROBENECID.

Contains: INDOMETHACIN.
Other preparations: Indocid Suspension, Indocid Suppositories, Indocid-R. IMBRILON (Berk), INDOLAR SR (Lagap), INDOMOD (Pharmacia).

Indolar SR *see* Indocid
(Lagap)

---

indomethacin *see* Flexin Continus, Indocid

Indomod *see* Indocid
(Pharmacia)

---

indoramin *see* Baratol, Doralese

Infacol *see* Asilone
(Pharmax)

Innovace
(MSD)

A round white tablet, a white scored, or red or peach, triangular tablet according to strengths of 2.5 mg, 5 mg, 10 mg, 20 mg and used as an ACE INHIBITOR to treat congestive heart failure, high blood pressure.

Dose: adults 2.5 mg at first in hospital, 10-20 mg thereafter. High blood pressure 5 mg a day at first, then 10-20 to a maximum of 40 mg once a day; elderly or patients suffering from kidney disease start with 2.5 mg a day.
Availability: NHS and private prescription.
Side effects: low blood pressure, kidney failure, swelling, rash, headache, tiredness, dizziness, stomach upset, and rarely a cough.

Caution: fluid depletion may cause a marked drop in blood pressure. Dose of diuretic given may need to be reduced. Care in patients suffering from some kidney diseases and in nursing mothers.
Not to be used for: children or pregnant women.
Not to be used with: other anti-hypertensives, LITHIUM, potassium supplements, potassium-sparing DIURETICS.
Contains: ENALAPRIL MALEATE.
Other preparations:

---

inosine pranobex *see* Munovir

---

inositol *see* Hexopal, Ketovite, Lipoflavonoid, Lipotriad

Intal
(Fisons)

A yellow/ clear spincap (delivery capsule) supplied at a strength of 20 mg and used as an anti-asthmatic drug for the prevention of bronchial asthma.

Dose: 4 a day at regular intervals in Spinhaler (delivery system) increasing if needed to 6-8 a day.
Availability: NHS and private prescription.
Side effects: passing cough, irritated throat, rarely bronchial spasm.
Caution:
Not to be used for:
Not to be used with:
Contains: SODIUM CROMOGLYCATE.
Other preparations: Intal Inhaler, Intal 5 Inhaler, Intal Nebuliser Solution.

Intal Compound
(Fisons)

An orange/clear Spincap (delivery capsule) used as an anti-asthmatic drug for the prevention of bronchial asthma.

Dose: 4 a day at regular intervals in Spinhaler (delivery system) up to 6-8 a day if needed. Treatment should be continuous.
Availability: NHS and private prescription.
Side effects: passing cough, irritated throat, headache, abnormal heart rhythms, rapid heart rate, dilation of the blood vessels, rarely bronchial spasm.
Caution: in patients suffering from diabetes, high blood pressure.
Not to be used for:
Not to be used with: MAOIS, SYMPATHOMIMETICS, TRICYCLICS.
Contains: SODIUM CROMOGLYCATE, ISOPRENALINE SULPHATE.
Other preparations:

Integrin
(Sterling Research Laboratories)

A white capsule or a white, scored tablet according to strengths of 10 mg, 40 mg and used as a sedative to treat anxiety, schizophrenia, mental disorders, delirium.

Dose: anxiety 1 10 mg capsule 3-4 times a day to a maximum of 6 capsules a day; others 1 tablet 2-3 times a day to a maximum of 300 mg a day.
Availability: NHS and private prescription.
Side effects: tremor, ANTI-CHOLERGENIC effects, low blood pressure episodes, changes in some blood tests.
Caution: in pregnant women. Your doctor may advise that blood and liver tests should be made regularly, and that your judgement and abilities may be reduced.
Not to be used for: children.
Not to be used with: MAOIS, alcohol, sedatives.
Contains: OXYPERTINE.
Other preparations:

Intralgin
(3M Riker)

A gel used as an analgesic rub to treat muscle strains, sprains.

Dose: massage gently into the affected area as needed.
Availability: NHS, private prescription, and over the counter.

Side effects: may be irritant.
Caution:
Not to be used for: areas near the eyes or on broken or inflamed skin or on membranes (such as the mouth).
Not to be used with:
Contains: SALICYLAMIDE, BENZOCAINE.
Other preparations:

Iodosorb
(Perstorp)

Powder in a sachet used as an absorbant, anti-bacterial treatment for leg ulcers.

Dose: apply a 3 mm coating and cover with a dressing; repeat the treatment before the dressing is saturated.
Availability: NHS and private prescription.
Side effects:
Caution: in patients having thyroid investigation.
Not to be used for: pregnant women or nursing mothers.
Not to be used with:
Contains: CADEXOMER IODINE.
Other preparations:

Ionamin
(Lipha)

A yellow/grey capsule or a yellow capsule according to strengths of 15 mg, 30 mg and used as an appetite suppressant to treat obesity.

Dose: adults 15-30 mg once a day at breakfast time; children 6-12 years 15 mg once a day at breakfast.
Availability: controlled drug.
Side effects: tolerance, addiction, mental disturbances, restlessness, nervousness, agitation, dry mouth, heart palpitations, raised blood pressure.
Caution: in patients suffering from angina, abnormal heart rhythms, high blood pressure.
Not to be used for: children under 6 years, pregnant women, nursing mothers, or for patients suffering from hardening of the arteries,

overactive thyroid gland, severe high blood pressure, or with a history of mental illness, alcoholism, or drug addiction.
Not to be used with: MAOIS, SYMPATHOMIMETICS, METHYLDOPA, GUANETHID-INE, sedatives.
Contains: PHENTERMINE.
Other preparations:

Ionax
(Alcon)

An gel used as an abrasive, anti-bacterial preparation to clean the skin in the treatment of acne.

Dose: wet the face, then rub in once a day, and rinse.
Availability: NHS, private prescription, over the counter.
Side effects:
Caution:
Not to be used for: for children under 12 years.
Not to be used with:
Contains: POLYETHYLENE GRANULES, BENZALKONIUM CHLORIDE.
Other preparations:

Ionil T
(Alcon)

A shampoo used as an anti-psoriatic treatment for seborrhoeic inflammation of the scalp.

Dose: shampoo once a day if needed.
Availability: NHS, private prescription, over the counter.
Side effects: irritation, sensitivity to light.
Caution:
Not to be used for: patients suffering from acute psoriasis.
Not to be used with:
Contains: SALICYLIC ACID, BENZALKONIUM CHLORIDE, COAL TAR SOLUTION.
Other preparations:

---

ipecacuanha *see* **Alophen**

Ipral *see* **Monotrim**
(Squibb)

---

ipratropium *see* **Atrovent, Duovent**

---

iprindole *see* **Prondol**

Irofol C
(Abbott)

A red oblong tablet used as an iron, folic acid, and vitamin supplement for the prevention and treatment of iron and folic acid deficiency in pregnancy where vitamin supplement is also needed.

Dose: 1 tablet a day before food.
Availability: private prescription and over the counter.
Side effects:
Caution: in patients suffering from slow bowel action.
Not to be used for: children or for patients suffering from megaloblastic anaemia, diverticular disease, intestinal blockage.
Not to be used with: TETRACYCLINES, Clinistix urine test.
Contains: FERROUS SULPHATE, FOLIC ACID, ASCORBIC ACID.
Other preparations:

Ismelin
(Ciba)

A white tablet or a pink tablet according to strengths of 10 mg, 25 mg and used as an anti-hypertensive treatment for high blood pressure.

Dose: adults 20 mg a day at first increasing by 10 mg at a time at weekly intervals if needed; children as advised by physician.
Availability: NHS and private prescription.
Side effects: low blood pressure on standing up, diarrhoea, failure of ejaculation.
Caution: in patients undergoing anaesthesia or suffering from kidney

disease or peptic ulcer.

Not to be used for: patients suffering from phaeochromocytoma (a disease of the adrenal glands).

Not to be used with: TRICYCLIC anti-depressants, SYMPATHOMIMETICS, MAOIS, DIURETICS, RESERPINE-like drugs.

Contains: GUANETHIDINE.

Other preparations:

Ismelin
(Zyma)

Drops used as a fluid balance altering drug to treat glaucoma.

Dose: 1 drop into the eye 1-2 times a day.

Availability: NHS and private prescription.

Side effects: swelling, redness, or inflammation of the eye.

Caution:

Not to be used for: children or patients suffering from narrow angle glaucoma or who wear soft contact lenses.

Not to be used with: MAOIS.

Contains: GUANETHIDINE monosulphate.

Other preparations:

ISMO
(MCP)

A white tablet or white, scored tablet according to strengths of 10 mg, 20 mg, 40 mg and used as a NITRATE treatment for angina, and in addition to other treatment for congestive heart failure etc.

Dose: 10 mg a day for 2 days, then 10 mg twice a day for 3 days, followed by 20 mg 2-3 times a day; no more than 120 mg a day.

Availability: NHS and private prescription.

Side effects: headache, flushes, dizziness.

Caution:

Not to be used for: children.

Not to be used with:

Contains: ISOSORBIDE MONONITRATE.

Other preparations:

Iso-Autohaler
(3M-Riker)

An aerosol supplied at a strength of 0.08 mg and used as a bronchodilator to treat bronchial spasm brought on by chronic bronchitis or bronchial asthma.

Dose: 1- 3 sprays and again after 30 minutes if needed up to a maximum of 24 sprays in 24 hours.
Availability: NHS and private prescription.
Side effects: headache, dilation of the blood vessels, rapid heart rate, abnormal heart rhythms.
Caution: in patients suffering from diabetes or high blood pressure.
Not to be used for: patients suffering from heart disease, cardiac asthma, or overactive thyroid gland.
Not to be used with: MAOIS, TRICYCLICS, SYMPATHOMIMETICS.
Contains: ISOPRENALINE sulphate.
Other preparations:

---

isoaminile linctus

A linctus supplied at a strength of 40 mg and used as an anti-tussive agent to treat cough.

Dose: adults 1 5 ml teaspoonful 3-5 times a day; children ½ -1 teaspoonful 3-5 times a day.
Availability: NHS and private prescription.
Side effects: constipation, dizziness, nausea.
Caution:
Not to be used for:
Not to be used with:
Contains: ISOAMINILE CITRATE.
Other preparations:

---

isocarboxazid *see* Marplan

---

isoconazole nitrate *see* Travogyn

---

isoetharine hydrochloride *see* Numotac

---

isoetharine mesylate see Bronchilator

Isogel
(A & H)

Granules supplied at a strength of 200 g and used as a bulking agent to treat constipation, diarrhoea, irritable colon, and for colostomy control.

Dose: adults 10 ml in water once or twice a day with meals, children half adult dose.
Availability: NHS and private prescription.
Side effects:
Caution:
Not to be used for:
Not to be used with:
Contains: ISPAGHULA husk.
Other preparations:

Isoket Retard
(Schwarz)

A yellow, scored tablet or an orange, scored tablet according to strengths of 20 mg, 40 mg and used as a NITRATE for the prevention of angina.

Dose: 20-40 mg every 12 hours to a maximum of 160 mg a day.
Availability: NHS and private prescription.
Side effects: headache, flushes, dizziness.
Caution:
Not to be used for: children or for patients suffering from uncompensated heart shock, severe high blood pressure, anaemia, brain haemorrhage.
Not to be used with:
Contains: ISOSORBIDE DINITRATE.
Other preparations: Isoket 0.1%.

isometheptene mucate *see* **Midrid**

---

isoniazid *see* **Mynah, Rifater, Rifinah**

---

isoprenaline *see* **Duo-Autohaler, Intal Compound, Iso-Autohaler, Medihaler-Duo, Medihaler-Iso, Saventrine**

---

isopropyl alcohol see Hibisol, Manusept

Isopto Alkaline
(Alcon)

Drops used to lubricate the eyes.

Dose: 1-2 drops into the eye 3 times a day.
Availability: NHS, private prescription, over the counter.
Side effects:
Caution:
Not to be used for: patients who wear soft contact lenses.
Not to be used with:
Contains: HYPROMELLOSE.
Other preparations:

Isopto Frin
(Alcon)

Drops to lubricate the eyes where no infection is present.

Dose: 1-2 drops into the eye 3 times a day.
Availability: NHS, private prescription, over the counter.
Side effects:
Caution: in infants and patients suffering from narrow angle glaucoma.
Not to be used for: patients who wear soft contact lenses.
Not to be used with:

Contains: PHENYLEPHRINE hydrochloride.
Other preparations:

Isopto Plain
(Alcon)

Drops used to moisten dry eyes.

Dose: 1-2 drops into the eye 3 times a day.
Availability: NHS, private prescription, over the counter.
Side effects:
Caution:
Not to be used for: patients who wear soft contact lenses.
Not to be used with:
Contains: HYPROMELLOSE.
Other preparations:

Isordil
(Wyeth)

A white, scored tablet supplied at strengths of 10 mg, 30 mg and used as a NITRATE for the prevention of angina, acute congestive heart failure.

Dose: 5-15 mg under the tongue every 2-3 hours at first, then 10-60 mg swallowed 4 times a day. 40-120 mg day for the prevention of angina.
Availability: NHS and private prescription.
Side effects: headache, flushes, dizziness, may make chest pain worse.
Caution: heart function should be checked in the case of heart failure.
Not to be used for: children.
Not to be used with:
Contains: ISOSORBIDE DINITRATE.
Other preparations: Isordil Sublingual, Isordil Tembids

---

isosorbide dinitrate *see* **Isoket Retard, Isordil, Soni-Slo, Sorbichew, Sorbid SA, Sorbitrate, Vascardin**

isosorbide mononitrate *see* Elantan, ISMO, Monit, Mono-

---

isotretinoin *see* Roaccutane

---

ispaghula *see* Colven, Fibogel, Isogel, Manevac, Regulan

---

isradipine *see* Prescal

---

itraconazole *see* Sporanox

Kalspare
(Rorer)

An orange, scored tablet used as a DIURETIC combination to treat high blood pressure, fluid retention.

Dose: high blood pressure 1 tablet a day in the morning increasing to 2 tablets if needed, fluid retention 1 tablet a day in the morning increasing to 2 a day after 7 days if the condition fails to respond.
Availability: NHS and private prescription.
Side effects: rash, sensitivity to light, blood changes, gout, cramps
Caution: in pregnant women, nursing mothers, and in patients suffering from diabetes, electrolyte changes, gout, kidney or liver disease.
Not to be used for: children, and for patients suffering from progressive or severe kidney failure, raised potassium levels.
Not to be used with: potassium supplements, potassium-sparing diuretics, LITHIUM, DIGITALIS, anti-hypertensives, ACE INHIBITORS.
Contains: CHLORTHALIDONE, TRIAMTERENE.
Other preparations:

K

Kalten
(Stuart)

A red and cream capsule used as a ß-BLOCKER and DIURETIC combination high blood pressure.

Dose: 1 capsule a day
Availability: NHS and private prescription.
Side effects: cold hands and feet, sleep disturbance, slow heart rate, tiredness, wheezing, heart failure, stomach upset, rash, sensitivity to light, blood changes, gout, cramps
Caution: in pregnant women, nursing mothers, and in patients suffering from diabetes, electrolyte changes, gout, kidney or liver disease, asthma.
Not to be used for: children, and for patients suffering from progressive or severe kidney failure, raised potassium levels, heart block or failure.
Not to be used with: potassium supplements, potassium-sparing diuretics, LITHIUM, DIGITALIS, anti-hypertensives, ACE INHIBITORS, VERAPAMIL, CLONIDINE withdrawal, some anti-arrhythmic drugs and anaesthetics, RESERPINE, ergot alkaloids, CIMETIDINE, sedatives, SYMPATHOMIMETICS, INDOMETHACIN.
Contains: ATENOLOL, HYDROCHLOROTHIAZIDE, AMILORIDE hydrochloride
Other preparations:

Keflex
(Eli Lilly)

A dark green/white capsule supplied at a strength of 250 mg and used as a cephalosporin antibiotic to treat respiratory, soft tissue, urine, and skin infections.

Dose: adults 4-16 capsules a day in divided doses; children 25-50 mg per kg body weight a day in divided doses.
Availability: NHS and private prescription.
Side effects: allergic reactions, stomach disturbances.
Caution: in patients suffering from kidney disease or who are very sensitive to penicillin.
Not to be used for:
Not to be used with: loop DIURETICS.
Contains: CEPHALEXIN.
Other preparations: Keflex Tablets, Keflex Chewable, Keflex Suspension.

K

Kelfizine W
(Farmitalia CE)

A white tablet supplied at a strength of 2 g and used as a sulphonamide to treat bronchitis, urine infections.

Dose: 1 tablet a week.
Availability: NHS and private prescription.
Side effects: anaemia, stomach disturbances, sore tongue, rash, blood changes when used for an extended period of treatment.
Caution: in patients suffering from liver or kidney disease, blood changes. Your doctor may advise that blood should be checked regularly for patients on extended periods of treatment.
Not to be used for: children, pregnant women, nursing mothers.
Not to be used with: TRIMETHOPRIM, anti-diabetics taken by mouth.
Contains: SULFAMETOPYRAZINE.
Other preparations:

Kemadrin
(Wellcome)

A white, scored tablet supplied at a strength of 5 mg and used as an ANTI-CHOLINERGIC to treat Parkinson's disease.

Dose: 1/2 tablet 3 times a day after meals at first, increasing every 2-3 days by 1/2 -1 tablet to a maximum of 6 tablets a day.
Availability: NHS and private prescription.
Side effects: anti-cholinergic effects, confusion at high doses.
Caution: in patients suffering from heart problems, stomach obstruction, glaucoma, enlarged prostate. Reduce dose slowly.
Not to be used for: children or patients suffering from movement disorders.
Not to be used with: phenothiazines, antihistamines, anti-depressants.
Contains: PROCYCLIDINE hydrochloride
Other preparations: Kemadrin Injection.

K

Keralyt
(Westwood)

A gel used as a skin softener to treat thickened skin.

Dose: wet the skin for 5 minutes and then apply once a day at night.
Availability: NHS, private prescription, over the counter.
Side effects:
Caution: keep out of the eyes, nose, and mouth.
Not to be used for:
Not to be used with:
Contains: SALICYLIC ACID.
Other preparations:

Kerecid
(Allergan)

Drops used as an anti-viral treatment for herpes infections of the cornea.

Dose: 1 drop into the eye every hour during the day and every 2 hours at night or 1 drop every minute for 5 minutes every 4 hours continuously for 5-7 days after the lesion stops staining but for no more th
Availability: NHS and private prescription.
Side effects: temporary irritation, swelling.
Caution: in pregnant women.
Not to be used for:
Not to be used with: corticosteroids, boric acid.
Contains: IDOXURIDINE, POLYVINYL ALCOHOL.
Other preparations: Kerecid Ointment.

Kerlone
(Lorex)

A white, scored tablet supplied at a strength of 20 mg and used as a ß-BLOCKER to treat high blood pressure.

Dose: 1 tablet a day; elderly $1/2$ tablet a day at first.
Availability: NHS and private prescription.
Side effects: cold hands and feet, sleep disturbance, slow heart rate, tiredness, wheezing, heart failure, stomach upset.
Caution: in pregnant women, nursing mothers, and in patients suffering from diabetes, kidney or liver disorders, asthma. May need to be withdrawn before surgery. Withdraw gradually. Your doctor may advise additional treatment with diuretics or digitalis.

Not to be used for: children or for patients suffering from heart block or failure.
Not to be used with: VERAPAMIL, CLONIDINE withdrawal, some anti-arrhythmic drugs and anaesthetics, RESERPINE, some anti-hypertensives, ergot alkaloids, CIMETIDINE, sedatives, SYMPATHOMIMETICS, IN-DOMETHACIN.
Contains: BETAXOLOL hydrochloride.
Other preparations:

Kest
(Rorer)

A white tablet used as a stimulant to treat constipation.

Dose: adults 1 tablet at night and 2 in the morning.
Availability: private prescription.
Side effects: allergic reactions to PHENOLPHTHALEIN.
Caution: in patients suffering from kidney problems.
Not to be used for: children
Not to be used with:
Contains: MAGNESIUM SULPHATE, PHENOLPHTHALEIN.
Other preparations:

---

ketazolam *see* Anxon

---

ketoconazole *see* Nizoral, Nizoral Cream

K

---

ketoprofen *see* Orudis

---

ketotifen *see* Zaditen

Ketovite
(Paines & Byrne)

A yellow tablet used as a multivitamin supplement in artificial diets.

Dose: 1 tablet 3 times a day plus 1 5 ml teaspoonful of Ketovite Liquid a day.
Availability: NHS and private prescription.
Side effects:
Caution:
Not to be used for:
Not to be used with: levodopa.
Contains: tablet: ACETOMENAPHTHONE, THIAMINE, RIBOFLAVINE, PYRIDOXINE, NICOTINAMIDE, CALCIUM PANTOTHENATE, ACSORBIC ACID, TOCOPHERYL ACETATE, INOSITOL, BIOTIN, FOLIC ACID; liquid: VITAMIN A, VITAMIN D, CHOLINE.
Other preparations: Ketovite Liquid.

Kiditard *see* Kinidin Durules
(Delandale)

Kinidin Durules
(Astra)

A white tablet supplied at a strength of 250 mg and used as an anti-arrhythmic drug to treat abnormal heart rhythm.

Dose: 1 tablet at first, then 2-5 tablets twice a day.
Availability: NHS
Side effects: allergies, liver disease, quinine excess, heart muscle toxicity.
Caution: in pregnant women, nursing mothers and in patients with congestive heart failure, low blood pressure, rapid heart rate.
Not to be used for: children or patients suffering from acute infection, myasthenia gravis (a muscle disorder), severe heart disease.
Not to be used with: DIGOXIN, anti-coagulants.
Contains: QUINIDINE bisulphate
Other preparations:

Kloref
(Cox)

A white, effervescent tablet used as a potassium supplement to treat potassium deficiency.

Dose: adults 1-2 tablets in water 3 times a day; children as advised by the physician.
Availability: NHS, private prescription, and over the counter.
Side effects:
Caution: in patients suffering from kidney disease.
Not to be used for: patients suffering from increased chloride levels or other rare metabolic disorders.
Not to be used with:
Contains: BETAINE HYDROCHLORIDE, POTASSIUM BENZOATE, POTASSIUM BICAR-BONATE, POTASSIUM CHLORIDE.
Other preparations: Kloref-S

---

kola liquid extract *see* Glykola

---

kola nut dried extract *see* Labiton

Kolanticon
(Merrell Dow)

A gel used as an antacid, anti-spasm, and ANTI-CHOLINERGIC treatment for bowel/stomach spasm, acidity, wind, ulcers.

Dose: adults 10-20 ml every 4 hours.
Availability: NHS and over the counter.
Side effects: occasionally constipation, blurred vision, confusion, dry mouth.
Caution:
Not to be used for: infants or patients suffering from glaucoma, inflammatory bowel disease, intestinal obstruction, or enlarged prostate.
Not to be used with: TETRACYCLINE antibiotics.

K

Contains: ALUMINIUM HYDROXIDE, MAGNESIUM OXIDE, DICYCLAMINE HYDRO-CHLORIDE, DIMETHICONE.
Other preparations:

---

l-cysteine *see* Cicatrin

---

labetalol *see* Trandate

Labiton
(LAB)

A liquid used as a tonic.

Dose: 2-4 5 ml teaspoonsful twice a day.
Availability: private prescription and over the counter.
Side effects:
Caution:
Not to be used for: children, or for patients suffering from hepatitis or who are taking sedatives.
Not to be used with:
Contains: THIAMINE hydrochloride, P-AMINOBENZOIC ACID, KOLA NUT DRIED EXTRACT, alcohol, CAFFEINE.
Other preparations:

Labosept
(LAB)

A red hexagonal-shaped pastille supplied at a strength of 0.25 mg and used as an antiseptic treatment for throat and mouth infections.

Dose: suck 1 pastille every 4 hours.
Availability: NHS, private prescription, over the counter.
Side effects:
Caution:
Not to be used for:
Not to be used with:

Contains: DEQUALINIUM CHLORIDE.
Other preparations:

Labrocol *see* **Trandate**

Lacri-Lube
(Allergan)

An ointment used for lubricating the eyes and protecting the cornea.

Dose: apply into the eye as needed.
Availability: NHS, private prescription, over the counter.
Side effects:
Caution:
Not to be used for:
Not to be used with:
Contains: LIQUID PARAFFIN, WOOL FAT.
Other preparations:

---

lactic acid *see* **Calmurid HC, Cuplex, Duofilm, Salactol, Tampovagan, Variclene**

---

lactose *see* **Logynon ED**

---

lactulose *see* **Duphalac**

Ladropen *see* **Floxapen**
(Berk)

---

laevulose *see* **Rehidrat**

Laractone *see* **Aldactone**
(Lagap)

Laraflex *see* **Naprosyn**
(Lagap)

Larapam *see* **Feldene**
(Lagap)

Laratrim *see* **Septrin**
(Lagap)

Largactil
(M & B)

A white tablet supplied at strengths of 10 mg, 25 mg, 50 mg, 100 mg and used as a sedative to treat brain disturbances needing sedation, premedication, inducing hypothermia, nausea, schizophrenia, mood change.

Dose: adults 25 mg 3 times a day at first increasing if needed by 25 mg a day to 75-300 mg a day; children as advised by physician.
Availability: NHS and private prescription.
Side effects: muscle spasms, restlessness, hands shaking, dry mouth, urine retention, palpitations, low blood pressure, weight gain, changes in libido, low body temperature, breast swelling, menstrual changes, jaundice, blood and skin changes, drowsiness, rarely fits.
Caution: in pregnant women, nursing mothers, and in patients suffering from liver disease, cardiovascular disease, epilepsy, or Parkinson's disease.
Not to be used for: unconscious patients or for patients suffering from bone marrow depression.
Not to be used with: alcohol, tranquillizers, pain killers, anti-hypertensives, anti-depressants, anti-convulsants, anti-diabetic drugs, LEVODOPA.

Contains: CHLORPROMAZINE hydrochloride.
Other preparations: Largactil Syrup, Largactil Forte Suspension, Largactil Injection.

Larodopa
(Roche)

A white, quarter-scored tablet supplied at a strength of 500 mg and used as an anti-parkinsonian drug to treat Parkinson's disease.

Dose: 1/4 tablet twice a day after meals at first increasing after 7 days to 1/4 tablet 4-5 times a day, then increasing every 7 days by 3/4 tablet a day to 5-16 tablets a day in 4-5 divided doses.
Availability: NHS and private prescription.
Side effects: nausea, vomiting anorexia, low blood pressure on standing up, involuntary movments, heart and brain disturbances, discoloration of urine.
Caution: in pregnant women and in patients suffering from heart, liver, kidney, lung, or endocrine disease and glaucoma.Your doctor may advise that blood and liver, kidney, and cardiovascular systems should be checked regularly.
Not to be used for: children or for patients suffering from severe mental disorder, glaucoma, or a history of malignant melanoma.
Not to be used with: MAOIS, PYRIDOXINE, anti-hypertensives, SYMPATH-OMIMETICS.
Contains: LEVODOPA.
Other preparations: BROCADOPA (Brocades)

Lasikal
(Hoechst)

A white/yellow, double-layered tablet used as a DIURETIC and potassium supplement to treat fluid retention where a potassium supplement is needed.

L

Dose: 2 tablets a day as a single dose in the morning, then either 4 tablets a day in 2 doses if needed, or 1 tablet a day.
Availability: NHS and private prescription.
Side effects: stomach upset, rash, gout.
Caution: in pregnant women, nursing mothers, or in patients suffering

from liver or kidney disease, enlarged prostate, or impaired urination.
Not to be used for: patients suffering from cirrhosis of the liver, raised potassium levels, or Addison's disease.
Not to be used with: potassium-sparing diuretics, DIGITALIS, LITHIUM, aminoglycosides, non-steroid anti-inflammatory drugs, cephalosporin antibiotics, anti-hypertensives.
Contains: frusemide, potassium chloride.
Other preparations:

Lasilactone
(Hoechst)

A blue/white capsule used as a DIURETIC combination to treat fluid retention, some types of high blood pressure.

Dose: 1-4 capsules a day.
Availability: NHS and private prescription.
Side effects: stomach upset, gout, rash, blood changes, breast swelling.
Caution: in pregnant women, nursing mothers, young patients, or in patients suffering from enlarged prostate, impaired urination, diabetes, kidney or liver disease.
Not to be used for: for patients suffering from severe or progressive kidney failure, liver cirrhosis, raised potassium levels, Addison's disease.
Not to be used with: potassium supplements, potassium-sparing diuretics, anti-hypertensives, DIGITALIS, LITHIUM, aminoglycoside and cephalosporin antibiotics.
Contains: FRUSEMIDE, SPIRONOLACTONE.
Other preparations:

Lasipressin
(Hoechst)

A white, oblong, scored tablet used as a ß-BLOCKER and DIURETIC to treat high blood pressure.

Dose: 1 tablet in the morning at first increasing to 2 tablets a day if needed.
Availability: NHS and private prescription.

Side effects: cold hands and feet, sleep disturbance, slow heart rate, tiredness, wheezing, heart failure, stomach upset, rash, gout.
Caution: pregnant women, nursing mothers, and in patients suffering from asthma, diabetes, kidney or liver disorders, gout, enlarged prostate, impaired urination.
Not to be used for: for patients suffering from heart block or failure, or liver cirrhosis.
Not to be used with: VERAPAMIL, CLONIDINE withdrawal, some anti-arrhythmic drugs and anaesthetics, RESERPINE, anti-hypertensives, ergot alkaloids, CIMETIDINE, sedatives, SYMPATHOMIMETICS, INDOMETHACIN, DIGITALIS, LITHIUM, aminoglycoside and cephalosporin antibiotics, NON-STEROID ANTI-INFLAMMATORY DRUGS.
Contains: FRUSEMIDE, PENBUTOLOL sulphate
Other preparations:

Lasix
(Hoechst)

A white, scored tablet supplied at strengths of 20 mg, 40 mg and used as a diuretic to treat fluid retention, high blood pressure.

Dose: 20-80 mg a day or every other day as one dose.
Availability: NHS and private prescription.
Side effects: stomach upset, rash, gout.
Caution: in pregnant women, nursing mothers, and in patients suffering from liver or kidney disease, gout, diabetes, enlarged prostate, impaired urination.
Not to be used for: patients suffering from liver cirrhosis.
Not to be used with: DIGITALIS, LITHIUM, aminoglycoside and cepha-losporin antibiotics, anti-hypertensives, NON-STEROID ANTI-INFLAMMATORY DRUGS.
Contains: frusemide.
Other preparations: Lasix 500, Lasix Paediatric Liquid, Lasix Injection, DIURESAL (Lagap), DRYPTAL (Berk), FRUSID (DDSA)

L

Lasix + K
(Hoechst)

Ten white, scored tablets plus 20 pale-yellow tablets supplied at strengths of 40 mg plus 750 mg and used as a DIURETIC and potassium supplement.

Dose: 1 white tablet a day in the morning and 2 pale-yellow tablets a day at noon and in the evening.
Availability: NHS and private prescription.
Side effects: stomach upset, rash, gout.
Caution: in pregnant women, nursing mothers, and in patients suffering from liver or kidney disease, enlarged prostate, diabetes, gout, impaired urination.
Not to be used for: patients suffering from liver cirrhosis, raised potassium levels, Addison's disease.
Not to be used with: potassium-sparing diuretics, DIGITALIS, LITHIUM, aminoglycoside and cephalosporin antibiotics, NON-STEROID ANTI-IN-FLAMMATORY DRUGS, anti-hypertensives.
Contains: FRUSEMIDE plus POTASSIUM CHLORIDE.
Other preparations:

Lasonil
(Bayer)

An ointment used as an anti-inflammatory preparation to treat haemorrhoids.

Dose: night and morning after passing motions.
Availability: NHS and private prescription.
Side effects:
Caution:
Not to be used for: if there are open or infected wounds.
Not to be used with:
Contains: HEPARINOID.
Other preparations:

Lasoride
(Hoechst)

A yellow tablet used as a potassium-sparing DIURETIC combination used for fast diuretic treatment where maintaining potassium is important.

Dose: adults 1-2 tablets a day in the morning; elderly according to

kidney function, response to treatment and potassium level.
Availability: NHS and private prescription.
Side effects: general feeling of being unwell, stomach upset, itch, blood changes, reduced alertness, calcium loss, rarely minor mental disturbances, altered liver function, ototoxicity, pancreatitis.
Caution: in the elderly, pregnant women, nursing mothers, and in patients suffering from enlarged prostate, impaired urination, diabetes, and gout.
Not to be used for: patients suffering from liver cirrhosis, severe or progressive kidney failure, raised potassium levels, Addison's disease (a disease of the adrenal glands), electrolyte imbalance.
Not to be used with: potassium supplements and potassium-sparing diuretics, LITHIUM, aminoglycoside or cephalosporin antibiotics, NON-STEROID ANTI-INFLAMMATORY DRUGS, DIGITALIS, anti-hypertensives, anti-diabetic drugs, non-depolarizing muscle relaxants.
Contains: FRUSEMIDE, AMILORIDE hydrochloride.
Other preparations:

---

laureth *see* Alcos-Anal

---

lauromacrogol *see* Anacal

Laxoberal
(Windsor)

A liquid used as a stimulant to treat constipation, and for evacuation of the bowels before surgery etc.

Dose: adults 5-15 ml at night, children under 5 years 2.5 ml at night, 5-10 years 2.5-5 ml at night.
Availability: NHS (when prescribed as a generic), private prescription.
Side effects:
Caution: in patients suffering from inflammatory bowel disease.
Not to be used for:
Not to be used with: antibiotics.
Contains: sodium picosulphate.
Other preparations:

L

Ledercort
(Lederle)

A blue, oblong, scored tablet or a white, oblong, scored tablet according to strengths of 2 mg, 4 mg and used as a corticosteroid treatment for rheumatoid arthritis, allergies.

Dose: as advised by physician.
Availability: NHS and private prescription.
Side effects: fluid retention, suppression of adrenal glands, thinning of the skin may occur.
Caution: use for short periods of time only.
Not to be used for: patients suffering from acne or any other skin infections caused by tuberculosis, ringworm, viruses, or fungi, or continuously especially in pregnant women.
Not to be used with:
Contains: TRIAMCINOLONE.
Other preparations:

Ledercort Cream
(Lederle)

A cream used as a steroid treatment for skin disorders where there is also inflammation.

Dose: apply a small quantity to the affected area 3-4 times a day.
Availability: NHS and private prescription.
Side effects: fluid retention, suppression of adrenal glands, thinning of the skin may occur.
Caution: use for short periods of time only.
Not to be used for: patients suffering from acne or any other skin infections caused by tuberculosis, ringworm, viruses, or fungi, or continuously especially in pregnant women.
Not to be used with:
Contains: TRIAMCINOLONE acetonide.
Other preparations: Ledercort Ointment.

Lederfen
(Lederle)

A blue, oblong tablet or a blue,oblong, scored tablet according to strengths of 300 mg, 450 mg and used as a NON-STEROID ANTI-INFLAMMATORY DRUG rheumatoid arthritis, osteoarthritis. ankylosing spondylitis, and acute muscle or bone problems.

Dose: either 300 mg in the morning and 600 mg at night or 450 mg twice a day.
Availability: NHS and private prescription.
Side effects: rash, stomach intolerance.
Caution: in pregnant women, nursing mothers, and in patients suffering from peptic ulcer or a history of gastro-intestinal lesions.
Not to be used for: children or for patients suffering from anti-inflammatory drug/ASPIRIN allergy.
Not to be used with: salicylates, anti-coagulants.
Contains: FENBUFEN.
Other preparations: Lederfen Capsules, Lederfen F

Ledermycin
(Lederle)

A dark-red/pale-red capsule tablet supplied at a strength of 150 mg and used as a TETRACYCLINE to treat respiratory and soft tissue infections.

Dose: 2 capsules twice a day or 1 capsule 4 times a day.
Availability: NHS and private prescription.
Side effects: stomach disturbances, sensitivity to light, additional infections.
Caution: in patients suffering from liver or kidney disease.
Not to be used for: children, nursing mothers, or women in the last half of pregnancy.
Not to be used with: milk, antacids, mineral supplements, contraceptive pill.
Contains: DEMECLOCYCLINE.
Other preparations: Ledermycin Tablets.

L

Lejfibre
(Britannia)

A 4.04 g biscuit used as a bulking agent to treat constipation.

Dose: 2 biscuits a day eaten with a drink.

Availability: NHS (when prescribed as a generic) and private prescription.
Side effects:
Caution:
Not to be used for: children.
Not to be used with:
Contains: OAT BRAN MEAL.
Other preparations:

---

lemon bioflavonoid complex *see* Lipoflavonoid

Lenium
(Winthrop)

An anti-dandruff preparation.

Dose: twice a week for the first two weeks, once a week for two further weeks, then once every 3-6 weeks.
Availability: NHS, private prescription, over the counter.
Side effects:
Caution: keep out of the eyes and any areas of broken skin; do not use within 48 hours of waving or colouring substances.
Not to be used for:
Not to be used with:
Contains: SELENIUM SULPHIDE.
Other preparations:

Lentizol
(Parke-Davis)

A pink capsule or pink/red capsule according to strengths of 25 mg, 50 mg and used as an anti-depressant to treat depression especially where sedation is needed.

Dose: adults usually 50 mg before going to bed, up to a maximum of 100 mg; elderly 25-75 mg a day at first.
Availability: NHS and private prescription.
Side effects: dry mouth, constipation, urine retention, blurred vision, palpitations, drowsiness, sleeplessness, dizziness, hands shaking,

low blood presure, weight change, skin reactions, jaundice or blood changes, loss of libido may occur.
Caution: in nursing mothers or in patients suffering from heart disease, thyroid disease, epilepsy, diabetes, some other psychiatric conditions. Your doctor may advise regular blood tests.
Not to be used for: children under 6 years, pregnant women, or for patients suffering from heart attacks, liver disease, heart block.
Not to be used with: alcohol, ANTI-CHOLINERGICS, ADRENALINE, MAOIS, barbiturates, other anti-depressants, anti-hypertensives.
Contains: AMITRYPTILINE hydrochloride.
Other preparations:

Leo K
(Leo)

A white, oval tablet used as a potassium supplement to treat potassium deficiency.

Dose: adults 3-5 tablets a day in divided doses; children as advised by the physician.
Availability: NHS, private prescription, over the counter.
Side effects: ulcers or blockage in the small bowel.
Caution: in patients suffering from kidney disease.
Not to be used for:
Not to be used with:
Contains: POTASSIUM CHLORIDE.
Other preparations:

Lergoban
(3M Riker)

An off-white tablet supplied at a strength of 5 mg and used as an anti-histamine treatment for allergies.

Dose: 1-2 tablets every 12 hours.
Availability: NHS, private prescription, over the counter.
Side effects: drowsiness, reduced reactions, dizziness, headache, flushing, anorexia, dry mouth.
Caution: in nursing mothers.
Not to be used for: children.
Not to be used with: sedatives, MAOIS, alcohol.

L

Contains: DIPHENYLPYRALINE HYDROCHLORIDE.
Other preparations:

---

levodopa *see* **Dalivit Drops, Larodopa, Madopar, Sinemet**

---

levonorgestrel *see* **Cyclo-Progynova 1mg Eugynon 30, Logynon, Logynon ED, Microgynon 30, Microval, Norgeston, Ovran, Ovranette**

---

levorphanol *see* **Dromoran**

Lexotan
(Roche)

A lilac, hexagonal, scored tablet or a pink, hexagonal, scored tablet according to strengths of 1.5 mg, 3 mg and used for the short-term treatment of anxiety.

Dose: elderly 1.5-9 mg a day in divided doses, adults 3-18 mg a day in divided doses.
Availability: private prescription only.
Side effects: drowsiness, confusion, unsteadiness, low blood pressure, rash, changes in vision, changes in libido, retention of urine. Risk of addiction increases with dose and length of treatment. May impair judgement.
Caution: in the elderly, pregnant women, nursing mothers, in women during labour, and in patients suffering from lung disorders, kidney or liver disorders. Avoid long-term use and withdraw gradually.
Not to be used for: children or for patients suffering from acute lung diseases, some chronic lung diseases, some obsessional and psychotic diseases.
Not to be used with: alcohol and other tranquillizers and anti-convulsants.
Contains: BROMAZEPAM.
Other preparations:

Lexpec
(RP Drugs)

A syrup used as a folic acid supplement to treat megaloblastic anaemia (anaemia with large red blood cells).

Dose: adults 4-8 5 ml teaspoonsful a day for 14 days then 2-4 teaspoonsful a day; children 2-6 5 ml teaspoonsful a day.
Availability: NHS and private prescription.
Side effects: nausea, constipation, mottled teeth.
Caution: mottled teeth can be minimized by drinking syrup through a straw.
Not to be used for: megaloblastic anaemia caused by vitamin B_{12} deficiency.
Not to be used with: TETRACYCLINES.
Contains: FOLIC ACID.
Other preparations: Lexpec with Iron, Lexpec with Iron-M.

Libanil *see* Daonil
(APS)

Librium
(Roche)

A yellow-green, light blue-green, or dark blue-green tablet according to strengths of 5 mg, 10, mg, 25 mg and used as a tranquillizer to treat anxiety, symptoms of acute alcohol withdrawal, short-term treatment of sleeplessness where sedation during the day does not cause difficulty.

Dose: elderly 10 mg a day at first; adults 30 mg a day at first; 40-100 mg a day in severe cases.
Availability: NHS (when prescribed as a generic) and private prescription.
Side effects: drowsiness, confusion, unsteadiness, low blood pressure, rash, changes in vision, changes in libido, retention of urine. Risk of addiction increases with dose and length of treatment. May impair judgement.
Caution: in the elderly, pregnant women, nursing mothers, in women during labour, and in patients suffering from lung disorders, kidney or liver disorders. Avoid long-term use and withdraw gradually.

L

Not to be used for: children or for patients suffering from acute lung diseases, some chronic lung diseases, some obsessional and psychotic diseases.
Not to be used with: alcohol and other tranquillizers and anti-convulsants.
Contains: CHLORDIAZEPOXIDE.
Other preparations: Librium Capsules, CHLORDIAZEPOXIDE, TROPIUM (DDSA)

Lidifen *see* **Brufen**
(Berk)

---

lidoflazine *see* **Clinium**

Lignocaine and Fluorescein
(SNP)

Drops used as a local anaesthetic and dye for carrying out procedures on the eye.

Dose: 1 or more drops into the eye as needed.
Availability: NHS and private prescription.
Side effects:
Caution:
Not to be used for:
Not to be used with:
Contains: LIGNOCAINE HYDROCHLORIDE, SODIUM FLUORESCEIN.
Other preparations:

---

lignocaine *see* **Betnovate Rectal, Lignocaine and Fluorescein, Xyloproct**

Limbitrol 5
(Roche)

A pink/green capsule used as an anti-depressant to treat depression and anxiety.

Dose: 1 tablet 3 times a day.
Availability: private prescription only.
Side effects: dry mouth, constipation, palpitations, sleeplessness, shaking hands, weight change, skin reactions, jaundice or blood changes, drowsiness, confusion, unsteadiness, low blood pressure, rash, changes in vision, changes in libido, retention of urine. Risk of addiction increases with dose and length of treatment. May impair judgement.
Caution: in the elderly, pregnant women, nursing mothers, in women during labour, and in patients suffering from lung disorders, kidney or liver disorders. Avoid long-term use and withdraw gradually.
Not to be used for: children, the elderly, or for patients suffering from acute lung diseases, some chronic lung diseases, some obsessional and psychotic diseases, heart disease, liver disease, thyroid disease, epilepsy.
Not to be used with: alcohol and other tranquillizers and anti-convulsants, ANTI-CHOLINERGICS, ADRENALINE, MAOIs, barbiturates, other anti-depressants, anti-hypertensives.
Contains: AMITRYPTILINE hydrochloride, CHLORDIAZEPOXIDE.
Other preparations: Limbitrol 10.

Lincocin
(Upjohn)

A dark-blue/pale-blue capsule tablet supplied at a strength of 500 mg and used as an antibiotic to treat severe infections.

Dose: 1 capsule 3-4 times a day.
Availability: NHS and private prescription.
Side effects: diarrhoea, colitis.
Caution: liver and blood should be checked regularly if the treatment is given over an extended period.
Not to be used for: children under 1 month or for patients suffering from kidney, liver, hormonal, or metabolic problems or who are sensitive to CLINDAMYCIN.
Not to be used with: neuromuscular blocking drugs.
Contains: LINCOMYCIN hydrochloride.
Other preparations: Lincocin Injection, Lincocin Syrup.

L

lincomycin see Lincocin

---

lindane see Lorexane, Quellada

Lingraine
(Winthrop)

A green tablet supplied at a strength of 2 mg and used as an ergot preparation to treat migraine, headache.

Dose: 1 tablet under the tongue at the beginning of a migraine attack, and repeat if needed $1/2$ -1 hour later to a maximum of 3 tablets in 24 hours or 6 tablets in a week.
Availability: NHS and private prescription.
Side effects: nausea, stomach pain, leg cramps.
Caution:
Not to be used for: children, pregnant women, nursing mothers, or for patients suffering from coronary, peripheral, or occlusive vascular disease, severe high blood pressure, kidney or liver disease, or sepsis.
Not to be used with: ERYTHROMYCIN, ß-BLOCKERS.
Contains: ERGOTAMINE tartrate.
Other preparations:

Lioresal
(Ciba)

A white, scored tablet supplied at a strength of 10 mg and used as a muscle relaxant to treat voluntary muscle spasticity caused by cerebrovascular accidents, cerebral palsy, meningitis, multiple sclerosis, spinal lesions.

Dose: adults $1/2$ tablet 3 times a day at first increasing as needed by $1/2$ tablet 3 times a day every 3 days to a maximum of 10 tablets a day; children under 8 years $1/2$ -1 tablet a day at first to a maximum of 6 tablets a day in divided doses.
Availability: NHS and private prescription.
Side effects: nausea, sedation, confusion, muscle tiredness, reduced alertness.

Caution: in the elderly and in patients suffering from epilepsy or mental disorders. Withdraw treatment gradually.
Not to be used for:
Not to be used with: anti-hypertensives.
Contains: BACLOFEN.
Other preparations: Lioresal Liquid.

Lipantil
(Bristol Myers)

A white capsule tablet supplied at a strength of 100 mg and used as a lipid-lowering agent to lower cholesterol or triglycerides.

Dose: 2-4 capsules a day.
Availability: NHS and private prescription.
Side effects: stomach upset, dizziness, headache, tiredness, rashes.
Caution: in patients suffering from kidney impairment.
Not to be used for: pregnant women, nursing mothers, or for patients suffering from severe kidney or liver problems.
Not to be used with: anti-coagulants, PHENYLBUTAZONE, anti-diabetic drugs taken by mouth.
Contains: FENOFIBRATE.
Other preparations:

Lipoflavonoid
(Lipomed)

A black/pink capsule used as a multivitamin treatment for vitamin B deficiency.

Dose: 3 capsules 3 times a day for 2-3 months reducing to 2 capsules 3 times a day.
Availability: private prescription and over the counter.
Side effects:
Caution:
Not to be used for: children.
Not to be used with:
Contains: CHOLINE BITARTRATE, INOSITOL, METHIONINE, ASCORBIC ACID, LEMON BIOFLAVONOID COMPLEX, THIAMINE, RIBOFLAVINE, NICOTINAMIDE, PYRIDOXINE, PANTHENOL, HYDROXOCOBALAMIN.
Other preparations:

L

Lipotriad
(Lipomed)

A clear pink capsule used as a multivitamin treatment for vitamin B deficiency.

Dose: 3 capsules 3 times a day for 2-3 months then reducing to 2 capsules 3 times a day.
Availability: private prescription and over the counter.
Side effects:
Caution:
Not to be used for: children.
Not to be used with: LEVODOPA.
Contains: CHOLINE BITARTRATE, INOSITOL, DI-METHIONINE, HYDROXOCOBALAMIN, THIAMINE, RIBOFLAVINE, NICOTINAMIDE, PYRIDOXINE, PANTHENOL.
Other preparations: Lipotriad Liquid.

---

liquid paraffin see Petrolagar No 1

Liquifilm Tears
(Allergan)

Drops used to lubricate dry eyes.

Dose: 1 drop into the eye as needed.
Availability: NHS, private prescription, over the counter.
Side effects:
Caution:
Not to be used for: patients who wear soft contact lenses.
Not to be used with:
Contains: POLYVINYL ALCOHOL.
Other preparations:

---

liquorice see Caved-S

---

lisinopril see Carace, Zestril

Liskonum
(S K B)

A white, scored, oblong tablet supplied at a strength of 450 mg and used as a sedative to treat mania, hypomania, manic depression.

Dose: as judged by blood tests to keep a constant level.
Availability: NHS and private prescription.
Side effects: nausea, diarrhoea, hand tremor, muscular weakness, brain and heart disturbances, weight gain, fluid retention, underactive or over active thyroid gland, thirst and frequent urination, kidney changes, skin reactions, intoxication.
Caution: treatment should be started in hospital and a careful check on the functioning of the kidneys and thyroid should be made, as well as ensuring that there is an adequate consumption of salt and fluid. Your doctor may advise blood tests to gauge dose.
Not to be used for: children, for pregnant women, nursing mothers, or for patients suffering from disturbed sodium balance, Addison's disease, kidney or heart disease, or underactive thyroid.
Not to be used with: DIURETICS, NON-STEROID ANTI-INFLAMMATORY DRUGS, CARBAMAZEPINE, PHENYTOIN, HALOPERIDOL, FLUPENTHIXOL, METHYLDOPA, PHENYTOIN.
Contains: LITHIUM CARBONATE.
Other preparations:

Litarex
(CP Pharmaceuticals)

A white, oval tablet supplied at a strength of 564 mg and used as a sedative to treat acute mania, and for the prevention of recurring mood changes.

Dose: 1 tablet morning and evening at first and then as advised by the physician.
Availability: NHS and private prescription.
Side effects: nausea, diarrhoea, hand tremor, muscular weakness, brain and heart disturbances, weight gain, fluid retention, underactive or overactive thyroid gland, thirst and frequent urination, skin reactions.
Caution: treatment should be started in hospital, thyroid function should be checked regularly, and there should be an adequate consumption of salt and fluid. Your doctor may advise frequent blood

L

tests to gauge dose.

Not to be used for: children, pregnant women, nursing mothers, or for patients suffering from Addison's disease, kidney or cardiovascular disease, underactive thyroid, in cases where there is a disturbed sodium balance.

Not to be used with: DIURETICS, NON-STEROID ANTI-INFLAMMATORY DRUGS, CARBAMAZEPINE, FLUPENTHIXOL, METHYLDOPA, PHENYTOIN, HALOPERIDOL.

Contains: LITHIUM CITRATE.

Other preparations:

---

lithium carbonate *see* Liskonum, Phasal, Priadel

---

lithium citrate *see* Litarex

---

lithium *see* Camcolit

Loasid
(Calmic)

A white tablet used as an antacid and anti-wind preparation to treat ulcers, oesophagitis, gastritis, hiatus hernia, heartburn.

Dose: 1-2 tablets when required.
Availability: over the counter and on private prescription.
Side effects: few; occasionally constipation.
Caution: kidney failure.
Not to be used for: infants.
Not to be used with: tetracycline antibiotics.
Contains: ALUMINIUM HYDROXIDE, DIMETHICONE.
Other preparations:

Lobak
(Sterling Research Laboratories)

A white, scored tablet used as a muscle relaxant and analgesic to relieve painful muscle spasm

Dose: adults 1-2 tablets 3 times a day to a maximum of 8 tablets a day; elderly half normal adult dose.
Availability: private prescription only.
Side effects: reduced alertness, drowsiness, dizziness, rash, dry mouth.
Caution: in patients suffering from kidney or liver disease.
Not to be used for: children.
Not to be used with: alcohol, sedatives.
Contains: CHLORMEZANONE, PARACETAMOL.
Other preparations:

Locabiotal
(Servier)

An aerosol tablet supplied at a strength of 125 micrograms and used as an anti-inflammatory, antibiotic treatment for infection, inflammation, of the nose, mouth, and throat.

Dose: adults 5 sprays into the mouth or 3 sprays into each nostril 5 times a day; children 3-5 years 2 sprays into the mouth 3 times a day or 1 spray into each nostril 5 times a day, 6-12 years 3 sprays into each nostril 5 times a day.
Availability: NHS and private prescription.
Side effects:
Caution:
Not to be used for: children under 3 years.
Not to be used with:
Contains: FUSAFUNGINE.
Other preparations:

Locoid *see* Hydrocortisone
(Brocades)

L

Lodine
(Wyeth)

A dark-grey/light-grey capsule marked with 2 red bands tablet supplied at a strength of 200 mg and used as a NON-STEROID ANTI-INFLAMMATORY DRUG to treat rheumatoid arthritis.

Dose: 1 capsule twice a day to a maximum of 3 capsules a day.
Availability: NHS and private prescription.
Side effects: nausea, stomach pain, headache, dizziness, tinnitus, rash, swelling.
Caution: in the elderly on long-term treatment and in patients suffering from kidney or liver disease.
Not to be used for: children, pregnant women, nursing mothers, or for patients suffering from peptic ulcer, a history of peptic ulcer or gastro-intestinal bleeding, allergy to anti-inflammatory drugs/aspirin.
Not to be used with: anti-coagulants, anti-diabetic drugs.
Contains: ETODOLAC.
Other preparations: Lodine Tablets.

Loestrin 20
(Parke-Davis)

A blue tablet used as an oestrogen, progestogen contraceptive.

Dose: 1 tablet a day for 21 days starting on day 5 of the period.
Availability: NHS and private prescription.
Side effects: enlarged breasts, bloating and fluid retention, cramps, leg pains, mood change, reduction in sexual desire, headaches, nausea, vaginal erosion, discharge, and bleeding, weight gain, skin changes.
Caution: in patients suffering from high blood pressure, diabetes, vascular disorders, asthma, depression, kidney disease, multiple sclerosis, womb diseases. Your doctor may advise you not to smoke, to have regular examinations. You should stop treatment at the first sign of serious symptoms such as severe headache or jaundice. Treatment should be stopped before surgery.
Not to be used for: pregnant women, or for patients suffering from sickle-cell anaemia, history of heart disease or thrombosis, liver disorders, some cancers, undiagnosed vaginal bleeding, some ear, skin, and kidney disorders.
Not to be used with: RIFAMPICIN, TETRACYCLINES, GRISEOFULVIN, barbiturates, PHENYTOIN, PRIMIDONE, CARBAMAZEPINE, ETHOSUXIMIDE, CHLORAL HYDRATE, DICHLORALPHENAZONE.
Contains: ETHINYLOESTRADIOL, NORETHISTERONE acetate.
Other preparations: Loestrin 30.

L

Iofepramine *see* **Gamanil**

Logynon
(Schering)

A brown tablet, or a white tablet and an ochre tablet used as an oestrogen, progestogen contraceptive.

Dose: 1 tablet a day for 21 days starting on day 1 of the period.
Availability: NHS and private prescription.
Side effects: enlarged breasts, bloating and fluid retention, cramps, leg pains, mood change, reduction in sexual desire, headaches, nausea, vaginal erosion, discharge, and bleeding, weight gain, skin changes.
Caution: in patients suffering from high blood pressure, diabetes, vascular disorders, asthma, depression, kidney disease, multiple sclerosis, womb diseases. Your doctor may advise you not to smoke, to have regular examinations. You should stop treatment at the first sign of serious symptoms such as severe headache or jaundice. Treatment should be stopped before surgery.
Not to be used for: pregnant women, or for patients suffering from sickle-cell anaemia, history of heart disease or thrombosis, liver disorders, some cancers, undiagnosed vaginal bleeding, some ear, skin, and kidney disorders.
Not to be used with: RIFAMPICIN, TETRACYCLINES, GRISEOFULVIN, barbiturates, PHENYTOIN, PRIMIDONE, CARBAMAZEPINE, ETHOSUXIMIDE, CHLORAL HYDRATE, DICHLORALPHENAZONE.
Contains: ETHINYLOESTRADIOL, LEVONORGESTREL.
Other preparations:

Logynon ED
(Schering)

A brown tablet, white tablet, and ochre tablet, or white and ochre tablet and white tablet used as an oestrogen, progestogen contraceptive

Dose: 1 tablet a day for 28 days starting on day 1 of the period.
Availability: NHS and private prescription.
Side effects: enlarged breasts, bloating and fluid retention, cramps, leg pains, mood change, reduction in sexual desire, headaches,

L

nausea, vaginal erosion, discharge, and bleeding, weight gain, skin changes.

Caution: in patients suffering from high blood pressure, diabetes, vascular disorders, asthma, depression, kidney disease, multiple sclerosis, womb diseases. Your doctor may advise you not to smoke, to have regular examinations. You should stop treatment at the first sign of serious symptoms such as severe headache or jaundice. Treatment should be stopped before surgery.

Not to be used for: pregnant women, or for patients suffering from sickle-cell anaemia, history of heart disease or thrombosis, liver disorders, some cancers, undiagnosed vaginal bleeding, some ear, skin, and kidney disorders.

Not to be used with: RIFAMPICIN, TETRACYCLINES, GRISEOFULVIN, barbiturates, PHENYTOIN, PRIMIDONE, CARBAMAZEPINE, ETHOSUXIMIDE, CHLORAL HYDRATE, DICHLORALPHENAZONE.

Contains: ETHINYLOESTRADIOL, LEVONORGESTREL, LACTOSE.

Other preparations:

Loniten
(Upjohn)

A white tablet supplied at strengths of 2.5 mg, 5 mg, 10 mg and used as a vasodilator to treat high blood pressure.

Dose: adults 5 mg a day at first increasing at 3-day intervals to up to 10 mg a day and then by 10 mg at a time to a maximum of 50 mg a day; children 0.2 mg per kg of bodyweight a day at first, increasing at 3-day intervals by 0.1-0.2 mg per kg bodyweight to a maximum of 1 mg per kg bodyweight a day.

Availability: NHS and private prescription.

Side effects: hair growth, swelling, rapid heart rate.

Caution: angina or heart attack patients need to be monitored carefully. Other anti-hypertensives need to be withdrawn (apart from ß-BLOCKERS and DIURETICS). Needs to be given in conjunction with some other anti-hypertensive drugs.

Not to be used for: patients suffering from phaeochromocytoma (a disease of the adrenal glands).

Not to be used with:

Contains: MINOXIDIL.

Other preparations: REGAINE (Upjohn) — local application for the treatment of male pattern baldness.

Lopid
(Parke-Davis)

A white/maroon capsule tablet supplied at a strength of 300 mg and used as a lipid-lowering agent to treat raised lipid levels.

Dose: usually 4 capsules a day to a maximum of 5 capsules a day.
Availability: NHS and private prescription.
Side effects: stomach upset, rashes, impotence, headache, dizziness, painful extremities, muscle aches, blurred vision.
Caution: your doctor may advise a lipid check; blood count, and liver function should be checked before treatment; eyes, blood, and serum should be checked regularly.
Not to be used for: pregnant women, nursing mothers, alcoholics, or patients suffering from gallstones or liver disease.
Not to be used with: anti-coagulants.
Contains: GEMFIBROZIL.
Other preparations:

---

loprazolam *see also* Dormonoct

A tablet supplied at a strength of 1 mg and used as a sleeping tablet for the short-term treatment of sleeplessness or waking at night.

Dose: elderly up to 1 tablet before going to bed; adults 1-2 tablets before going to bed.
Availability: NHS and private prescription.
Side effects: drowsiness, confusion, unsteadiness, low blood pressure, rash, changes in vision, changes in libido, retention of urine. Risk of addiction increases with dose and length of treatment. May impair judgement.
Caution: in the elderly, pregnant women, nursing mothers, in women during labour, and in patients suffering from lung disorders, kidney or liver disorders. Avoid long-term use and withdraw gradually.
Not to be used for: children, or for patients suffering from acute lung diseases, some chronic lung diseases, some obsessional and psychotic diseases.
Not to be used with: alcohol, other tranquillizers, anti-convulsants.
Contains: LOPRAZOLAM mesylate.
Other preparations:

L

Lopresor
(Geigy)

A pink, scored tablet or a pale-blue, scored tablet according to strengths of 50 mg, 100 mg and used as a ß-BLOCKER to treat angina, for the prevention of heart muscle damage, high blood pressure, and as an additional treatment in thyrotoxicosis, migraine.

Dose: angina 50-100 mg 2-3 times a day. High blood pressure 100 mg a day at first increasing to 400 mg a day if needed. Thyrotoxicosis 50 mg 4 times a day. Migraine 100-200 mg a day in divided doses.
Availability: NHS and private prescription.
Side effects: cold hands and feet, sleep disturbance, slow heart rate, tiredness, wheezing, heart failure, stomach upset.
Caution: in pregnant women, nursing mothers, and in patients suffering from diabetes, kidney or liver disorders, asthma. May need to be withdrawn before surgery. Withdraw gradually. Your doctor may advise additional treatment with diuretics or digitalis.
Not to be used for: children, or for patients suffering from heart block or failure.
Not to be used with: VERAPAMIL, CLONIDINE withdrawal, some anti-arrhythmic drugs and anaesthetics, RESERPINE, some anti-hypertensives, ergot alkaloids, CIMETIDINE, sedatives, SYMPATHOMIMETICS, INDOMETHACIN.
Contains: METOPROLOL tartrate
Other preparations: Lopresor Injection, Lopresor SR

Lopresoretic
(Geigy)

An off-white, scored tablet used as a ß-BLOCKER/thiazide DIURETIC combination to treat high blood pressure.

Dose: 1 tablet a day in the morning at first, increasing to 3-4 tablets a day as needed.
Availability: NHS and private prescription.
Side effects: cold hands and feet, sleep disturbance, slow heart rate, tiredness, wheezing, heart failure, stomach upset, low blood potassium, rash, sensitivity to light, blood changes, gout.
Caution: in pregnant women, nursing mothers, and in patients suffering from diabetes, kidney or liver disorders, gout, asthma. May need to be withdrawn before surgery. Withdraw gradually. Your doctor

L

may advise potassium supplements, blood tests.
Not to be used for: children, or for patients suffering from heart block or failure, severe kidney failure.
Not to be used with: VERAPAMIL, CLONIDINE withdrawal, some anti-arrhythmic drugs and anaesthetics, RESERPINE, some anti-hypertensives, ergot alkaloids, CIMETIDINE, sedatives, SYMPATHOMIMETICS, INDOMETHACIN, LITHIUM, DIGITALIS, other diuretics.
Contains: METOPROLOL tartrate, CHLORTHALIDONE.
Other preparations:

---

loratadine *see* Clarityn

---

lorazepam *see also* Ativan

A tablet supplied at strengths of 1 mg, 2.5 mg and used as a sedative to treat anxiety.

Dose: elderly 0.5-2 mg a day in divided doses; adults 1-4 mg a day in divided doses.
Availability: NHS and private prescription.
Side effects: drowsiness, confusion, unsteadiness, low blood pressure, rash, changes in vision, changes in libido, retention of urine. Risk of addiction increases with dose and length of treatment. May impair judgement.
Caution: in the elderly, pregnant women, nursing mothers, in women during labour, and in patients suffering from lung disorders, kidney or liver disorders. Avoid long-term use and withdraw gradually.
Not to be used for: children, or for patients suffering from acute lung diseases, some chronic lung diseases, some obsessional and psychotic diseases.
Not to be used with: alcohol, other tranquillizers, anti-convulsants.
Contains:
Other preparations:

L

Lorexane
(Care)

A cream used as a scabicide and pediculicide to treat scabies and lice.

Dose: apply to the affected areas as directed.
Availability: NHS, private prescription, over the counter.
Side effects:
Caution: keep out of the eyes.
Not to be used for:
Not to be used with:
Contains: LINDANE.
Other preparations: Lorexane Medicated Shampoo.

---

lormetazepam

A tablet supplied at strengths of 0.5 mg, 1 mg and used as a sedative to treat sleeplessness.

Dose: elderly 0.5 mg before going to bed; adults 1 mg before going to bed.
Availability: NHS and private prescription.
Side effects: drowsiness, confusion, unsteadiness, low blood pressure, rash, changes in vision, changes in libido, retention of urine. Risk of addiction increases with dose and length of treatment. May impair judgement.
Caution: in the elderly, pregnant women, nursing mothers, in women during labour, and in patients suffering from lung disorders, kidney or liver disorders. Avoid long-term use and withdraw gradually.
Not to be used for: children, or for patients suffering from acute lung diseases, some chronic lung diseases, some obsessional and psychotic diseases.
Not to be used with: alcohol, other tranquillizers, anti-convulsants.
Contains:
Other preparations:

Lorocorten-Vioform
(Zyma)

Drops used as an antibacterial, corticosteroid treatment for inflammation of the outer ear where secondary infections may be present.

Dose: 2-3 drops into the ear twice a day.
Availability: NHS and private prescription.
Side effects: additional infection.

Caution:
Not to be used for: patients suffering from perforated ear drum or primary infections of the outer ear.
Not to be used with:
Contains: CLIOQUINOL, FLUMETHASONE PIVALATE.
Other preparations:

Losec
(Astra)

A pink/brown capsule tablet supplied at a strength of 20 mg and used as an anti-ulcer drug for ulcers which are difficult to treat.

Dose: usually 1-2 capsules a day for up to 8 weeks; rarely up to 6 capsules a day.
Availability: NHS and private prescription.
Side effects: constipation, diarrhoea, headache, nausea, rashes.
Caution: your doctor may advise endoscopic checks of the stomach.
Not to be used for: pregnant women or nursing mothers.
Not to be used with: DIAZEPAM, PHENYTOIN, WARFARIN.
Contains: OMEPRAZOLE.
Other preparations:

Lotriderm *see* Betnovate
(Kirby-Warrick)

Lotussin
(Searle)

A linctus used as an antihistamine, antussive treatment for cough.

Dose: adults 2 5 ml teaspoonsful 3 times a day; children 1-5 years $^1/_2$ -1 teaspoonful 3 times a day, 5-12 years 1-2 teaspoonsful 3 times a day.
Availability: private prescription and over the counter.
Side effects: drowsiness, reduced reactions, constipation, rarely skin eruptions.
Caution: in patients suffering from kidney disease, asthma.

L

Not to be used for: infants under 1 year, or for patients suffering from liver disease.
Not to be used with: alcohol, sedatives, some anti-depressants (MAOIS)
Contains: DIPHENHYDRAMINE HYDROCHLORIDE, DEXTROMETHORPHAN HYDROBROMIDE.
Other preparations:

Lotycin *see* Erythrocin
(Eli Lilly)

Ludiomil
(Ciba)

A peach tablet, greyish red tablet, pale-orange tablet, or brownish orange tablet according to strengths of 10 mg, 25 mg, 50 mg, 75 mg and used as a tetracyclic anti-depressant to treat depression.

Dose: adults 25-75 mg a day at first usually at night or in 3 divided doses, then adjusted as needed after 1-2 weeks; elderly 30 mg a day at first at night or in 3 divided doses.
Availability: NHS and private prescription.
Side effects: convulsions, rash, reduced reactions, anti-cholinergic effects.
Caution: in the elderly, in pregnant women, nursing mothers, and in patients suffering from cardiovascular disease.
Not to be used for: children or for patients suffering from mania, severe kidney or liver disease, history of epilepsy, narrow-angle glaucoma, recent heart attack, retention of urine.
Not to be used with: MAOIS, anti-hypertensives, SYMPATHOMIMETICS, barbiturates, anti-psychotics, alcohol, anaesthetics.
Contains: MAPROTILINE hydrochloride.
Other preparations:

Lurselle
(Merrell Dow)

A white, scored tablet supplied at a strength of 250 mg and used as a lipid-lowering agent to treat elevated lipids.

Dose: 2 tablets twice a day with morning and evening meals.
Availability: NHS and private prescription.
Side effects: diarrhoea, stomach upset.
Caution: cease treatment 6 months before a planned pregnancy.
Not to be used for: children, pregnant women, or nursing mothers.
Not to be used with:
Contains: PROBUCOL.
Other preparations:

---

lynoestrenol *see* **Minilyn**

---

lyothyronine sodium *see* **Tertroxin**

---

lypressin *see* **Syntopressin**

Maalox
(Rorer)

A white tablet used as an antacid to treat gastric and duodenal ulcer, gastritis, heartburn, acidity.

Dose: adults 1-2 tablets after meals and at bedtime.
Availability: NHS and over the counter (except for Maalox Plus tablets).
Side effects: few; occasionally constipation.
Caution:
Not to be used for: infants.
Not to be used with: TETRACYCLINE antibiotics.
Contains: ALUMINIUM HYDROXIDE, MAGNESIUM HYDROXIDE.
Other preparations: Maalox suspension, Maalox Plus suspension and tablets (with DIMETHICONE), Maalox TC (higher-dose ALUMINIUM HYDROXIDE suspension and tablets). MUCOGEL (Pharmax).

M

Macrodantin
(Norwich Eaton)

A yellow/white capsule or a white capsule according to strengths of 50 mg, 100 mg and used as an antiseptic to treat infection of the urinary tract.

Dose: adults treatment 100 mg 4 times a day with food or milk, prevention 100-200 mg a day; children 2$\frac{1}{2}$ -6 years 50 mg twice a day, 6-11 years 50 mg 4 times a day, 11-14 years 100 mg 3 times a day.
Availability: NHS and private prescription.
Side effects: stomach upset, allergy, blood disorders, nerve damage, jaundice, possible liver damage.
Caution:
Not to be used for: children under 21/2 years or for patients suffering from kidney failure.
Not to be used with:
Contains: NITROFURANTOIN.
Other preparations:

Madopar
(Roche)

A blue/grey capsule, blue/pink capsule, or blue/caramel capsule according to strengths of 62.5 mg, 125 mg, 250 mg and used as an anti-parkinsonian combination to treat Parkinson's disease.

Dose: adults over 25 years 1 low-dose capsule 3-4 times a day after meals at first increasing by 2 low-dose capsules a day 1-2 times a week up to 8-12 low dose capsules a day in divided doses or as advised by the physician; elderly 1 low-dose capsule twice a day at first increasing by 1 low-dose capsule every 3-4 days.
Availability: NHS and private prescription.
Side effects: nausea, vomiting, anorexia, low blood pressure on standing, involuntary movements, heart and brain disturbances, discoloration of urine, rarely haemolytic anaemia.
Caution: in patients suffering from cardiovascular, liver, lung, endocrine or kidney disease, peptic ulcer, mental disturbance, glaucoma, bone changes. Your doctor may advise that blood, liver, kidney, and cardiovascular systems should be checked regularly.
Not to be used for: children, pregnant women, nursing mothers, or

for patients suffering from severe mental disorders, glaucoma, history of malignant melanoma.
Not to be used with: MAOIS, anti-hypertensives, SYMPATHOMIMETICS.
Contains: LEVODOPA, BENSERAZIDE HYDROCHLORIDE.
Other preparations: Madopar Dispersible

Magnapen
(S K B)

A turquoise/black capsule used as a penicillin to treat serious infections.

Dose: adults1 capsule 4 times a day $\frac{1}{2}$ -1 hour before food; under 2 years $\frac{1}{2}$ 5 ml teaspoonful syrup 4 times a day, 2-10 years 1 5 ml teaspoonful 4 times a day .
Availability: NHS and private prescription.
Side effects: allergies, stomach disturbances.
Caution: in patients suffering from glandular fever.
Not to be used for: for patients suffering from penicillin allergy.
Not to be used with:
Contains: AMPICILLIN, FLUCLOXACILLIN.
Other preparations: Magnapen Syrup, Magnapen Injection.

magnesium alginate *see* Algicon

magnesium carbonate *see* Algicon, APP, Bellocarb, Caved-S, Nulacin, Roter, Topal

magnesium chloride *see* Glandosane

magnesium citrate *see* Picolax

M

magnesium hydroxide *see* **Actonorm, Andursil, Carbellon, Diovol, Maalox, Mucaine, Octovit**

---

magnesium oxide *see* **Asilone, Kolanticon, Nulacin, Polyalk**

---

magnesium sulphate mixture

An osmotic laxative used to evacuate the bowels quickly.

Dose: adults 10-20 ml on an empty stomach; children 5-10 ml on an empty stomach.
Availability: NHS and private prescription.
Side effects:
Caution: in patients suffering from kidney disease.
Not to be used for:
Not to be used with:
Contains:
Other preparations: MAGNESIUM SULPHATE crystals.

---

magnesium sulphate *see* **Kest, magnesium sulphate mixture**

---

magnesium trisilicate mixture

A white liquid used as an antacid to treat acidity, dyspepsia.

Dose: 10-20 ml as required.
Availability:
Side effects: diarrhoea.
Caution: in patients suffering from kidney impairment.
Not to be used for: children.
Not to be used with:
Contains: MAGNESIUM TRISILICATE.
Other preparations: magnesium trisilicate tablets co., magnesium trisilicate powder.

---

magnesium trisilicate *see* **Aluhyde, Bellocarb, Droxalin,**

Gastrocote, Gastron, Genusil, magnesium trisilicate mixture, Nulacin

---

Malatex
(Norton)

A solution used as an anti-inflammatory preparation to treat varicose and indolent ulcers, bed sores, burns.

Dose: cleanse the affected area with the solution and then apply the cream twice a day.
Availability: NHS, private prescription, over the counter.
Side effects:
Caution:
Not to be used for:
Not to be used with:
Contains: PROPYLENE GLYCOL, MALIC ACID, BENZOIC ACID, SALICYLIC ACID.
Other preparations: Malatex Solution.

---

malathion *see* Derbac-M, Prioderm, Suleo-M

---

malic acid *see* Aserbine, Malatex

Malinal
(Robins)

A scored, white, chewable tablet supplied at a strength of 500 mg and used as an antacid to treat indigestion, ulcers, hyperacidity.

Dose: adults 2 tablets at mealtimes and at bedtime.
Availability: over the counter and private prescription.
Side effects:
Caution:
Not to be used for: children.
Not to be used with: TETRACYCLINE antibiotics.
Contains: ALMASILATE.
Other preparations: Malinal suspension.

M

Malix see Daonil
(Lagap)

Maloprim
(Wellcome)

A white, scored tablet used as a sulphone preparation for the prevention of malaria.

Dose: adults and children over 10 years 1 tablet a week; children 5-10 years half adult dose.
Availability: NHS and private prescription.
Side effects: blood disorders, sensitive skin.
Caution: in pregnant women, nursing mothers, and in patients suffering from liver or kidney disease.
Not to be used for:
Not to be used with: FOLATE INHIBITORS such as TRIMETHOPRIM.
Contains: DAPSONE, PYRIMETHAMINE.
Other preparations:

---

maltose see Nulacin

Manevac
(Galen)

Granules used as a stimulant and bulking agent to treat constipation.

Dose: adults 5-10 ml at night and before breakfast if needed; children over 5 years 5 ml daily.
Availability: NHS and private prescription.
Side effects: wind, distension, diarrhoea.
Caution:
Not to be used for: infants, or patients suffering from obstruction of the intestine, coeliac disease, spastic bowel conditions, enterocolitis.
Not to be used with:
Contains: ISPAGHULA, SENNOSIDES.
Other preparations:

M

manganese glycerophosphate *see* Tonivitan A & D, Tonivitan B, Verdiviton

manganese *see* Metatone

manganese sulphate *see* Folicin

Manusept
(Hough, Hoseason)

A solution used as a disinfectant for cleansing and disinfecting skin and hands before surgery.

Dose: rub into the skin until dry.
Availability: NHS, private prescription, over the counter.
Side effects:
Caution: keep out of the eyes.
Not to be used for:
Not to be used with:
Contains: TRICLOSAN, ISOPROPYL ALCOHOL.
Other preparations:

MAOI (mono-amine oxidase inhibitor)

An anti-depressant agent which may interact with some foods and other drugs. Example ISOCARBOXAZID *see* Marplan.

maprotiline *see* Ludiomil

M

Marevan
(Duncan, Flockhart)

A brown tablet, blue tablet, or pink tablet according to strengths of 1 mg, 3 mg, 5 mg and used as an anti-coagulant to thin the blood.

Dose: 10-15 mg a day.
Availability: NHS and private prescription.
Side effects: alopecia, rash, diarrhoea, blood changes.
Caution: in the elderly or very ill patients, and for patients suffering from high blood pressure, weight changes, kidney disease, or potassium deficiency.
Not to be used for: children, pregnant women, within 24 hours of surgery or labour, or for patients suffering from kidney or liver disease, or haemorrhagic conditions.
Not to be used with: NON-STEROID ANTI-INFLAMMATORY DRUGS, oral hypoglycaemics, sulphonamides, QUINIDINE, antibiotics, PHENFORMIN, CIMETIDINE, drugs affecting liver chemistry, corticosteroids, IMIDAZOLE anti-fungal drugs,
Contains: sodium WARFARIN.
Other preparations:

Marplan
(Roche)

A pink, scored tablet supplied at a strength of 150 mg and used as an MAOI to treat depression.

Dose: adults 3 tablets a day at first, then 1-2 tablets a day; elderly half adult dose.
Availability: NHS and private prescription.
Side effects: severe high blood pressure reactions with certain foods, sleeplessness, low blood pressure, dizziness, drowsiness, weakness, dry mouth, constipation, stomach upset, blurred vision, urinary difficulties, ankle swelling, rash, jaundice, weight gain, confusion, sexual desire changes.
Caution: in the elderly and in patients suffering from epilepsy.
Not to be used for: children, or for patients suffering from liver disease, blood changes, heart disease, phaeochromocytoma, overactive thyroid, brain artery disease.
Not to be used with: amphetamines or similar SYMPATHOMIMETIC drugs, TRICYCLIC antidepressants, PETHIDINE and other narcotics, some cough mixtures and appetite suppressants containing sympathomimetics. Barbiturates, sedatives, alcohol, and anti-diabetics may be enhanced. Anti-cholinergic side effects are increased. Cheese, Bovril, Oxo, meat extracts, broad beans, banana, Marmite, yeast extracts, wine, beer,

other alcohol, pickled herrings, vegetable proteins. (Up to 14 days after cessation.)
Contains: ISOCARBOXAZID.
Other preparations:

Marvelon
(Organon)

A white tablet used as an oestrogen, progestogen contraceptive.

Dose: 1 tablet a day for 21 days starting on day 1 or day 5 of the period.
Availability: NHS and private prescription.
Side effects: enlarged breasts, bloating and fluid retention, cramps, leg pains, mood change, reduction in sexual desire, headaches, nausea, vaginal erosion, discharge, and bleeding, weight gain, skin changes.
Caution: in patients suffering from high blood pressure, diabetes, vascular disorders, asthma, depression, kidney disease, multiple sclerosis, womb diseases. Your doctor may advise you not to smoke, to have regular examinations. You should stop treatment at the first sign of serious symptoms such as severe headache or jaundice. Treatment should be stopped before surgery.
Not to be used for: pregnant women, or for patients suffering from sickle-cell anaemia, history of heart disease or thrombosis, liver disorders, some cancers, undiagnosed vaginal bleeding, some ear, skin, and kidney disorders.
Not to be used with: RIFAMPICIN, TETRACYCLINES, GRISEOFULVIN, barbiturates, PHENYTOIN, PRIMIDONE, CARBAMAZEPINE, ETHOSUXIMIDE, CHLORAL HYDRATE, DICHLORALPHENAZONE.
Contains: ETHINYLOESTRADIOL, DESOGESTREL.
Other preparations:

Maxepa
(Duncan, Flockhart)

A clear, soft capsule used as a lipid-lowering agent to treat elevated lipids.

M

Dose: 5 capsules twice a day with food.
Availability: NHS and private prescription.

Side effects: nausea, belching
Caution: in patients suffering from bleeding disorders.
Not to be used for: children.
Not to be used with: anti-coagulants
Contains: EICOSAPENTAENOIC ACID, DOCOSAHEXAENOIC ACID.
Other preparations: Maxepa Liquid.

Maxidex
(Alcon)

Drops used as a corticosteroid, lubricant treatment for inflammation of the front of the eye.

Dose: 1-2 drops every hour for 3-4 days then every 2-3 hours for 7-14 days.
Availability: NHS and private prescription.
Side effects: cataract, thinning cornea, fungal infection, rise in eye pressure.
Caution: in pregnant women and infants — do not use for extended periods.
Not to be used for: patients suffering from viral, fungal, tubercular, or weeping infections, glaucoma, or for patients who wear soft contact lenses.
Not to be used with:
Contains: DEXAMETHASONE, HYPROMELLOSE.
Other preparations:

Maxitrol
(Alcon)

Drops used as a corticosteroid, aminoglycoside antibiotic, lubricant, and protein treatment for infected inflammation of the eye.

Dose: 1-2 drops into the eye 4-6 times a day.
Availability: NHS and private prescription.
Side effects: rise in eye pressure, fungal infection, thinning cornea, cataract.
Caution: in pregnant women and infants— do not use for extended periods.
Not to be used for: patients suffering from glaucoma, viral, fungal,

M

tubercular, or weeping infections, or for patients who wear soft contact lenses.
Not to be used with:
Contains: DEXAMETHASONE, NEOMYCIN sulphate, HYPROMELLOSE, POLYMYXIN B SULPHATE.
Other preparations: Maxitrol Ointment.

Maxolon
(S K B)

A white tablet supplied at a strength of 10 mg and used as an anti-sickness (anti-dopaminergic), anti-spasm drug to treat nausea, vomiting, dyspepsia, wind, heartburn, and other symptoms related to stomach and bowels, intolerance to cytotoxic drugs, congestive heart failure, after operations, deep X-ray or cobalt treatment.

Dose: adults over 20 years 10 mg 3 times a day; children and young adults use only for special circumstances such as in sickness caused by cancer treatment.
Availability: NHS and private prescription.
Side effects: occasionally parkinsonian-type symptoms, extra-pyramidal reactions (tremor, rigidity).
Caution: in pregnant women, nursing mothers, and in patients suffering from liver and kidney problems.
Not to be used for: where recent gastric or bowel surgery has occurred. Some rare tumours such as phaeochromocytoma (a disease of the adrenal glands) or prolactin-dependent breast cancers.
Not to be used with: ANTI-CHOLINERGICS, PHENOTHIAZINES, BUTYROPHE-NONES.
Contains: METOCLOPRAMIDE.
Other preparations: syrup and injectable preparations, slow-release preparations such as Maxolon SR, Maxolon High Dose. GASTROBID CONTINUS (Napp), GASTROMAX (Farmitalia CE), METOX (Steinhard), METRAMID (Nicholas), parmid (Lagap).

mazindol *see* Teronac

M

mebendazole *see* Vermox

mebeverine *see* Colofac, Colven

---

mebhydrolin *see* Fabahistine

---

medazepam *see* Nobrium

Medicoal
(Lundbeck)

Effervescent granules used as an adsorbent to treat poisoning and overdosing with drugs.

Dose: 5-10 g in 100 ml of water, repeat up to a maximum of 50 g.
Availability: NHS, private prescription, over the counter.
Side effects:
Caution:
Not to be used for: poisoning where there is a known antidote or for poisoning by acids, alkalis, iron salts, cyanides, MALATHION, DDT, sulphonylureas.
Not to be used with: drugs taken by mouth.
Contains: activated CHARCOAL.
Other preparations:

Medihaler-Duo
(3M-Riker)

An aerosol used as a broncho-dilator to treat bronchial spasm brought on by bronchial asthma or chronic bronchitis.

Dose: 1-3 sprays and again after 30 minutes if needed up to a maximum of 24 sprays in 24 hours.
Availability: NHS and private prescription.
Side effects: headache, dry mouth, dilation of the blood vessels, rapid or abnormal heart rhythms.
Caution: in patients suffering from diabetes.
Not to be used for: patients suffering from heart disease, high blood

M

pressure, cardiac asthma, overactive thyroid.
Not to be used with: MAOIS, SYMPATHOMIMETICS, TRICYCLICS.
Contains: ISOPRENALINE hydrochloride, PHENYLEPHRINE bitartrate.
Other preparations:

Medihaler-EPI
(3M-Riker)

An aerosol supplied at a strength of 0.28 mg and used as a SYMPATH-OMIMETIC additional treatment for sensitivity to drugs or stings due to previous exposure.

Dose: adults at least 20 sprays; children 10-15 sprays.
Availability: NHS and private prescription.
Side effects: nervousness, shaking hands, dry mouth, stomach pain, abnormal rhythms.
Caution: in patients suffering from diabetes.
Not to be used for: patients suffering from heart disease, cardiac asthma, high blood pressure, overactive thyroid.
Not to be used with: MAOIS, TRICYCLICS, other sympathomimetics.
Contains: ADRENALINE ACID TARTRATE.
Other preparations:

Medihaler-Ergotamine
(3M Riker)

An aerosol used to treat migraine, recurring headache, histamine headache, neuralgia.

Dose: 1 dose repeated if needed after 5 minutes up to a maximum of 6 doses in 24 hours or 15 doses in a week.
Availability: NHS and private prescription.
Side effects: nausea, muscular pain.
Caution:
Not to be used for: children under 10 years, pregnant women, nursing mothers, or for patients suffering from coronary, peripheral, or occlusive vascular disease, severe high blood pressure, kidney or liver disease, or sepsis.
Not to be used with: ERYTHROMICIN, ß-BLOCKERS.
Contains: ERGOTAMINE TARTRATE.
Other preparations:

M

Medihaler-Iso
(3M Riker)

An aerosol supplied at a strength of 0.08 mg and used as a ß-agonist to treat bronchial asthma, chronic bronchitis.

Dose: 1-3 sprays and again after 30 minutes if needed, to a maximum of 24 sprays in 24 hours.
Availability: NHS and private prescriptions.
Side effects: dilation of the blood vessels, headache, rapid or abnormal heart rate.
Caution: in patients suffering from diabetes, high blood pressure.
Not to be used for: patients suffering from heart disease, overactive thyroid, cardiac asthma.
Not to be used with: MAOIS, SYMPATHOMIMETICS, TRICYCLICS.
Contains: ISOPRENALINE sulphate.
Other preparations:

Medilave
(Martindale)

A gel used as an antiseptic and local anaesthetic to treat abrasions or ulcers in the mouth, teething.

Dose: apply to the affected area without rubbing in 3-4 times a day.
Availability: NHS, private prescription, over the counter.
Side effects:
Caution:
Not to be used for: infants under 6 months.
Not to be used with:
Contains: BENZOCAINE, CETYLPYRIDINIUM.
Other preparations:

Medised Suspension
(Panpharma)

A suspension used as an analgesic, antihistamine treatment to relieve pain and fever associated with congestion, chicken pox.

Dose: children 3 months-1 year 1 5 ml teaspoonful up to 4 times a day, 1-6 years 2 5 ml teaspoonsful up to 4 times a day, 6-12 year 4 5 ml tea-

spoonsful up to 4 times a day.
Availability: private prescription only.
Side effects: drowsiness.
Caution: in patients with liver or kidney disease.
Not to be used for: infants under 3 months.
Not to be used with: alcohol, sedatives.
Contains: paracetamol, PROMETHAZINE hydrochloride.
Other preparations: Medised Tablets.

Meditar
(Brocades)

A waxy stick used as an anti-psoriatic treatment for psoriasis, eczema.

Dose: apply to the affected area 1-2 times a day.
Availability: NHS, private prescription, over the counter.
Side effects: irritation, sensitivity to light.
Caution:
Not to be used for: patients suffering from acute psoriasis.
Not to be used with:
Contains: COAL TAR.
Other preparations:

Medocodene
(Medo)

An yellow, scored tablet used as an analgesic to relieve pain.

Dose: adults 1-2 tablets every 4 hours to a maximum of 8 in 24 hours; children 6-12 years half adult dose.
Availability: NHS (when prescribed as generic), and private prescription.
Side effects: constipation.
Caution: in patients suffering from kidney or liver disease.
Not to be used for: children under 6 years.
Not to be used with:
Contains: PARACETAMOL, CODEINE phosphate.
Other preparations:

M

Medomet *see* Aldomet
(DDSA)

Medrone
(Upjohn)

A pink, quarter-scored, oval tablet, a white, quarter-scored, oval tablet, or a white, quarter-scored tablet according to strengths of 2 mg, 4 mg, 16 mg and used as a corticosteroid treatment for rheumatoid arthritis, inflammatory conditions, allergies.

Dose: as advised by the physician.
Availability: NHS and private prescription.
Side effects: high blood sugar, thin bones, mood changes, ulcers.
Caution: pregnant women, or for patients who have had recent bowel surgery, or who are suffering from inflamed veins, psychiatric disorders, virus infections, some cancers, some kidney diseases, thinning of the bones, ulcers, tuberculosis, other infections, high blood pressure, glaucoma, epilepsy, diabetes, underactive thyroid, liver disease, stress. Withdraw gradually.
Not to be used for: infants under 1 year.
Not to be used with: PHENYTOIN, PHENOBARBITONE, EPHEDRINE, RIFAMPICIN, DIURETICS, ANTI-CHOLINESTERASES, DIGITALIS, anti-diabetic agents, anti-coagulants, NON-STEROID ANTI-INFLAMMATORY DRUGS.
Contains: METHYLPREDNISOLONE.
Other preparations:

Medrone Lotion
(Upjohn)

A lotion used as a corticosteroid and skin softener to treat acne, dermatitis.

Dose: apply a small amount to the affected area 1-2 times a day.
Availability: NHS and private prescription.
Side effects: fluid retention, suppression of adrenal glands, thinning of the skin may occur.
Caution: in pregnant women. Use for short periods of time only.
Not to be used for: patients suffering from acne or any other skin infections caused by tuberculosis, ringworm, viruses, or fungi, or con-

M

tinuously especially in pregnant women.
Not to be used with:
Contains: METHYLPREDNISOLONE acetate, SULPHUR, ALUMINIUM CHLORHY-
DROXIDE.
Other preparations:

---

medroxyprogesterone *see* Provera

---

mefenamic acid *see* Ponstan, Ponstan Forte

---

mefruside *see* Baycaron

Megace
(Bristol-Myers)

A white, scored tablet or an off-white, oval, scored tablet according to
strengths of 40 mg, 160 mg and used as a progestogen treatment for
breast cancer.

Dose: 160 mg a day for at least 2 months.
Availability: NHS and private prescription.
Side effects: gain in weight, skin allergies, nausea.
Caution: in patients suffering from thrombophlebitis.
Not to be used for: children or pregnant women.
Not to be used with:
Contains: MEGESTROL ACETATE.
Other preparations:

Megaclor
(Pharmax)

A red, oblong capsule tablet supplied at a strength of 170 mg and used
as a tetracycline treatment for respiratory, ear, nose, and throat, and
soft tissue infections, acne.

M

393

Dose: 1-2 capsules 3-4 times a day.
Availability: NHS and private prescription.
Side effects: stomach disturbances, allergy, additional infections.
Caution: in patients suffering from liver or kidney disease.
Not to be used for: children, nursing mothers, or women in the last half of pregnancy.
Not to be used with: milk, antacids, mineral supplements, the contraceptive pill.
Contains: *clomocycline.*
Other preparations:

---

megestrol *see* **Megace**

Melleril
(Sandoz)

A white tablet supplied at strengths of 10 mg, 25 mg, 50 mg, 100 mg and used as a sedative to treat schizophrenia, manic mental disorders, senile confusion, behavioural disorders in children.

Dose: adults 30-100 mg a day at first increasing to 600 mg a day if needed; children under 5 years 1 mg per kg body weight a day, 5-12 years 75-150 mg a day, to a maximum of 300 mg a day.
Availability: NHS and private prescription.
Side effects: muscle spasms, restlessness, hands shaking, dry mouth, urine retention, palpitations, low blood pressure, weight gain, changes in libido, low body temperature, breast swelling, menstrual changes, jaundice, blood and skin changes, drowsiness, rarely fits.
Caution: in pregnant women, nursing mothers, and in patients suffering from liver disease, or cardiovascular disease.
Not to be used for: severely depressed or unconscious patients or for patients suffering from bone marrow depression .
Not to be used with: alcohol, tranquillizers, pain killers, anti-hypertensives, anti-depressants, anti-convulsants, anti-diabetic drugs, LEVODOPA.
Contains: THIORIDAZINE hydrochloride.
Other preparations:

M

---

menadiol diphosphate *see* **Synkavit**

Menophase
(Syntex)

Five pink tablets, 8 orange tablets, 2 yellow tablets, 3 green tablets, 6 blue tablets, and 4 lavender tablets used as an oestrogen, progestogen treatment for symptoms associated with the menopause.

Dose: 1 tablet a day.
Availability: NHS and private prescription.
Side effects: enlarged breasts, bloating and fluid retention, cramps, leg pains, mood change, reduction in sexual desire, headaches, nausea, vaginal erosion, discharge, and bleeding, weight gain, skin changes.
Caution: in patients suffering from high blood pressure, diabetes, vascular disorders, asthma, depression, kidney disease, multiple sclerosis, womb diseases. Your doctor may advise you not to smoke, to have regular check-ups.
Not to be used for: children, pregnant women, or for patients suffering from sickle-cell anaemia, history of heart disease or thrombosis, liver disorders, some cancers, undiagnosed vaginal bleeding, some ear, skin, and kidney disorders.
Not to be used with: DIURETICS, anti-hypertensives, and drugs that change liver enzymes, RIFAMPICIN, TETRACYCLINES, GRISEOFULVIN, barbiturates, phenytoin, PRIMIDONE, CARBAMAZEPINE, ETHOSUXIMIDE, CHLORAL HYDRATE, DICHLORALPHENAZONE.
Contains: MESTRANOL, MESTRANOL and NORETHISTERONE,
Other preparations:

---

menthol *see* **Aradolene, Aspellin, Balmosa, Benylin Expectorant, Copholco, Copholcoids, Expurhin, Guanor, Histalix, Phytocil, Rowachol, Salonair, Tercoda, Terpoin**

M

menthone *see* **Rowachol**

---

mepenzolate *see* Cantil

---

meprobamate *see* Equagesic, Equanil, Tenavoid

---

meptazinol *see* Meptid

Meptid
(Wyeth)

An orange, oval tablet tablet supplied at a strength of 200 mg and used as an analgesic to relieve pain.

Dose: 1 tablet every 3-6 hours as needed.
Availability: NHS and private prescription.
Side effects: dizziness, nausea.
Caution: in patients with liver or kidney disease or respiratory depression.
Not to be used for: children.
Not to be used with:
Contains: MEPTAZINOL.
Other preparations:

---

mequitazine *see* Primalan

Merbentyl
(Merrell Dow)

A white tablet supplied at strengths of 10 mg, 20 mg and used as an anti-spasm, ANTI-CHOLINERGIC treatment for bowel and stomach spasm.

Dose: children 6 months-2 years 5-10 mg 3-4 times a day before feeds, over 2 years 10 mg 3 times a day, adults 10-20 mg 3 times a day between meals.
Availability: NHS and private prescription.

Side effects: blurred vision, confusion, dry mouth.
Caution: glaucoma, inflammatory bowel disease, intestinal obstruction, enlarged prostate.
Not to be used for:
Not to be used with:
Contains: DICYCLOMINE.
Other preparations: Merbentyl syrup.

Mercilon
(Organon)

A white tablet used as an oestrogen, progestogen contraceptive.

Dose: 1 tablet a day for 21 days starting on day 1 or day 5 of the period.
Availability: NHS and private prescription.
Side effects: enlarged breasts, bloating and fluid retention, cramps, leg pains, mood change, reduction in sexual desire, headaches, nausea, vaginal erosion, discharge, and bleeding, weight gain, skin changes.
Caution: in patients suffering from high blood pressure, diabetes, vascular disorders, asthma, depression, kidney disease, multiple sclerosis, womb diseases. Your doctor may advise you not to smoke, to have regular examinations. You should stop treatment at the first sign of serious symptoms such as severe headache or jaundice. Treatment should be stopped before surgery.
Not to be used for: pregnant women, or for patients suffering from sickle-cell anaemia, history of heart disease or thrombosis, liver disorders, some cancers, undiagnosed vaginal bleeding, some ear, skin, and kidney disorders.
Not to be used with: RIFAMPICIN, TETRACYCLINES, GRISEOFULVIN, barbiturates, PHENYTOIN, PRIMIDONE, CARBAMAZEPINE, ETHOSUXIMIDE, CHLORAL HYDRATE, DICHLORALPHENAZONE.
Contains: ETHINYLOESTRADIOL, DESOGESTREL.
Other preparations:

Merocaine
(Merrell Dow)

A green lozenge tablet supplied at a strength of 1.4 mg and used as an antiseptic and local anaesthetic to treat painful infections of the

M

throat and mouth, and as an additional treatment for tonsillitis and pharyngitis.

Dose: 1 lozenge allowed to dissolve in the mouth every 2 hours up to a maximum of 8 lozenges in 24 hours.
Availability: NHS, private prescription, over the counter.
Side effects:
Caution:
Not to be used for: children.
Not to be used with:
Contains: CETYLPYRIDINIUM CHLORIDE, BENZOCAINE.
Other preparations:

Merocet
(Merrell Dow)

A solution used as an antiseptic to treat infections of the throat and mouth.

Dose: rinse the mouth or gargle with the solution diluted or undiluted every 3 hours or as needed.
Availability: NHS, private prescription, over the counter.
Side effects:
Caution:
Not to be used for: children under 6 years.
Not to be used with:
Contains: CETYLPYRIDINIUM CHLORIDE.
Other preparations: Merocets Lozenge

---

mesalazine *see* Asacol

---

mesterolone *see* Pro-Viron

M

Mestinon
(Roche)

A white tablet tablet supplied at a strength of 60 mg and used as a nerve conduction enhancer to treat paralytic ileus, myasthenia gravis (muscular disorders).

Dose: for paralytic ileus adults 1-4 tablets as required; children 1/4-1 tablet as required. For myasthenia gravis adults 5-20 tablets a day in divided doses; infants 5-10 mg every 4 hours, under 6 years 3
Availability: NHS and private prescription.
Side effects: nausea, salivation, diarrhoea, colic.
Caution: in patients suffering from bronchial asthma, heart disease, epilepsy, Parkinson's disease.
Not to be used for: patients with bowel or urinary obstruction.
Not to be used with: depolarizing muscle relaxants, CYCLOPROPANE, HALOTHANE.
Contains: PYRIDOSTIGMINE BROMIDE.
Other preparations:

---

mestranol *see* **Menophase, Norinyl-1, Ortho-Novin 1/50**

Metatone
(Warner-Lambert)

A liquid used as a source of vitamin B_1 and minerals and used as a tonic.

Dose: adults 1-2 5 ml teaspoonsful 2-3 times a day; children 6-12 years half adult dose.
Availability: private prescription and over the counter.
Side effects:
Caution:
Not to be used for: children under 6 years.
Not to be used with:
Contains: THIAMINE hydrochloride, CALCIUM GLYCEROPHOSPHATE, MANGA-NESE, POTASSIUM, SODIUM.
Other preparations:

M

Metenix
(Hoechst)

A blue tablet tablet supplied at a strength of 5 mg and used as a

DIURETIC to treat high blood pressure, fluid retention, swollen abdomen, or toxaemia of pregnancy.

Dose: high blood pressure 5 mg a day at first, then reduce to 5 mg every other day after 3-4 weeks; fluid retention 5-10 mg as a single dose; no more than 80 mg in 24 hours.
Availability: NHS and private prescription.
Side effects: low potassium levels, headache, stomach upset, cramps, rash.
Caution: in pregnant women, nursing mothers, and in patients suffering from liver disease, gout, or diabetes. Potassium supplements may be needed.
Not to be used for: patients suffering from liver cirrhosis or kidney failure.
Not to be used with: DIGITALIS, LITHIUM, hypertensives.
Contains: METOLAZONE.
Other preparations:

Meterfolic
(Sinclair)

A grey tablet used as an iron and folic acid supplement in the prevention of iron and folic acid deficiencies in pregnancy.

Dose: 1 tablet 1-2 times a day.
Availability: NHS and private prescription.
Side effects: nausea, constipation.
Caution: in patients suffering from haemolytic anaemia, or with a history of peptic ulcer.
Not to be used for: children or for patients suffering from vitamin B_{12} deficiency.
Not to be used with: TETRACYCLINES.
Contains: FERROUS FUMARATE, FOLIC ACID.
Other preparations:

M

metformin *see* **Glucophage**

---

methadone *see* **Physeptone**

methionine *see* **Lipoflavonoid, Pameton**

---

methixene hydrochloride *see* **Tremonil**

---

methocarbamol *see* **Robaxin, Robaxisal Forte**

---

methoserpidine *see* **Decaserpyl, Decaserpyl Plus**

---

methotrimeprazine *see* **Veractil**

---

methyclothiazide *see* **Enduron**

---

methyl nicotinate *see* **Cremalgin, Dubam**

---

methyl salicylate *see* **Aspellin, Balmosa, Dubam, Monphytol, Phytex**

---

methyl undecoanate *see* **Monphytol**

---

methylcellulose granules

A bulking agent used to treat constipation.

M

Dose: adults 2.5-10 ml with water; children in proportion to dosage for 70 kg adult.
Availability: NHS and private prescription.

Side effects: may cause dehydration in children.
Caution:
Not to be used for:
Not to be used with:
Contains:
Other preparations: METHYLCELLULOSE mixture.

---

methylcellulose *see* **Celevac, Cologel, methylcellulose granules, Nilstim**

---

methylcysteine hydrochloride *see* **Visclair**

---

methyldopa *see* **Aldomet, Cytacon, Hydromet**

---

methylphenobarbitone *see* **Prominal**

---

methylprednisolone *see* **Medrone, Medrone Lotion, Neo-Medrone Cream, Neo-Medrone Lotion**

---

methyprylone *see* **Noludar**

---

methysergide *see* **Deseril**

Metipranolol
(SNP)

Drops used as a ß-BLOCKER to treat high eye pressure.

Dose: 1 drop into the eye twice a day.
Availability: NHS and private prescription.
Side effects: slight smarting, temporary headache.
Caution: in patients suffering from heart block.
Not to be used for: children, pregnant women, or for patients suffering from heart failure or blocked airways disease, or for those who wear contact lenses.
Not to be used with: VERAPAMIL, other ß-blockers.
Contains: METIPRANOLOL.
Other preparations:

---

metipranolol *see* **Metipranolol**

---

metoclopramide *see* **Maxolon, Migravess Forte, Paramax**

---

metolazone *see* **Metenix**

---

metoprolol *see* **Betaloc**

Metopirone
(Ciba)

A cream capsule tablet supplied at a strength of 250 mg and used as a hormone blocker to treat Cushing's syndrome, and with glucocorticoids to treat resistant oedema caused by increased aldosterone secretion (adrenal gland disorder).

Dose: Cushing's syndrome 1-24 tablets a day; oedema 10-18 tablets a day.
Availability: NHS and private prescription.
Side effects: nausea, vomiting, low blood pressure, allergies.
Caution: in patients suffering from underactive pituitary gland.
Not to be used for: children, pregnant women, or nursing mothers.

M

Not to be used with:
Contains: METYRAPONE.
Other preparations:

---

metoprolol *see* **Co-Betaloc, Lopresor, Lopresoretic, Metoros**

Metoros
(Geigy)

A white tablet tablet supplied at a strength of 190 mg and used as a ß-BLOCKER to treat high blood pressure.

Dose: 1-2 tablets with water every morning.
Availability: NHS and private prescription.
Side effects: cold hands and feet, sleep disturbance, slow heart rate, tiredness, wheezing, heart failure, stomach upset.
Caution: in pregnant women, nursing mothers, and in patients suffering from diabetes, kidney or liver disorders, asthma. May need to be withdrawn before surgery. Withdraw gradually. Your doctor may advise additional treatment with diuretics or digitalis.
Not to be used for: children or for patients suffering from heart block or failure.
Not to be used with: VERAPAMIL, CLONIDINE withdrawal, some anti-arrhythmic drugs and anaesthetics, RESERPINE, some anti-hypertensives, ergot alkaloids, CIMETIDINE, sedatives, SYMPATHOMIMETICS, INDOMETHACIN.
Contains: METOPROLOL fumarate.
Other preparations: Metoros LS.

Metosyn
(Stuart)

A cream used as a steroid treatment for allergic and other skin conditions where there is also inflammation.

Dose: massage into the affected area 3-4 times a day at first and then reduce to 1-2 times a day as soon as possible.

Availability: NHS and private prescription.
Side effects: fluid retention, suppression of adrenal glands, thinning of the skin may occur.
Caution: use for short periods of time only.
Not to be used for: patients suffering from acne or any other skin infections caused by tuberculosis, ringworm, viruses, or fungi, or continuously especially in pregnant women.
Not to be used with:
Contains: FLUOCINONIDE.
Other preparations: Metosyn Ointment, Metosyn Scalp Lotion.

Metox *see* **Maxolon**
(Steinhard)

Metramid *see* **Maxolon**
(Nicholas)

Metrolyl *see* **Flagyl**
(Lagap)

---

metronidazole *see* **Flagyl**

---

metyrapone *see* **Metopirone**

---

mexiletene *see* **Mexitil**

M

Mexitil
(Boehringer Ingelheim)

A red/purple capsule or a red capsule according to strengths of 50 mg,

200 mg and used as an anti-arrhythmic treatment for abnormal heart rhythm.

Dose: 400-600 mg at first, then 2 hours later and thereafter 200-250 mg 3-4 times a day.
Availability: NHS and private prescription.
Side effects: stomach and brain disorders, low blood pressure.
Caution: in patients suffering from nerve conduction defects in the heart, low blood pressure, heart, liver, or kidney failure, Parkinson's disease.
Not to be used for: children.
Not to be used with:
Contains: MEXILETENE hydrochloride.
Other preparations: Mexitil Perlongets, Mexitil Injection

mianserin hydrochloride *see* Norval

mianserin *see* Bolvidon, Norval

Micolette
(Wyeth)

A micro-enema used as a faecal softener and lubricant to treat constipation, and for the evacuation of bowels before surgery.

Dose: adults and children over 3 years 1-2 enemas.
Availability: NHS and private prescription.
Side effects:
Caution:
Not to be used for: children under 3 years or patients suffering from inflammatory or ulcerative bowel disease, or acute stomach conditions.
Not to be used with:
Contains: SODIUM LAURYL SULPHOACETATE, SODIUM CITRATE, GLYCEROL.
Other preparations:

M

miconazole *see* **Acnidazil, Daktacort, Daktarin, Daktarin Cream, Daktarin Oral Gel, Dermonistat, Gyno-Daktarin 1, Monistat**

Micralax
(S K B)

A disposable enema used as a faecal softener and lubricant to treat constipation, and for evacuation of bowels

Dose: adults and children over 3 years 1 enema.
Availability: NHS
Side effects:
Caution:
Not to be used for: for children or patients suffering from inflammatory bowel disease.
Not to be used with:
Contains: SODIUM CITRATE, SODIUM ALKYLSULPHOACETATE, SORBIC ACID.
Other preparations:

---

microfurantoin *see* **Macrodantin**

Microgynon 30
(Schering)

A beige tablet used as an oestrogen, progestogen contraceptive.

Dose: 1 tablet a day starting on day 5 of the period.
Availability: NHS and private prescription.
Side effects: enlarged breasts, bloating and fluid retention, cramps, leg pains, mood change, reduction in sexual desire, headaches, nausea, vaginal erosion, discharge, and bleeding, weight gain, skin changes.
Caution: in patients suffering from high blood pressure, diabetes, vascular disorders, asthma, depression, kidney disease, multiple sclerosis, womb diseases. Your doctor may advise you not to smoke, to have regular examinations. You should stop treatment at the first sign of serious symptoms such as severe headache or jaundice.

M

Treatment should be stopped before surgery.

Not to be used for: pregnant women, or for patients suffering from sickle-cell anaemia, history of heart disease or thrombosis, liver disorders, some cancers, undiagnosed vaginal bleeding, some ear, skin, and kidney disorders.

Not to be used with: RIFAMPICIN, TETRACYCLINES, GRISEOFULVIN, barbiturates, PHENYTOIN, PRIMIDONE, CARBAMAZEPINE, ETHOSUXIMIDE, CHLORAL HYDRATE, DICHLORALPHENAZONE.

Contains: ETHINYLOESTRADIOL, LEVONORGESTREL.

Other preparations:

Micronor
(Cilag)

A white tablet used as a progesterone contraceptive.

Dose: 1 tablet at the same time every day starting on day 1 of the period.

Availability: NHS and private prescription.

Side effects: irregular bleeding, breast discomfort, acne, headache.

Caution: in patients suffering from high blood pressure, tendency to thrombosis, migraine, liver abnormalities, ovarian cysts. Your doctor may advise regular check-ups.

Not to be used for: pregnant women, or for patients suffering from severe heart or artery disease, benign liver tumours, vaginal bleeding, previous ectopic pregnancy.

Not to be used with: barbiturates, PHENYTOIN, PRIMIDONE, CARBAMAZEPINE, CHLORAL HYDRATE, DICHLORALPHENAZONE, ETHOSUXIMIDE, RIFAMPICIN, GLUTETHIMIDE, CHLORPROMAZINE, MEPROBAMATE, GRISEOFULVIN.

CONTAINS: NORETHISTERONE.

Other preparations:

Microval
(Wyeth)

A white tablet used as a progesterone contraceptive.

Dose: 1 tablet at the same time every day starting on day 1 of the period.

Availability: NHS and private prescription.

Side effects: irregular bleeding, breast discomfort, acne, headache.
Caution: in patients suffering from high blood pressure, tendency to thrombosis, migraine, liver abnormalities, ovarian cysts. Your doctor may advise regular check-ups.
Not to be used for: pregnant women, or for patients suffering from severe heart or artery disease, benign liver tumours, vaginal bleeding, previous ectopic pregnancy.
Not to be used with: barbiturates, PHENYTOIN, PRIMIDONE, CARBAMAZEPINE, CHLORAL HYDRATE, DICHLORALPHENAZONE, ETHOSUXIMIDE, RIFAMPICIN, GLUTETHIMIDE, CHLORPROMAZINE, MEPROBAMATE, GRISEOFULVIN.
Contains: LEVONORGESTREL.
Other preparations:

Mictral
(Sterling Research Laboratories)

Granules in a sachet used as an antiseptic to treat cystitis and some infections of the urinary tract.

Dose: the contents of 1 sachet dissolved in water 3 times a day for 3 days.
Availability: NHS and private prescription.
Side effects: stomach problems, disturbed vision, rash, seizures, anaemia, blood changes.
Caution: in pregnant women and in patients suffering from liver disease. Keep out of sunlight.
Not to be used for: children or patients suffering from kidney disease or with a history of convulsions.
Not to be used with: anti-coagulants, anti-bacterials.
Contains: NALIDIXIC ACID, SODIUM CITRATE, CITRIC ACID, SODIUM BICARBONATE.
Other preparations:

Micturin
(KabiVitrum)

A white tablet supplied at a strength of 12.5 mg and used as an antihistamine-type drug to treat abnormally frequent or urgent urination, incontinence.

M

Dose: adults 2 tablets twice a day; infirm elderly 1 tablet twice a day.

Availability: NHS and private prescription.
Side effects: dry mouth, disturbed vision, constipation, dizziness, rapid heart rate.
Caution: in patients suffering from fever, thyrotoxicosis, heart disease, gastric retention, gastro-intestinal tract obstruction, liver disease.
Not to be used for: children or for patients suffering from bladder obstruction, flaccid bladder or large amount of residual urine, severe liver or biliary tract failure, glaucoma.
Not to be used with: ANTI-CHOLINERGICS, calcium antagonists.
Contains: TERODILINE hydrochloride.
Other preparations: Terolin (former name).

Midrid
(Carnrick)

A red capsule used as an analgesic to treat migraine.

Dose: 2 capsules at the beginning of the migraine attack, then 1 capsule every hour to a maximum of 5 capsules in 12 hours.
Availability: NHS, private prescription, over the counter.
Side effects: dizziness.
Caution: in pregnant women and nursing mothers.
Not to be used for: children, or for patients suffering from severe kidney, liver, or heart disease, gastritis, severe hhigh blood pressure, or glaucoma.
Not to be used with: MAOIS.
Contains: ISOMETHEPTENE MUCATE, PARACETAMOL.
Other preparations:

Migraleve
(International)

A pink tablet and a yellow tablet according to strength and contents and used as an analgesic, antihistamine treatment for migraine.

M

Dose: adults and children over 10 years 2 pink tablets at the beginning of the attack, and then 2 yellow tablets every 4 hours if needed to a maximum of 2 pink tablets and 6 yellow tablets in 24 hours.
Availability: NHS, private prescription, over the counter.

Side effects: drowsiness.
Caution: in patients suffering from kidney or liver disease.
Not to be used for: children under 10 years.
Not to be used with:
Contains: pink: BUCLIZINE hydrochloride, PARACETAMOL, CODEINE phosphate; yellow: PARACETAMOL, CODEINE phosphate.
Other preparations:

Migravess Forte
(Bayer)

A white, scored, effervescent tablet used as an anti-emetic and analgesic to treat migraine.

Dose: adults 2 tablets dissolved in water at the beginning of the attack, then up to a maximum of 6 tablets in 24 hours; children 10-15 years half adult dose.
Availability: NHS and private prescription.
Side effects: extrapyramidal reactions (shaking and rigidity).
Caution: in pregnant women or in patients suffering from anti-inflammatory induced allergy, kidney or liver disease, asthma.
Not to be used for: children under 10 years or for patients suffering from peptic ulcer or haemophilia.
Not to be used with: ANTI-CHOLINERGICS, phenothiazines, butyrophenones, anti-coagulants, anti-diabetics and uric acid lowering agents.
Contains: metoclopramide hydrochloride, aspirin.
Other preparations:

Migril
(Wellcome)

A white, scored tablet used as an ergot preparation to treat migraine.

Dose: 1-2 tablets at the beginning of an attack, then $1/2$ to 1 tablet every $1/2$ hour if needed to a maximum of 4 tablets for any 1 attack and 6 tablets in any 1 week.
Availability: NHS and private prescription.
Side effects: rebound headache, poor circulation, abdominal pain, drowsiness, dry mouth.
Caution: in patients suffering from sepsis, anaemia, overactive

M

thyroid.

Not to be used for: children, pregnant women, nursing mothers, or for patients suffering from coronary, peripheral, or occlusive vascular disease, severe high blood pressure, kidney or liver disease.

Not to be used with: ERYTHROMYCIN, ß-BLOCKERS, sedatives.

Contains: ERGOTAMINE tartrate, CYCLIZINE hydrochloride, CAFFEINE hydrate.

Other preparations:

Mildison Lipocream
(Brocades)

A cream used as a steroid treatment for eczema and other skin disorders.

Dose: apply a small quantity to the affected area 2-3 times a day.

Availability: NHS and private prescription.

Side effects: fluid retention, suppression of adrenal glands, thinning of the skin may occur.

Caution: do not use for children or for facial conditions for longer than 5 days.

Not to be used for: with covering dressings or for patients suffering from bacterial, fungal, or viral infections, or for extended treatments in pregnant women.

Not to be used with:

Contains: HYDROCORTISONE.

Other preparations:

Minamino
(Chancellor)

A syrup used as a source of aminoacids, B vitamins, and minerals to treat vitamin and mineral deficiencies.

Dose: adults 4 5 ml teaspoonsful 3 times a day; children half adult dose.

Availability: private prescription and over the counter.

Side effects:

Caution:

Not to be used for:

M

412

Not to be used with: LEVODOPA.
Contains: multivitamins and minerals.
Other preparations:

Minilyn
(Organon)

A white tablet used as an oestrogen, progestogen contraceptive.

Dose: 1 tablet a day for 21 days starting on day 1 of the period.
Availability: NHS and private prescription.
Side effects: enlarged breasts, bloating and fluid retention, cramps, leg pains, mood change, reduction in sexual desire, headaches, nausea, vaginal erosion, discharge, and bleeding, weight gain, skin changes.
Caution: in patients suffering from high blood pressure, diabetes, vascular disorders, asthma, depression, kidney disease, multiple sclerosis, womb diseases. Your doctor may advise you not to smoke, to have regular examinations. You should stop treatment at the first sign of serious symptoms such as severe headache or jaundice. Treatment should be stopped before surgery.
Not to be used for: pregnant women, or for patients suffering from sickle-cell anaemia, history of heart disease or thrombosis, liver disorders, some cancers, undiagnosed vaginal bleeding, some ear, skin, and kidney disorders.
Not to be used with: RIFAMPICIN, TETRACYCLINES, GRISEOFULVIN, barbiturates, PHENYTOIN, PRIMIDONE, CARBAMAZEPINE, ETHOSUXIMIDE, CHLORAL HYDRATE, DICHLORALPHENAZONE.
Contains: ETHINYLOESTRADIOL, LYNOESTRENOL.
Other preparations:

Minims Saline
(SNP)

Drops used to irrigate the eyes.

Dose: use as needed.
Availability: NHS, private prescription, over the counter.
Side effects:
Caution:

M

Not to be used for:
Not to be used with:
Contains: SODIUM CHLORIDE.
Other preparations:

Minocin 50
(Lederle)

A beige tablet supplied at a strength of 50 mg and used as an antibiotic treatment for acne.

Dose: 1 tablet twice a day for at least 6 weeks.
Availability: NHS and private prescription.
Side effects: stomach disturbances, allergies, additional infections.
Caution: in patients suffering from liver disease.
Not to be used for: children, nursing mothers, or women in the last half of pregnancy.
Not to be used with: antacids, mineral supplements.
Contains: MINOCYCLINE hydrochloride.
Other preparations:

Minocin *see* Tetracycline

minocycline *see* Minocin 50

Minodiab
(Farmitalia CE)

A white tablet supplied at strengths of 2.5 mg, 5 mg and used as an anti-diabetic treatment for diabetes.

Dose: 2.5-5 mg a day in divided doses at first titrating by 2.5 or 5 mg a day every 7 days, then usually 2.5-30 mg a day to a maximum of 40 mg a day, taken in divided doses 15-20 minutes before food.
Availability: NHS and private prescription.
Side effects: allergy, including skin rash.

M

Caution: in the elderly and in patients suffering from kidney failure.
Not to be used for: children, pregnant women, nursing mothers, during surgery, or for patients suffering from juvenile diabetes, liver or kidney disorders, stress, infections.
Not to be used with: ß-BLOCKERS, MAOIS, steroids, DIURETICS, alcohol, anti-coagulants, lipid-lowering agents, ASPIRIN, some antibiotics (RIFAMPICIN, sulphonamides, CHLORAMPHENICOL), GLUCAGON, CYCLOPHOSPHAMIDE.
Contains: GLIPIZIDE.
Other preparations:

---

minoxidil *see* Loniten

Mintec
(Bridge)

A green/ivory capsule used as an anti-spasm treatment for irritable bowel syndrome, spastic colon.

Dose: adults 1-2 tablets 3 times a day before meals.
Availability: NHS and over the counter.
Side effects:
Caution:
Not to be used for:
Not to be used with:
Contains: PEPPERMINT OIL.
Other preparations:

Mintezol
(MSD)

A pink, scored, chewable tablet supplied at a strength of 500 mg and used to treat worms and other associated conditions and infections.

Dose: under 60 kg body weight 25 mg per kg twice a day with food; over 60 kg body weight 1.5 g twice a day with food.
Availability: NHS, private prescription, over the counter.
Side effects: reduced alertness, stomach and brain disturbances,

M

allergy, liver damage, changes to sight and hearing, low blood pressure, bed wetting.
Caution: in patients suffering from liver or kidney disease.
Not to be used for:
Not to be used with: xanthine derivatives (such as THEOPHYLLINE).
Contains: THIABENDAZOLE.
Other preparations:

Minulet
(Wyeth)

A white tablet used as an oestrogen, progestogen contraceptive.

Dose: 1 tablet a day for 21 days starting on day 1 of the period.
Availability: NHS and private prescription.
Side effects: enlarged breasts, bloating and fluid retention, cramps, leg pains, mood change, reduction in sexual desire, headaches, nausea, vaginal erosion, discharge, and bleeding, weight gain, skin changes.
Caution: in patients suffering from high blood pressure, diabetes, vascular disorders, asthma, depression, kidney disease, multiple sclerosis, womb diseases. Your doctor may advise you not to smoke, to have regular examinations. You should stop treatment at the first sign of serious symptoms such as severe headache or jaundice. Treatment should be stopped before surgery.
Not to be used for: pregnant women, or for patients suffering from sickle-cell anaemia, history of heart disease or thrombosis, liver disorders, some cancers, undiagnosed vaginal bleeding, some ear, skin, and kidney disorders.
Not to be used with: RIFAMPICIN, TETRACYCLINES, GRISEOFULVIN, barbiturates, PHENYTOIN, PRIMIDONE, CARBAMAZEPINE, ETHOSUXIMIDE, CHLORAL HYDRATE, DICHLORALPHENAZONE.
Contains: ETHINYLOESTRADIOL, GESTODENE.
Other preparations:

Miraxid
(Fisons)

A white tablet supplied at a strength of 125 mg and used as a penicillin treatment for respiratory, ear, and urinary infections.

Dose: 2-4 tablets twice a day with food or drink.
Availability: NHS and private prescription.
Side effects: allergy, stomach disturbances.
Caution: in patients suffering from lymphatic leukaemia. Your doctor may advise regular liver and kidney checks.
Not to be used for: children or patients suffering from glandular fever or penicillin allergy.
Not to be used with:
Contains: PIVAMPICILLIN.
Other preparations: Miraxid Paediatric Syrup, Miraxid 450.

---

misoprostol *see* Cytotec

Mobiflex
(Roche)

A brown, five-sided tablet supplied at a strength of 20 mg and used as a NON-STEROID ANTI-INFLAMMATORY DRUG to treat osteoarthritis, rheumatoid arthritis.

Dose: 1 tablet a day.
Availability: NHS and private prescription.
Side effects: stomach disturbances, swelling, headache, rash, blood changes, liver changes, disturbances of the eyesight.
Caution: in the elderly or in patients suffering from liver or kidney disease.
Not to be used for: children, pregnant women, patients with a history of or suffering from peptic ulcer, gastro-intestinal bleeding, gastritis, allergy to aspirin or anti-inflammatory drugs.
Not to be used with: anti-coagulants, anti-diabetics taken by mouth, other non-steroid anti-inflammatory drugs, LITHIUM.
Contains: TENOXICAM.
Other preparations:

M

Moditen
(Squibb)

A pink tablet, yellow tablet, or white tablet according to strengths of 1 mg, 2.5 mg, 5 mg and used as a sedative to treat schizophrenia, behavioural problems, anxiety, tension, senile disorders.

Dose: adults 1-2 mg a day at first up to 2-4 mg a day if needed; senile elderly 1 mg a day adjusted as needed.
Availability: NHS and private prescription.
Side effects: muscle spasms, restlessness, hands shaking, dry mouth, urine retention, palpitations, low blood pressure, weight gain, changes in libido, low body temperature, breast swelling, menstrual changes, jaundice, blood and skin changes, drowsiness, rarely fits.
Caution: in the elderly, pregnant women, nursing mothers, and reduce or change to anti-Parkinson's disease drugs in patients showing tremor or rigidity.
Not to be used for: children or for patients suffering from phaeochromocytoma, kidney or liver failure, poor brain circulation, or severe heart weakness.
Not to be used with: alcohol, tranquillizers, pain killers, anti-hypertensives, anti-depressants, anti-convulsants, anti-diabetic drugs, LEVODOPA.
Contains: FLUPHENAZINE hydrochloride.
Other preparations: Moditen Enanthate

Modrasone
(Kirby-Warrick)

A cream used as a steroid treatment for skin disorders.

Dose: apply to the affected area 2-3 times a day.
Availability: NHS and private prescription.
Side effects: fluid retention, suppression of adrenal glands, thinning of the skin may occur.
Caution: use for short periods of time only.
Not to be used for: patients suffering from acne or any other skin infections caused by tuberculosis, ringworm, viruses, or fungi, or continuously especially in pregnant women.
Not to be used with:
Contains: ALCLOMETASONE DIPROPRIONATE.
Other preparations: Modrasone Ointment.

M

Modrenal
(Sterling Research Laboratories)

A pink/black capsule supplied at a strength of 60 mg and used as an adrenal inhibitor and hormone blocker.

Dose: 1 capsule 4 times a day for the first 3 days, then adjust as needed usually to 2-8 capsules a day up to a maximum of 16 capsules a day.
Availability: NHS and private prescription.
Side effects: flushing, nausea, running nose, diarrhoea.
Caution: in patients suffering from kidney or liver disease, stress. Your doctor may wish to ensure there is no tumour of the adrenal glands.
Not to be used for: children, pregnant women, or for patients suffering from severe kidney or liver disease.
Not to be used with: ALDOSTERONE antagonists (another hormone blocker), AMILORIDE, TRIAMTERENE.
Contains: TRILOSTANE.
Other preparations:

Moducren
(Morson)

A blue, scored, square tablet used as a ß-BLOCKER/DIURETIC/ potassium-sparing diuretic combination to treat high blood pressure.

Dose: 1-2 tablets a day.
Availability: NHS and private prescription.
Side effects: cold hands and feet, sleep disturbance, slow heart rate, tiredness, wheezing, heart failure, stomach upset, rash, sensitivity to light, blood changes, gout, cramps
Caution: in pregnant women, nursing mothers, and in patients suffering from diabetes, electrolyte changes, gout, kidney or liver disease, asthma.
Not to be used for: children, and for patients suffering from progressive or severe kidney failure, raised potassium levels, heart block or failure.
Not to be used with: potassium supplements, potassium-sparing diuretics, LITHIUM, DIGITALIS, anti-hypertensives, ACE INHIBITORS, VERAPAMIL, CLONIDINE withdrawal, some anti-arrhythmic drugs and anaesthetics, RESERPINE, ergot alkaloids, CIMETIDINE, sedatives, SYMPATHOMIMETICS, INDOMETHACIN.

M

Contains: HYDROCHLOROTHIAZIDE, AMILORIDE hydrochloride, TIMOLOL maleate.
Other preparations:

Moduret 25
(Morson)

A near-white, diamond-shaped tablet used as a potassium-sparing DIURETIC to treat high blood pressure.

Dose: 1-4 tablets a day in divided doses.
Availability: NHS and private prescription.
Side effects: rash, sensitivity to light, blood changes, gout.
Caution: in patients suffering from diabetes, electrolyte changes, gout, liver or kidney disease.
Not to be used for: children, pregnant women, nursing mothers, or for patients suffering from raised potassium levels, progressive or severe kidney failure.
Not to be used with: potassium supplements, potassium-sparing diuretics, DIGITALIS, LITHIUM, anti-hypertensives, ACE INHIBITORS.
Contains: AMILORIDE hydrochloride, HYDROCHLOROTHIAZIDE.
Other preparations:

Moduretic
(MSD)

A peach-coloured, diamond-shaped, scored tablet used as a potassium-sparing DIURETIC to treat high blood pressure, congestive heart failure, liver cirrhosis with fluid retention.

Dose: 1-2 tablets a day increasing to up to 4 tablets a day if needed.
Availability: NHS and private prescription.
Side effects: rash, sensitivity to light, blood changes, gout.
Caution: in patients suffering from diabetes, electrolyte changes, gout, kidney or liver damage
Not to be used for: children, pregnant women, nursing mothers, or for patients suffering from raised potassium levels, progressive or severe kidney failure.
Not to be used with: potassium supplements, potassium-sparing diuretics, DIGITALIS, LITHIUM, anti-hypertensives, ACE INHIBITORS.

M

Contains: AMILORIDE hydrochloride, HYDROCHLOROTHIAZIDE.
Other preparations: Moduretic Solution.

Mogadon
(Roche)

A white, scored tablet supplied at a strength of 5 mg and used as a sleeping tablet for the short-term treatment of sleeplessness where sedation during the day does not cause difficulty.

Dose: elderly ¹/₂ -1 tablet before going to bed; adults 1-2 tablets before going to bed.
Availability: NHS (when prescribed as a generic) and private prescription.
Side effects: drowsiness, confusion, unsteadiness, low blood pressure, rash, changes in vision, changes in libido, retention of urine. Risk of addiction increases with dose and length of treatment. May impair judgement.
Caution: in the elderly, pregnant women, nursing mothers, in women during labour, and in patients suffering from lung disorders, kidney or liver disorders. Avoid long-term use and withdraw gradually.
Not to be used for: children, or for patients suffering from acute lung diseases, some chronic lung diseases, some obsessional and psychotic diseases.
Not to be used with: alcohol, other tranquillizers, anti-convulsants.
Contains: NITRAZEPAM.
Other preparations: Mogadon Capsules, NITRAZEPAM, REMNOS (DDSA), SOMNITE (Norgine), SUREM (Galen), UNISOMNIA (Unigreg).

Molcer
(Wallace)

Drops as a wax softener to soften ear wax.

Dose: fill ear with the drops and plug with cotton wool; leave for 2 nights and then clean out.
Availability: NHS, private prescription, over the counter.
Side effects:
Caution:
Not to be used for: patients suffering from perforated ear drum.

M

Not to be used with:
Contains: sodium DOCUSATE.
Other preparations:

Molipaxin
(Roussel)

A pink, scored tablet supplied at a strength of 150 mg and used as a sedative to treat depression and anxiety.

Dose: adults 1 tablet a night at first or as divided doses daily after meals, then increase to 2 tablets a day after 1 week if needed, up to a maximum of 4 tablets a day; elderly $^2/_3$ tablet at night at first or as divided doses daily after meals up to a maximum of 2 tablets a day.
Availability: NHS and private prescription.
Side effects: drowsiness, dizziness, headache, penile erection.
Caution: in patients suffering from epilepsy, severe kidney or liver disease.
Not to be used for: children.
Not to be used with: muscle relaxants, anaesthetics, alcohol, sedatives, MAOIS, CLONIDINE.
Contains: TRAZODONE hydrochloride.
Other preparations: Molipaxin Capsules, Molipaxin Liquid.

Monistat
(Cilag)

A cream with applicator used as an anti-fungal treatment for thrush of the vulva, vagina, or penis.

Dose: 1 5 g application into the vagina for 14 nights in a row.
Availability: NHS and private prescription.
Side effects: mild burning or irritation.
Caution:
Not to be used for: children.
Not to be used with:
Contains: MICONAZOLE nitrate.
Other preparations: Monistat Pessaries.

M

Monit
(Stuart)

A white, scored tablet supplied at a strength of 20 mg and used as a nitrate for the prevention of angina.

Dose: 10 mg twice a day at first, then usually 20 mg 2-3 times a day.
Availability: NHS and private prescription.
Side effects: headache, flushes, dizziness.
Caution:
Not to be used for: children.
Not to be used with:
Contains: ISOSORBIDE MONONITRATE.
Other preparations: Monit LS.

Mono-Cedocard
(Tillotts)

An orange, scored tablet or a white, scored tablet according to strengths of 10 mg, 20 mg, 40 mg and used as a nitrate for the prevention of angina.

Dose: 20-120 mg a day in divided doses.
Availability: NHS and private prescription.
Side effects: headache, flushes, dizziness.
Caution:
Not to be used for: children.
Not to be used with:
Contains: ISOSORBIDE MONONITRATE.
Other preparations:

Monocor
(Cyanamid)

A pink tablet or a white tablet according to strengths of 5 mg, 10 mg and used as a ß-BLOCKER to treat angina, high blood pressure.

Dose: 10 mg once a day to a maximum of 20 mg a day.
Availability: NHS and private prescription.
Side effects: cold hands and feet, sleep disturbance, slow heart rate, tiredness, wheezing, heart failure, stomach upset.

M

Caution: in pregnant women, nursing mothers, and in patients suffering from diabetes, kidney or liver disorders, asthma. May need to be withdrawn before surgery. Withdraw gradually. Your doctor may advise additional treatment with diuretics or digitalis.

Not to be used for: children or for patients suffering from heart block or failure..

Not to be used with: VERAPAMIL, CLONIDINE withdrawal, some anti-arrhythmic drugs and anaesthetics, RESERPINE, some anti-hypertensives, ergot alkaloids, CIMETIDINE, sedatives, SYMPATHOMIMETICS, IN-DOMETHACIN.

Contains: BISOPROLOL fumarate.

Other preparations:

---

monosulfiram *see* Tetmosol

Monotrim
(Duphar)

A white, scored tablet supplied at strengths of100 mg, 200 mg and used as an antibiotic to treat infections, urine infections.

Dose: adults 200 mg twice a day, children 6 weeks-5 months 25 mg twice a day, 6 months-5 years 50 mg twice a day, 6-12 years 100 mg twice a day.

Availability: NHS and private prescription.

Side effects: stomach disturbances, skin reactions.

Caution: in the elderly and in patients suffering from kidney disease from folate deficiency (vitamin deficiency). Your doctor may advise regular blood tests.

Not to be used for: infants under 6 weeks, pregnant women, or for patients suffering from severe kidney disease where regular blood tests cannot be made.

Not to be used with:

Contains: TRIMETHOPRIM.

Other preparations: Monotrim Suspension, Monotrim Injection, IPRAL (Squibb), TIEMPE (DDSA), TRIMOGAL (Lagap).

M

Monovent
(Lagap)

A tablet supplied at a strength of 5 mg and used as a broncho-dilator to treat bronchial spasm brought on by asthma, bronchitis, or emphysema.

Dose: adults 1 tablet twice a day or every 8 hours; children under 7 years use syrup, 7-15 years half adult dose.
Availability: NHS and private prescription.
Side effects: shaking of the hands, dilation of the blood vessels, tension, headache.
Caution: in pregnant women and in diabetics, or in patients suffering from high blood pressure, abnormal heart rhythms, heart muscle disorders, overactive thyroid gland, angina.
Not to be used for:
Not to be used with: SYMPATHOMIMETICS.
Contains: TERBUTALINE sulphate.
Other preparations: Monovent SA, Monovent Syrup.

Monphytol
(LAB)

A paint used as an anti-fungal treatment for athlete's foot.

Dose: paint on to the affected area twice a day at first then once a week.
Availability: NHS, private prescription, over the counter.
Side effects:
Caution:
Not to be used for: children or pregnant women.
Not to be used with:
Contains: CHLORBUTOL, METHYL UNDECOANATE, SALICYLIC ACID, METHYL SALICYLATE, PROPYL SALICYLATE, PROPYL UNDECOANATE.
Other preparations:

---

morphine *see* **MST Continus, Nepenthe, Oramorph**

M

Motilium
(Janssen)

A white tablet supplied at a strength of 10 mg and used as an anti-emetic drug to treat acute nausea and vomiting.

Dose: adults 10-20 mg every 4-8 hours; elderly 10 mg every 4-8 hours at first then as adult dose; children use in rare situations in reduced doses.
Availability: NHS and private prescription.
Side effects: raised serum prolactin.
Caution:
Not to be used for: pregnant women.
Not to be used with:
Contains: DOMPERIDONE.
Other preparations: MOTILIUM SUSPENSION, MOTILIUM SUPPOSITORIES.

Motipress
(Squibb)

A yellow, triangular tablet used as a sedative to treat anxiety/depression.

Dose: 1 tablet a day at bedtime for up to 3 months.
Availability: NHS and private prescription.
Side effects: muscle spasms, restlessness, sleeplessness, dizziness, hands shaking, dry mouth, constipation, blurred vision, urine retention, palpitations, low blood pressure, weight change, changes in libido, low body temperature, breast swelling, menstrual changes, jaundice, blood and skin changes, drowsiness, rarely fits.
Caution: in patients with a history of epilepsy or brain damage, nursing mothers, and in patients suffering from heart disease, thyroid disease, epilepsy, diabetes, some other psychiatric conditions. Your doctor may advise regular blood and liver tests.
Not to be used for: children, pregnant women or for patients suffering from Parkinson's disease, heart attacks, liver disease, heart block.
Not to be used with: alcohol, ANTI-CHOLINERGICS, ADRENALINE, MAOIS, barbiturates tranquillizers, pain killers, anti-hypertensives, anti-depressants, anti-convulsants, anti-diabetic drugs, LEVODOPA.
Contains: FLUPHENAZINE hydrochloride, NORTRIPTYLINE
Other preparations:

M

Motival
(Squibb)

A triangular, pink tablet used as a sedative to treat anxiety/depression

Dose: 1 tablet 2-3 times a day for up to 3 months.
Availability: NHS and private prescription.
Side effects: muscle spasms, restlessness, sleeplessness, dizziness, hands shaking, dry mouth, constipation, blurred vision, urine retention, palpitations, low blood pressure, weight change, changes in libido, low body temperature, breast swelling, menstrual changes, jaundice, blood and skin changes, drowsiness, rarely fits.
Caution: in patients with a history of epilepsy or brain damage, nursing mothers, and in patients suffering from heart disease, thyroid disease, epilepsy, diabetes, some other psychiatric conditions. Your doctor may advise regular blood and liver tests.
Not to be used for: children, pregnant women or for patients suffering from Parkinson's disease, heart attacks, liver disease, heart block.
Not to be used with: alcohol, ANTI-CHOLINERGICS, ADRENALINE, MAOIS, barbiturates tranquillizers, pain killers, anti-hypertensives, anti-depressants, anti-convulsants, anti-diabetic drugs, LEVODOPA.
Contains: FLUPHENAZINE hydrochloride, NORTRIPTYLINE hydrochloride.
Other preparations:

Motrin *see* Brufen
(Upjohn)

Movelat
(Panpharma)

A cream and a gel used as an anti-inflammatory rub to relieve arthritis, fibrositis, soft tissue pain.

Dose: massage gently into the affected area up to 4 times a day.
Availability: NHS and private prescription.
Side effects: fluid retention, suppression of adrenal glands, thinning of the skin may occur.
Caution: use for short periods of time only.
Not to be used for: patients suffering from acne or any other skin infections caused by tuberculosis, ringworm, viruses, or fungi, or con-

M

tinuously especially in pregnant women.
Not to be used with:
Contains: STEROID EXTRACT, HEPARINOID, SALICYLIC ACID.
Other preparations:

MST Continus
(Napp)

A brown tablet, purple tablet, orange tablet, or grey tablet according to strengths of 10 mg, 30 mg, 60 mg, 100 mg and used as an opiate for the prolonged relief of severe pain.

Dose: 10-20 mg twice a day at first, then as advised by physician.
Availability: controlled drug.
Side effects: tolerance, addiction, constipation, nausea, vomiting.
Caution: in the elderly and in patients suffering from kidney or liver disease and underactive thyroid.
Not to be used for: children, pregnant women, or patients suffering from respiratory depression or blocked airways.
Not to be used with: MAOIS, sedatives, alcohol.
Contains: MORPHINE sulphate.
Other preparations:

Mucaine
(Wyeth)

A white liquid used as an antacid plus local anaesthetic to treat oesophagitis and hiatus hernia.

Dose: adults 5-10 ml 3-4 times a day before meals.
Availability: NHS and private prescription.
Side effects: occasional constipation.
Caution:
Not to be used for: children.
Not to be used with: TETRACYCLINE antibiotics.
Contains: OXETHAZAINE, ALUMINIUM HYDROXIDE, MAGNESIUM HYDROXIDE.
Other preparations:

M

Mucodyne
(Rorer)

A syrup supplied at a strength of 250 mg and used as a mucus softener to clear phlegm, running nose, glue ear in children.

Dose: adults 3 5 ml teaspoonsful 3 times a day reducing to 2 teaspoonsful; children over 2 years use paediatric syrup.
Availability: private prescription only.
Side effects: stomach disturbance, nausea, rash.
Caution: in pregnant women and in patients with a history of peptic ulcer.
Not to be used for: children under 2 years or for patients suffering from peptic ulcer.
Not to be used with:
Contains: CARBOCISTEINE.
Other preparations: Mucodyne Capsules, Mucodyne Paediatric.

Mucogel *see* Maalox
(Pharmax)

Multilind
(Squibb)

An ointment used as an anti-fungal treatment for skin and mucous membrane thrush, especially that associated with nappy rash.

Dose: apply freely to the affected area 2-4 times a day.
Availability: NHS and private prescription.
Side effects:
Caution:
Not to be used for:
Not to be used with:
Contains: NYSTATIN, ZINC OXIDE.
Other preparations:

M

Multivite
(Duncan, Flockhart)

A brown pellet used as a multivitamin treat ment for vitamin deficiencies.

Dose: adults 2 pellets a day; children 1 pellet a day.
Availability: private prescription, over the counter.
Side effects:
Caution:
Not to be used for:
Not to be used with:
Contains: VITAMIN A, THIAMINE, ASCORBIC ACID, CALCIFEROL.
Other preparations:

Munovir
(Burgess)

A white tablet supplied at a strength of 500 mg and used as an antiviral treatment for genital herpes and warts.

Dose: herpes 8 tablets a day for 7-14 days; warts 6 tablets a day for 14-28 days.
Availability: NHS and private prescription.
Side effects: increased levels of uric acid.
Caution: in patients suffering from kidney disease, gout, raised uric acid levels.
Not to be used for: children.
Not to be used with:
Contains: INOSINE PRANOBEX.
Other preparations:

Munovir
(Leo)

A white tablet supplied at a strength of 500 mg and used to treat herpes-type infections

Dose: 8 tablets a day for 7-14 days.
Availability: NHS
Side effects: raised levels of uric acid.
Caution: care in patients suffering from gout, kidney disease, or hyperuricaemia.

M

Not to be used for: for children.
Not to be used with:
Contains: INOSINE PRANOBEX.
Other preparations:

---

mupirocin *see* Bactroban Nasal

Muripsin
(Norgine)

An oblong, orange tablet used as a source of hydrochloric acid/proteolytic enzyme to treat low stomach acid.

Dose: adults 1-2 with meals; children as advised.
Availability: NHS and private prescription
Side effects:
Caution:
Not to be used for:
Not to be used with:
Contains: GLUTAMIC ACID HYDROCHLORIDE, PEPSIN.
Other preparations:

Myambutol
(Lederle)

A yellow tablet or a grey tablet according to strengths of 100 mg, 400 mg and used as an anti-tubercular, additional treatment and preventive drug for tuberculosis.

Dose: adults 15 mg per kg body weight once a day; children treatment 25 mg per kg body weight once a day for 60 days, then 15 mg per kg body weight once a day; prevention 15 mg per kg body weight once a day.
Availability: NHS and private prescription.
Side effects: visual changes, eye inflammation.
Caution: in nursing mothers and in patients suffering from kidney disease. Eyes should be checked regularly.
Not to be used for: patients suffering from inflamation of the optic

M

nerve.
Not to be used with:
Contains: ETHAMBUTOL.
Other preparations:

Mycardol
(Winthrop)

A white, scored tablet supplied at a strength of 30 mg and used as a nitrate in addition to glyceryl trintrate in the treatment of angina.

Dose: 2 tablets 3-4 times a day.
Availability: NHS and private prescription.
Side effects: headache, flushes, dizziness.
Caution:
Not to be used for: children.
Not to be used with:
Contains: PENTAERYTHRITOL TETRANITRATE.
Other preparations:

Mycifradin
(Upjohn)

A powder in a vial supplied at a strength of 350 mg and used as an aminoglycoside antibiotic to treat skin and mucous membrane infections.

Dose: as advised by the physician.
Availability: NHS and private prescription.
Side effects: hearing damage, sensitization.
Caution: in patients with large areas of affected skin.
Not to be used for:
Not to be used with:
Contains: NEOMYCIN sulphate.
Other preparations:

M

Myciguent *see* Neomycin
(Upjohn)

Mydriacyl
(Alcon)

Drops used as an ANTI-CHOLINERGIC pupil dilator.

Dose: 1-2 drops into the eye with 1-5 minutes between each drop, then a further drop into the eye after 30 minutes if needed.
Availability: NHS and private prescription.
Side effects: temporary smarting, dry mouth, blurred vision, aversion to light, rapid heart rate, headache, mental and behavioural changes, stinging.
Caution: in infants and in patients where the eye pressure is not known.
Not to be used for: patients suffering from narrow angle glaucoma or who wear soft contact lenses.
Not to be used with:
Contains: TROPICAMIDE.
Other preparations:

Mydrilate
(Boehringer Ingelheim)

Drops used as an ANTI-CHOLINERGIC pupil dilator

Dose: adults 1 drop into the eye; children reduced dose.
Availability: NHS and private prescription.
Side effects: systemic anti-cholinergic effects.
Caution: in patients suffering from raised eye pressure, enlarged prostate, or with coronary insufficiency.
Not to be used for: patients suffering from bowel paralysis.
Not to be used with:
Contains: CYCLOPENTOLATE HYDROCHLORIDE.
Other preparations:

Mynah
(Lederle)

A white tablet, yellow tablet, orange tablet, or pink tablet according to strengths and used as an anti-tuberculous drug combination for the prevention and treatment of tuberculosis.

Dose: 15 mg per kg body weight of ETHAMBUTOL plus 300 mg ISONIAZID once a day.
Availability: NHS and private prescription.
Side effects: visual changes, eye inflammation, hepatitis, sleeplessness, restlessness, rheumatic disorders.
Caution: in nursing mothers, in patients with a history of epilepsy, or patients suffering kidney or liver disease, chronic alcoholism. Eyes should be tested regularly.
Not to be used for: children or or patients suffering from inflammation of the optic nerve.
Not to be used with: alcohol.
Contains: ETHAMBUTOL, ISONIAZID.
Other preparations:

Myotonine
(Glenwood)

A pale-blue tablet supplied at strengths of 10 mg, 25 mg and used as a cholinergic drug to treat bowel paralysis or partial paralysis, urinary retention.

Dose: adults 10-25 mg 3-4 times a day; children in proportion to a 70 kg adult.
Availability: NHS and private prescription.
Side effects: nausea, vomiting, urination, abdominal cramps, blurred vision, sweating.
Caution:
Not to be used for: pregnant women or for patients suffering from asthma, overactive thyroid, urinary or gastro-intestinal blockage, marked vagotonia, slow heart rate, recent heart attacks, epilepsy, Parkinson's disease.
Not to be used with:
Contains: BETHANECHOL CHLORIDE.
Other preparations:

M Mysoline
(ICI)

A white, scored tablet supplied at a strength of 250 mg and used as an anti-convulsant to treat epilepsy

Dose: $1/2$ a tablet at night at first, increasing every 3 days by $1/2$ a tablet to 2 tablets a day, then increase by 1 tablet at a time to 6 tablets a day; children same as adults at first increasing by $1/2$ tablet a day. Lower maximum doses for children.

Availability: NHS and private prescription.

Side effects: drowsiness, hangover, dizziness, allergies, headache, confusion, excitement.

Caution: in patients suffering from kidney or lung disease. Dependence (addiction) may develop.

Not to be used for: children, young adults, pregnant women, nursing mothers, the elderly, patients with a history of drug or alcohol abuse, or suffering from porphyria (a rare blood disorder), or in the management of pain.

Not to be used with: anti-coagulants (blood-thinning drugs), alcohol, other tranquillizers, steroids, the contraceptive pill, GRISEOFULVIN, RIFAMPICIN, PHENYTOIN, METRONIDAZOLE, CHLORAMPHENICOL.

Contains: PRIMIDONE.

Other preparations: Mysoline Suspension.

Mysteclin *see* Tetracycline
(Squibb)

---

n-hexyl nicotinate *see* Transvasin

---

nabilone *see* Cesamet

---

nabumetone *see* Relifex

Nacton Forte
(Bencard)

An orange tablet supplied at a strength of 4 mg and used as an antispasm, ANTI-CHOLINERGIC treatment for spasm, acidity, ulcers.

N

Dose: 4 mg 3 times a day and at bedtime.
Availability: NHS and private prescription.
Side effects: blurred vision, confusion, dry mouth.
Caution:
Not to be used for: children, or for patients suffering from glaucoma, inflammatory bowel disease, intestinal obstruction, enlarged prostate.
Not to be used with:
Contains: POLDINE METHYLSULPHATE.
Other preparations: Nacton 2 mg.

---

nadolol *see* Corgard, Corgaretic 40

---

naftidrofuryl oxalate *see* Praxilene

Nalcrom
(Fisons)

A clear capsule supplied at a strength of 100 mg and used as an anti-allergy drug to treat allergies to foods.

Dose: adults 2 capsules 4 times a day before meals; children over 2 years 1 capsule 4 times a day before meals.
Availability: NHS and private prescription.
Side effects: rash, pain in the joints, nausea.
Caution:
Not to be used for: for infants under 2 years.
Not to be used with:
Contains: SODIUM CROMOGLYCATE.
Other preparations:

---

nalidixic acid *see* Mictral, Negram

N

Nalorex
(Du Pont)

A mottled, orange, scored tablet supplied at a strength of 50 mg and used as a narcotic antagonist as a treatment for patients who have been detoxified from opioid dependency.

Dose: ¹/₂ tablet a day at first, then 1 tablet a day for 3 months.
Availability: NHS and private prescription.
Side effects: vomiting, drowsiness, dizziness, stomach cramps, joint and muscle pain.
Caution: in patients suffering from liver or kidney disease.
Not to be used for: patients suffering from acute liver disease, liver failure, or current dependence on opiates.
Not to be used with:
Contains: NALTREXONE HYDROCHLORIDE.
Other preparations:

---

naltrexone hydrochloride *see* Nalorex

---

naphozoline hydrochloride *see* Vasocon-A

Naprosyn
(Syntex)

A yellow, scored tablet or a yellow, oblong, scored tablet according to strengths of 250 mg, 500 mg and used as a NON-STEROID ANTI-INFLAMMATORY DRUG to treat rheumatoid arthritis, osteoarthritis, ankylosing spondylitis, acute gout.

Dose: adults 250-500 mg twice a day at first; for gout 750 mg at first then 250 mg every 8 hours. Children 5-12 years 10 mg per kg body weight a day in 2 divided doses.
Availability: NHS and private prescription.
Side effects: rash, stomach intolerance, headache, tinnitus, vertigo, blood changes.
Caution: in the elderly, pregnant women, nursing mothers, and in patients suffering from kidney or liver disease, asthma, or a history of

N

gastro-intestinal lesions.

Not to be used for: children under 5 years, or for patients suffering from peptic ulcer or allergy to aspirin or non-steroid anti-inflammatory drugs.

Not to be used with: anti-coagulants, hydantoins, sulphonyureas, LITHIUM, ß-BLOCKERS, METHOTREXATE, PROBENECID, FRUSEMIDE.

Contains: naproxen.

Other preparations: Naprosyn Suspension, Naprosyn Granules, Naprosyn Suppositories, LARAFLEX (Lagap)

---

naproxen *see* **Naprosyn, Synflex**

Nardil
(Parke-Davis)

An orange tablet supplied at a strength of 15 mg and used as an MAOI to treat depression, phobias.

Dose: 1 tablet 3 times a day at first reducing gradually according to response.

Availability: NHS and private prescription.

Side effects: severe high blood pressure reactions with certain foods, sleeplessness, low blood pressure, dizziness, drowsiness, weakness, dry mouth, constipation, stomach upset, blurred vision, urinary difficulties, ankle swelling, rash, jaundice, weight gain, confusion, sexual desire changes.

Caution: in the elderly and in patients suffering from epilepsy.

Not to be used for: children, or for patients suffering from liver disease, blood changes, heart disease, phaeochromocytoma, overactive thyroid, brain artery disease.

Not to be used with: amphetamines or similar SYMPATHOMIMETIC drugs, TRICYCLIC antidepressants, PETHIDINE and other narcotics, some cough mixtures and appetite supressants containing sympathomimetics. Barbiturates, sedatives, alcohol, and anti-diabetics may be enhanced. ANTI-CHOLINERGIC side effects are increased. Cheese, Bovril, Oxo, meat extracts, broad beans, banana, Marmite, yeast extracts, wine, beer, other alcohol, pickled herrings, vegetable proteins. (Up to 14 days after cessation.)

Contains: PHENELZINE SULPHATE.

Other preparations:

N

Narphen
(SNP)

A white, scored tablet supplied at a strength of 5 mg and used as an opiate to control severe, prolonged pain including biliary and pancreatic pain.

Dose: 1 tablet every 4-6 hours either swallowed or under the tongue. No single dose should exceed 4 tablets.
Availability: controlled drug.
Side effects: tolerance, addiction, nausea, dizziness, constipation.
Caution: in the elderly, pregnant women, women in labour, or patients suffering from underactive thyroid, or liver or kidney disease.
Not to be used for: children or for patients in coma, or suffering from respiratory depression. blocked airways, acute alcoholism, epilepsy.
Not to be used with: MAOIS, sedatives, alcohol.
Contains: PHENAZOCINE HYDROBROMIDE.
Other preparations:

Naseptin
(ICI)

A cream used as an antibacterial treatment for infections of the nose.

Dose: apply into each nostril 2-4 times a day.
Availability: NHS and private prescription.
Side effects: sensitive skin.
Caution:
Not to be used for:
Not to be used with:
Contains: CHLORHEXIDINE HYDROCHLORIDE, NEOMYCIN sulphate.
Other preparations:

---

natamycin *see* **Pimafucin, Pimaficin 2¹/2%, Pimafucin Cream**

Natrilix
(Servier)

A pink tablet supplied at a strength of 2.5 mg and used as a vasorelaxant to treat high blood pressure.

Dose: 1 tablet in the morning.
Availability: NHS and private prescription.
Side effects: low potassium level, nausea, headache.
Caution: in pregnant women and in patients suffering from severe kidney or liver disease.
Not to be used for: children.
Not to be used with: DIURETICS.
Contains: INDAPAMIDE HEMIHYDRATE.
Other preparations:

Navidrex
(Ciba)

A white, scored tablet supplied at a strength of 0.5 mg and used as a DIURETIC to treat heart failure, toxaemia of pregnancy, fluid retention, high blood pressure.

Dose: adults 1/2 -2 tablets a day, up to 3 tablets a day if needed; children as advised by physician.
Availability: NHS and private prescription.
Side effects: low potassium level, rash, sensitivity to light, blood changes, gout, tiredness.
Caution: in pregnant women, nursing mothers, and in patients suffering from diabetes, kidney or liver disease, gout. Potassium supplements may be needed.
Not to be used for: in patients suffering from anuria or severe kidney failure.
Not to be used with: DIGITALIS, LITHIUM, anti-hypertensives.
Contains: CYCLOPENTHIAZIDE.
Other preparations:

Navidrex-K
(Ciba)

An reddish-yellow tablet used as a DIURETIC with potassium supplement to treat heart failure, toxaemia of pregnancy, fluid retention, high blood pressure where a potassium supplement is needed.

N

Dose: adults usually 1-4 tablets a day, up to 6 tablets a day; children as advised by the physician.
Availability: NHS and private prescription.
Side effects: rash, sensitivity to light, blood changes, gout, tiredness.
Caution: in pregnant women, nursing mothers, and in patients suffering from diabetes, kidney or liver disease, gout.
Not to be used for: patients suffering from severe kidney failure, raised potassium levels, Addison's disease.
Not to be used with: DIGITALIS, LITHIUM, potassium-sparing diuretics, anti-hypertensives.
Contains: CYCLOPENTHIAZIDE, POTASSIUM CHLORIDE.
Other preparations:

Naxogin 500
(Farmitalia CE)

A white, scored tablet supplied at a strength of 500 mg and used as an anti-protozoal treatment for trichomonal inflammation of the vagina, acute ulcerative gingivitis.

Dose: 2 g with the main meal of the day as a single dose; for gingivitis 1 tablet twice a day for 2 days.
Availability: NHS, private prescription, and over the counter.
Side effects: stomach upset.
Caution: in pregnant women.
Not to be used for: children, nursing mothers, or for patients suffering from kidney weakness or brain disease.
Not to be used with: alcohol.
Contains: NIMORAZOLE.
Other preparations:

---

nefopam hydrochloride *see* Acupan

Negram
(Sterling Research Laboratories)

A pale-brown tablet supplied at a strength of 500 mg and used as an antiseptic to treat urinary and stomach infections.

N

Dose: adults acute infections 2 tablets 4 times a day for at least 7 days, chronic infections 1-2 tablets 4 times a day; children 3 months-12 years up to 50 mg per kg body weight a day.
Availability: NHS and private prescription.
Side effects: stomach upset, disturbed vision, rash, blood changes, seizures.
Caution: in nursing mothers and in patients suffering from liver or kidney disease. Keep out of the sunlight.
Not to be used for: infants under 3 months or for patients with a history of convulsions.
Not to be used with: anti-coagulants, PROBENECID.
Contains: NALIDIXIC ACID.
Other preparations: Negram Suspension, URIBEN (RP Drugs).

Neo-Cortef
(Upjohn)

Drops used as an antibiotic, corticosteroid, and aminoglycoside antibiotic treatment for inflamation of the outer ear or infected inflammation of the eye.

Dose: 1-2 drops into the ear or eye at least 3 times a day.
Availability: NHS and private prescription.
Side effects: additional infection, sensitization, fungal infection, thinning cornea, cataract, rise in eye pressure.
Caution: in pregnant women and infants — avoid using over extended periods.
Not to be used for: patients suffering from perforated ear drum, or viral, tubercular, fungal, or acute weeping infections, glaucoma.
Not to be used with:
Contains: NEOMYCIN sulphate, HYDROCORTISONE acetate.
Other preparations: Neo-Cortef Ointment.

Neo-Medrone Cream
(Upjohn)

A cream used as an anti-bacterial, steroid treatment for allergic and other skin disorders where there is also inflammation and infection.

Dose: apply to the affected area 1-3 times a day.

N

Availability: NHS and private prescription.
Side effects: fluid retention, suppression of adrenal glands, thinning of the skin may occur.
Caution: use for short periods of time only.
Not to be used for: patients suffering from acne or any other skin infections caused by tuberculosis, ringworm, viruses, or fungi, or continuously especially in pregnant women.
Not to be used with:
Contains: METHYLPREDNISOLONE acetate, NEOMYCIN sulphate.
Other preparations:

Neo-Medrone Lotion
(Upjohn)

A lotion used as a corticosteroid, anti-bacterial, skin softener. to treat acne, dermatitis.

Dose: apply a little of the lotion to the affected area 1-2 times a day.
Availability: NHS
Side effects: hearing damage, sensitization, fluid retention, suppression of adrenal glands, thinning of the skin may occur..
Caution: care in pregnant women — use for short periods of time only.
Not to be used for: patients suffering from acne or any other skin infections caused by tuberculosis, ringworm, viruses, or fungi, or continuously especially in pregnant women.
Not to be used with:
Contains: METHYLPREDNISOLONE acetate, NEOMYCIN sulphate, ALUMINIUM CHLORHYDROXIDE, SULPHUR.
Other preparations:

Neo-Mercazole
(Nicholas)

A pink tablet supplied at strengths of 5 mg, 20 mg and used as an anti-thyroid treatment for thyrotoxicosis.

Dose: adults 20-60 mg a day at first in 2-3 divided doses, then 5-15 mg a day for 6-18 months, or continue with 20-60 mg a day with thyroxine; children 5-15 mg a day at first in divided doses.
Availability: NHS and private prescription.

N

Side effects: rash, headache, nausea, joint pain, bone marrow depression; inform the physician of sore throat, mouth ulcer.
Caution: in pregnant women. Your doctor may advise regular blood tests.
Not to be used for: nursing mothers or patients with a blocked trachea.
Not to be used with:
Contains: CARBIMAZOLE.
Other preparations:

Neo-Naclex
(Duncan, Flockhart)

A white, scored tablet supplied at a strength of 5 mg and used as a DIURETIC to treat fluid retention, high blood pressure, congestive heart failure, nephrotic syndrome (a kidney disease).

Dose: adults fluid retention 1-2 tablets once a day at first then $^1/_2$ -1 tablet from time to time, high blood pressure $^1/_2$-1 tablet a day; children fluid retention in proportion to the dose for a 70 kg adult.
Availability: NHS and private prescription.
Side effects: low potassium levels, rash, sensitivity to light, blood changes, gout, impotence.
Caution: in pregnant women, nursing mothers, and in patients suffering from diabetes, kidney or liver disease, gout. Potassium supplements may be needed.
Not to be used for: patients suffering from severe kidney failure, raised calcium levels.
Not to be used with: DIGITALIS, LITHIUM, anti-hypertensives.
Contains: BENDROFLUAZIDE.
Other preparations:

Neo-Naclex-K
(Duncan, Flockhart)

A double-layered pink/white tablet used as a DIURETIC with potassium supplement to treat high blood pressure, chronic fluid retention.

Dose: adults high blood pressure 1-4 tablets a day, fluid retention 2 tablets a day increasing to 4 tablets a day if needed then 1-2 tablets

N

from time to time; children fluid retention in proportion to dose for 70 kg adult.
Availability: NHS and private prescription.
Side effects: rash, sensitivity to light, blood changes gout, impotence.
Caution: in pregnant women, nursing mothers, and in patients suffering from diabetes, liver or kidney disease, gout.
Not to be used for: patients suffering from severe kidney failure, raised calcium or potassium levels, Addison's disease.
Not to be used with: DIGITALIS, LITHIUM, potassium sparing diuretics, antihypertensives, anti-diabetic drugs.
Contains: BENDROFLUAZIDE, POTASSIUM CHLORIDE.
Other preparations:

Neocon 1/35
(Cilag)

A peach-coloured tablet used as an oestrogen, progestogen contraceptive.

Dose: 1 tablet a day for 21 days starting on day 5 of the period.
Availability: NHS and private prescription.
Side effects: enlarged breasts, bloating and fluid retention, cramps, leg pains, mood change, reduction in sexual desire, headaches, nausea, vaginal erosion, discharge, and bleeding, weight gain, skin changes.
Caution: in patients suffering from high blood pressure, diabetes, vascular disorders, asthma, depression, kidney disease, multiple sclerosis, womb diseases. Your doctor may advise you not to smoke, to have regular examinations. You should stop treatment at the first sign of serious symptoms such as severe headache or jaundice. Treatment should be stopped before surgery.
Not to be used for: pregnant women, or for patients suffering from sickle-cell anaemia, history of heart disease or thrombosis, liver disorders, some cancers, undiagnosed vaginal bleeding, some ear, skin, and kidney disorders.
Not to be used with: RIFAMPICIN, TETRACYCLINES, GRISEOFULVIN, barbiturates, PHENYTOIN, PRIMIDONE, CARBAMAZEPINE, ETHOSUXIMIDE, CHLORAL HYDRATE, DICHLORALPHENAZONE.
Contains: ETHINYLOESTRADIOL, NORETHISTERONE.
Other preparations:

N

Neogest
(Schering)

A brown tablet used as a progesterone contraceptive.

Dose: 1 tablet at the same time every day starting on day 1 of the period.
Availability: NHS and private prescription.
Side effects: irregular bleeding, breast discomfort, acne, headache.
Caution: in patients suffering from high blood pressure, tendency to thrombosis, migraine, liver abnormalities, ovarian cysts. Your doctor may advise regular check-ups.
Not to be used for: pregnant women, or for patients suffering from severe heart or artery disease, benign liver tumours, vaginal bleeding, previous ectopic pregnancy.
Not to be used with: barbiturates, PHENYTOIN, PRIMIDONE, CARBAMAZEPINE, CHLORAL HYDRATE, DICHLORALPHENAZONE, ETHOSUXIMIDE, RIFAMPICIN, GLUTETHIMIDE, CHLORPROMAZINE, MEPROBAMATE, GRISEOFULVIN.
Contains: NORGESTREL.
Other preparations:

Neomycin
(SNP)

Drops used as a aminoglycoside antibiotic to treat bacterial infections of the eye.

Dose: adults 1 or more drops into the eye as needed; children 1 drop into the eye as needed.
Availability: NHS and private prescription.
Side effects:
Caution:
Not to be used for:
Not to be used with:
Contains: NEOMYCIN sulphate.
Other preparations: MYCIGUENT (Upjohn).

---

neomycin *see* **Audicort, Cicatrin, Dexa-Rhinaspray, Gregoderm, Graneodin, Hydroderm, Maxitrol, Mycifradin, Myciguent, Naseptin, Neo-Cortef, Neo-Medrone Cream, Neo-**

Medrone Lotion, Neomycin, Neosporin, Nivemycin, Oto-sporin, Polybactrin, Tri-Adcortyl, Tri-Adcortyl Otic, Tricicatrin, Tribiotic, Uniroid, Vibrocil

Neophryn
(Winthrop)

A spray or drops used as a SYMPATHOMIMETIC to clear blocked nose.

Dose: adults 2-3 drops or 2 sprays into each nostril every 3-4 hours; children over 7 years1-2 drops into each nostril every 3-4 hours..
Availability: private prescription and over the counter.
Side effects:
Caution: in patients suffering from cardiovascular disease or overactive thyroid. Do not use for longer than 7 days.
Not to be used for: children under 7 years.
Not to be used with: MAOIS.
Contains: PHENYLEPHRINE hydrochloride.
Other preparations:

Neosporin
(Calmic)

Drops used as a peptide and aminoglycoside antibiotic to treat eye infections, prevention of eye infections before and after eye operations, removal of foreign bodies from the eye.

Dose: 1-2 drops 2-4 times a day or more often if needed.
Availability: NHS and private prescription.
Side effects:
Caution:
Not to be used for:
Not to be used with:
Contains: POLYMYXIN B SULPHATE, NEOMYCIN sulphate, GRAMICIDIN.
Other preparations:

neostigmine *see* **Prostigimin**

N

Nepenthe
(Evans)

An opiate solution used as an additional treatment for the relief of severe pain.

Dose: adults 1-2 ml not more often than every 4 hours; children 1-5 years 0.25-0.5 ml, 6-12 years 0.5-1 ml not more often than every 4 hours.
Availability: controlled drug.
Side effects: tolerance, addiction, nausea, vomiting, constipation.
Caution: in the elderly,pregnant women, women in labour, and in patients suffering from liver disease or underactive thyroid. The solution should be stored in a tightly sealed container in a cool place.
Not to be used for: children under 1 year, or for patients suffering from respiratory depression or blocked airways.
Not to be used with: other opiates, MAOIS, sedatives, alcohol.
Contains: anhydrous MORPHINE in solution.
Other preparations: Nepenthe Injection

Nephril
(Pfizer)

A white, scored tablet supplied at a strength of 1 mg and used as a DIURETIC to treat fluid retention, high blood pressure.

Dose: 1-4 tablets a day.
Availability: NHS and private prescription.
Side effects: low potassium levels, rash, sensitivity to light, blood changes, gout, tiredness.
Caution: in pregnant women, nursing mothers, and in patients suffering from diabetes, liver or kidney disease, gout. Potassium supplement may be needed.
Not to be used for: children or patients suffering from kidney failure.
Not to be used with: DIGITALIS, LITHIUM, anti-hypertensives.
Contains: POLYTHIAZIDE.
Other preparations:

Nericur
(Schering)

N

A gel used as an anti-bacterial, skin softener to treat acne.

Dose: wash and dry the affected area, then apply the gel once a day.
Availability: NHS, private prescription, over the counter.
Side effects: irritation, peeling.
Caution: keep out of the eyes, nose, mouth.
Not to be used for: children.
Not to be used with:
Contains: BENZOYL PEROXIDE.
Other preparations:

Nerisone
(Schering)

A cream used as a steroid treatment for skin disorders.

Dose: apply to the affected area 2-3 times a day reducing to once a day as soon as possible.
Availability: NHS and private prescription.
Side effects: fluid retention, suppression of adrenal glands, thinning of the skin may occur.
Caution: do not use for longer than 3 weeks for children under 4 years; do not use for prolonged periods for other patients.
Not to be used for: patients suffering from acne or any other skin infections caused by tuberculosis, ringworm, viruses, or fungi, or continuously especially in pregnant women.
Not to be used with:
Contains: DIFLUCORTOLONE VALERATE.
Other preparations: Nerisone Oily Cream, Nerisone Ointment, Nerisone Forte.

Neulactil
(M & B)

A yellow, scored tablet supplied at strengths of 2.5 mg, 10 mg, 25 mg and used as a sedative to treat behavioural and character problems, schizophrenia, anxiety, tension, agitation.

Dose: elderly 15-30 mg a day at first; adults 15-75 mg a day at first; children as advised by physician.

N

Availability: NHS and private prescription.
Side effects: muscle spasms, restlessness, hands shaking, dry mouth, urine retention, palpitations, low blood pressure, weight gain, changes in libido, low body temperature, breast swelling, menstrual changes, jaundice, blood and skin changes, drowsiness, rarely fits.
Caution: in pregnant women, nursing mothers, and in patients suffering from liver disease, Parkinson's disease, cardiovascular disease.
Not to be used for: unconscious patients or for patients suffering from bone marrow depression
Not to be used with: alcohol, tranquillizers, pain killers, anti-hypertensives, anti-depressants, anti-convulsants, anti-diabetic drugs, LEVODOPA.
Contains: PERICYAZINE.
Other preparations: Neulactil Forte Syrup.

---

nicardipine *see* Cardene

---

niclosamide *see* Yomesan

---

nicofuranose *see* Bradilan

Nicorette
(Lundbeck)

Chewing gum supplied at strengths of 2 mg, 4 mg and used as an alkaloid to end smoking addiction.

Dose: 1 when required.
Availability: private prescription only.
Side effects: addiction, hiccoughs, indigestion, irritated throat.
Caution: in patients suffering from coronary disease, angina, gastritis, peptic ulcer.
Not to be used for: children or pregnant women.
Not to be used with:

Contains: NICOTINE.
Other preparations:

---

nicotinamide *see* Abidec, Allbee with C, Apisate, BC 500, BC 500 with Iron, Becosym, Calcimax, Concavit, Fefol-Vit Spansule, Fesovit Spansule, Fesovit Z Spansule, Galfervit, Givitol, Ketovite, Lipoflavonoid, Lipotriad, Octovit, Orovite, Orovite 7, Polyvite, Pregnavite Forte F, Surbex T, Tonivitan B, Verdiviton, Villescon

---

nicotine *see* Nicorette

---

nicotinic acid *see* Tonivitan

---

nicotinyl alcohol tartrate *see* Ronicol

---

nicoumalone *see* Sinthrome

---

nifedipine *see* Adalat, Adalat Retard, Beta Adalat, Tenif

Niferex
(Tillotts)

An elixir used as an iron supplement to treat iron-deficiency anaemia.

Dose: adults treatment 1 5 ml teaspoonful 1-2 times a day, prevention $1/2$ teaspoonful a day; children 0-2 years 1 drop per 0.45 kg bodyweight a day, 2-6 years $1/2$ 5 ml teaspoonful a day, 6-12 years 1 teaspoonful a day.

N

Availability: NHS, private prescription, and over the counter.
Side effects:
Caution: in patients with a history of peptic ulcer.
Not to be used for:
Not to be used with: TETRACYCLINES.
Contains: POLYSACCHARIDE-IRON COMPLEX.
Other preparations: Niferex Tablets, Niferex-150.

Nilstim
(De Witt)

A green tablet used as a bulking agent to treat obesity.

Dose: 2 tablets to be broken into pieces and taken with liquid 15 minutes before meals.
Availability: NHS, private prescription, and over the counter.
Side effects:
Caution:
Not to be used for: children or for patients suffering from blocked intestine.
Not to be used with:
Contains: CELLULOSE, METHYLCELLULOSE.
Other preparations:

---

nimorazole *see* Naxogin 500

Nitoman
(Roche)

A yellow/buff, scored tablet supplied at a strength of 25 mg and used as a sedative to treat Huntington's chorea, hemiballismus, senile chorea (movement disorders)

Dose: 1 tablet 3 times a day at first increasing if needed by 1 tablet a day every 3-4 days to a maximum of 8 tablets a day.
Availability: NHS and private prescription.
Side effects: drowsiness, depression, low blood presure on standing, tremor, rigidity.

N

Caution: in pregnant women.
Not to be used for: children or for nursing mothers.
Not to be used with: RESERPINE, LEVOPODA, MAOIS.
Contains: TETRABENAZINE.
Other preparations:

Nitrados
(Berk)

A white, scored tablet supplied at a strength of 5 mg and used as a sleeping tablet. for the short-term treatment of sleeplessness where sedation during the day does not cause difficulty.

Dose: elderly ¹/₂ -1 tablet before going to bed; adults 1-2 tablets before going to bed.
Availability: NHS (when prescribed as a generic) and private prescription.
Side effects: drowsiness, confusion, unsteadiness, low blood pressure, rash, changes in vision, changes in libido, retention of urine. Risk of addiction increases with dose and length of treatment. May impair judgement.
Caution: in the elderly, pregnant women, nursing mothers, in women during labour, and in patients suffering from lung disorders, kidney or liver disorders. Avoid long-term use and withdraw gradually.
Not to be used for: children, or for patients suffering from acute lung diseases, some chronic lung diseases, some obsessional and psychotic diseases.
Not to be used with: alcohol, other tranquillizers, anti-convulsants.
Contains: NITRAZEPAM.
Other preparations:

---

nitrate

a drug used to treat poor blood supply to the heart muscle (angina). Nitrates reduce the work which the heart has to do. Example GLYCERYL TRINITRATE *see* Trinitrin.

---

nitrazepam *see* **Mogadon, Nitrados**

N

Nitrocontin Continus
(Degussa)

A pink tablet supplied at strengths of 2.6 mg, 6.4 mg and used as a NITRATE to treat angina.

Dose: 2.6-6.4 mg a day.
Availability: NHS and private prescription.
Side effects: passing headache.
Caution:
Not to be used for: children.
Not to be used with:
Contains: GLYCERYL TRINITRATE.
Other preparations:

---

nitrofurantoin *see* Furadantin

---

nitrofurazone *see* Furacin

Nitrolingual
(Lipha)

An aerosol used as a NITRATE for the prevention and treatment of angina.

Dose: 1-2 sprays on to tongue for each attack up to a maximum of 3 sprays.
Availability: NHS and private prescription.
Side effects: headache, flushes, dizziness
Caution: do not inhale spray.
Not to be used for: children.
Not to be used with:
Contains: GLYCERYL TRINITRATE.
Other preparations:

N

Nivaquine
(M & B)

A yellow tablet supplied at a strength of 200 mg and used as an anti-malarial drug for the prevention and treatment of malaria.

Dose: adults prevention 2 tablets on the same day once a week; treatment as advised by the physician; children use Nivaquine Syrup.
Availability: NHS, private prescription, and over the counter.
Side effects: headache, stomach upset, skin eruptions, hair loss, eye disorders, blood disorders, loss of pigment.
Caution: in pregnant women, nursing mothers, or in patients suffering from porphyria (a rare blood disorder), kidney or liver disease, psoriasis. The eyes should be tested before and during prolonged treatment.
Not to be used for:
Not to be used with:
Contains: CHLOROQUINE sulphate.
Other preparations: Nivaquine Syrup, Nivaquine Injection.

Nivemycin
(Boots)

A tablet supplied at a strength of 500 mg and used as an aminoglycoside antibiotic for preparation before bowel surgery, and as an additional treatment in liver disease coma.

Dose: adults 2 tablets every hour for 4 hours, then 2 tablets every 4 hours for 2-3 days; children under 5 years use elixir, 6-12 years 1/2 -1 tablet every 4 hours for 2-3 days, over 12 years 2 tablets every 4 hours for 2-3 days.
Availability: NHS and private prescription.
Side effects: stomach disturbances.
Caution: kidney damage, damaged hearing.
Not to be used for: patients suffering from a blockage of the intestine.
Not to be used with:
Contains: NEOMYCIN sulphate.
Other preparations: Nivemycin Elixir.

---

nizatidine *see* Axid

N

Nizoral
(Janssen)

A white scored tablet supplied at a strength of 200 mg and used as an anti-fungal treatment for severe fungus infections, chronic vaginal thrush which does not respond to other treatment.

Dose: adults 1-2 tablets a day with meals for 5-7 days; children 3 mg per kg body weight a day.
Availability: NHS and private prescription
Side effects: hepatitis, hypersensitivity, stomach upset, rash, head-ache, blood changes, rarely breast enlargement.
Caution: liver should be checked regularly.
Not to be used for: pregnant women, patients with any form of liver disorder, or hypersensitivity to ketoconazole or other imidazoles.
Not to be used with: ANTI-CHOLINERGICS, antacids, HYDROGEN ION AN-TAGONISTS, anti-coagulants, PHENYTOIN, RIFAMPICIN, CYCLOSPORIN A.
Contains: KETOCONAZOLE.
Other preparations: Nizoral Suspension, Nizoral Cream.

Nizoral Cream
(Janssen)

A cream used as an anti-fungal treatment for fungus infections, skin thrush, seborrhoeic dermatitis.

Dose: apply to the affected area 1-2 times a day.
Availability: NHS and private prescription.
Side effects: irritation.
Caution:
Not to be used for:
Not to be used with:
Contains: KETOCONAZOLE.
Other preparations: Nizoral Shampoo.

Nobrium
(Roche)

A yellow/orange capsule or an orange/black capsule according to strengths of 5 mg, 10 mg and used as a sleeping tablet for the short-term treatment of anxiety.

Dose: elderly 5-20 mg a day in divided doses; adults 15-40 mg a day in divided doses.
Availability: private prescription only.
Side effects: drowsiness, confusion, unsteadiness, low blood pressure, rash, changes in vision, changes in libido, retention of urine. Risk of addiction increases with dose and length of treatment. May impair judgement.
Caution: in the elderly, pregnant women, nursing mothers, in women during labour, and in patients suffering from lung disorders, kidney or liver disorders. Avoid long-term use and withdraw gradually.
Not to be used for: children, or for patients suffering from acute lung diseases, some chronic lung diseases, some obsessional and psychotic diseases.
Not to be used with: alcohol, other tranquillizers, anti-convulsants.
Contains: MEDAZEPAM.
Other preparations:

Noctec
(Squibb)

A liquid-filled, red capsule supplied at a strength of 500 mg and used as a sedative to treat sleeplessness.

Dose: usually 1-2 capsules taken with water 15-30 minutes before going to bed; maximum dose 4 capsules a day.
Availability: NHS and private prescription.
Side effects: stomach irritation, headache, excitement, delirium, skin allergies, ketones in the urine.
Caution: in nursing mothers and for patients suffering from porphyria (a rare blood disorder). Patients should be warned of reduced judgement and abilities.
Not to be used for: children, pregnant women, or for patients suffering from severe heart, liver, or kidney disease, or gastric inflammation.
Not to be used with: alcohol, sedatives, anti-coagulants.
Contains: CHORAL HYDRATE.
Other preparations:

Noltam *see* Nolvadex-D
(Lederle)

N

Noludar
(Roche)

A white, quarter-scored tablet supplied at a strength of 200 mg and used as a sedative for the short-term treatment of sleeplessness.

Dose: elderly ¹/₂ -1 tablet before going to bed; adults 1-2 tablets before going to bed.
Availability: NHS and private prescription.
Side effects: brain and stomach disturbances, itch, rash, low blood pressure, tolerance or dependence.
Caution: in patients suffering from kidney or liver disease. Patients should be warned of reduced judgement and abilities.
Not to be used for: for children.
Not to be used with: alcohol, sedatives, contraceptive pill, anti-co-agulants.
Contains: METHYPRYLONE.
Other preparations:

Nolvadex-D
(ICI)

A white, eight-sided tablet supplied at a strength of 20 mg and used as an anti-oestrogen treatment for infertility in women caused by failure of ovulation or breast cancer.

Dose: 1 tablet a day for 4 days beginning on the fourth day of the period. If needed increase to 2 tablets a day then 4 tablets a day for further courses. For breast cancer 1 tablet a day increasing to 4 tablets a day if needed.
Availability: NHS and private prescription.
Side effects: hot flushes, bleeding from the vagina, stomach upset, dizziness, disturbed vision.
Caution:
Not to be used for: children or pregnant women.
Not to be used with: WARFARIN.
Contains: TAMOXIFEN citrate.
Other preparations: Nolvadex Forte, Nolvadex, NOLTAM (Lederle), TAMOFEN (Tillotts).

N

non-steroidal anti-inflammatory drug (NSAID)

an anti-rheumatic preparation which has pain-killing properties. An NSAID may cause stomach upsets. Example IBUPROFEN *see* Brufen.

---

nonivamide *see* Finalgon

Noradran
(Norma)

A syrup used as an anti-tussive to treat bronchitis, bronchial asthma.

Dose: adults 2 5 ml teaspoonsful every four hours; children over 5 years 1 5 ml teaspoonful every four hours.
Availability: private prescription and over the counter.
Side effects: sedation, dry mouth, nervousness, restlessness, hands shaking, abnormal heart rhythm, stomach upset.
Caution: in patients suffering from heart or liver disease, diabetes.
Not to be used for: children under 5 years, or for patients suffering from high blood pressure, overactive thyroid, coronary disease, cardiac asthma.
Not to be used with: MAOIS, SYMPATHOMIMETICS, TRICYCLICS, alcohol, CIMETIDINE, ERYTHOMYCIN, INTERFERON, CIPROFLOXACIN.
Contains: GUAIPHENESIN.
Other preparations:

Nordox *see* Vibramycin
(Panpharma)

---

norethisterone *see* BiNovum, Brevinor, Controvlar, Estra-pak, Loestrin 20, Menophase, Micronor, Neocon 1/35, Noriday, Norimin, Norinyl-1, Ortho-Novin 1/50, Primolut N, Synphase, Trisequens, Utovlan

---

N

Norgeston
(Schering)

A white tablet used as a progesterone contraceptive.

Dose: 1 tablet at the same time every day starting on day 1 of the period.
Availability: NHS and over the counter.
Side effects: irregular bleeding, breast discomfort, acne, headache.
Caution: in patients suffering from high blood pressure, tendency to thrombosis, migraine, liver abnormalities, ovarian cysts. Your doctor may advise regular check-ups.
Not to be used for: pregnant women, or for patients suffering from severe heart or artery disease, benign liver tumours, vaginal bleeding, previous ectopic pregnancy.
Not to be used with: barbiturates, PHENYTOIN, PRIMIDONE, CARBAMAZEP-INE, CHLORAL HYDRATE, DICHLORALPHENAZONE, ETHOSUXIMIDE, RIFAMPICIN, GLUTETHIMIDE, CHLORPROMAZINE, MEPROBAMATE, GRISEOFULVIN.
Contains: LEVONORGESTREL.
Other preparations:

---

norgestrel *see* Neogest, Ovysmen, PC4, Prempak-C

Noriday
(Syntex)

A white tablet used as a progesterone contraceptive.

Dose: 1 tablet at the same time every day starting on day 1 of the period.
Availability: NHS and private prescription.
Side effects: irregular bleeding, breast discomfort, acne, headache.
Caution: in patients suffering from high blood pressure, tendency to thrombosis, migraine, liver abnormalities, ovarian cysts. Your doctor may advise regular check-ups.
Not to be used for: pregnant women, or for patients suffering from severe heart or artery disease, benign liver tumours, vaginal bleeding, previous ectopic pregnancy.
Not to be used with: barbiturates, PHENYTOIN, PRIMIDONE, CARBAMAZEP-INE, CHLORAL HYDRATE, DICHLORALPHENAZONE, ETHOSUXIMIDE, RIFAMPICIN, GLUTETHIMIDE, CHLORPROMAZINE, MEPROBAMATE, GRISEOFULVIN.

N

Contains: NORETHISTERONE.
Other preparations:

Norimin
(Syntex)

A yellow tablet used as an oestrogen, progestogen contraceptive.

Dose: 1 tablet a day for 21 days starting on day 5 of the period.
Availability: NHS and private prescription.
Side effects: enlarged breasts, bloating and fluid retention, cramps, leg pains, mood change, reduction in sexual desire, headaches, nausea, vaginal erosion, discharge, and bleeding, weight gain, skin changes.
Caution: in patients suffering from high blood pressure, diabetes, vascular disorders, asthma, depression, kidney disease, multiple sclerosis, womb diseases. Your doctor may advise you not to smoke, to have regular examinations. You should stop treatment at the first sign of serious symptoms such as severe headache or jaundice. Treatment should be stopped before surgery.
Not to be used for: pregnant women, or for patients suffering from sickle-cell anaemia, history of heart disease or thrombosis, liver disorders, some cancers, undiagnosed vaginal bleeding, some ear, skin, and kidney disorders.
Not to be used with: RIFAMPICIN, TETRACYCLINES, GRISEOFULVIN, barbiturates, PHENYTOIN, PRIMIDONE, CARBAMAZEPINE, ETHOSUXIMIDE, CHLORAL HYDRATE, DICHLORALPHENAZONE.
CONTAINS: ETHINYLOESTRADIOL, NORETHISTERONE.
Other preparations:

Norinyl-1
(Syntex)

A white tablet used as an oestrogen, progestogen contraceptive.

Dose: 1 tablet a day for 21 days starting on day 5 of the period.
Availability: NHS and private prescription.
Side effects: enlarged breasts, bloating and fluid retention, cramps, leg pains, mood change, reduction in sexual desire, headaches, nausea, vaginal erosion, discharge, and bleeding, weight gain, skin changes.

Caution: in patients suffering from high blood pressure, diabetes, vascular disorders, asthma, depression, kidney disease, multiple sclerosis, womb diseases. Your doctor may advise you not to smoke, to have regular examinations. You should stop treatment at the first sign of serious symptoms such as severe headache or jaundice. Treatment should be stopped before surgery.

Not to be used for: pregnant women, or for patients suffering from sickle-cell anaemia, history of heart disease or thrombosis, liver disorders, some cancers, undiagnosed vaginal bleeding, some ear, skin, and kidney disorders.

Not to be used with: RIFAMPICIN, TETRACYCLINES, GRISEOFULVIN, barbiturates, PHENYTOIN, PRIMIDONE, CARBAMAZEPINE, ETHOSUXIMIDE, CHLORAL HYDRATE, DICHLORALPHENAZONE.

Contains: MESTRANOL, NORETHISTERONE.

Other preparations:

Normacol
(Norgine)

White granules in 7 g sachets or supplied as as 500 g and used as a bulking agent. to treat constipation caused by lack of fibre in the diet.

Dose: adults 1-2 sachets or 1-2 heaped 5 ml spoonsful once or twice a day after meals swallowed with liquid; children half adult dose.

Availability: NHS and private prescription.

Side effects:

Caution:

Not to be used for:

Not to be used with:

Contains: STERCULIA.

Other preparations: Normacol Plus.

Normasol
(Seton-Prebbles)

A solution in a sachet used for washing out eyes, burns, wounds.

Dose: use as needed.

Availability: NHS, private prescription, over the counter.

Side effects:

Caution:

N

Not to be used for:
Not to be used with:
Contains: SODIUM CHLORIDE.
Other preparations:

Normax
(Bencard)

A brown capsule used as a stimulant and faecal softener to treat constipation in the elderly, in patients being treated with pain-killers, those with heart failure or coronary thrombosis, or in terminally ill patients.

Dose: adults 1-3 capsules at night as required; children over 6 years 1 capsule at night.
Availability: NHS (when prescribed as a generic) and private prescription.
Side effects:
Caution: in nursing mothers.
Not to be used for: children under 6 years or for patients suffering from an obstruction of the intestine.
Not to be used with:
Contains: DANTHRON, DOCUSATE sodium.
Other preparations:

Normetic
(Abbott)

A pale-peach, scored tablet used as a potassium-sparing DIURETIC to treat high blood pressure, congestive heart failure, liver cirrhosis with fluid retention.

Dose: 1-2 tablets a day up to a maximum of 4 tablets a day if needed.
Availability: NHS and private prescription.
Side effects: rash, sensitivity to light, blood changes, gout.
Caution: in patients suffering from diabetes, electrolyte changes, gout, kidney or liver disease.
Not to be used for: children, pregnant women, nursing mothers or for patients suffering from raised potassium levels, or progressive or severe kidney failure.
Not to be used with: potassium supplements, potassium-sparing diuretics, DIGITALIS, LITHIUM, anti-hypertensives.

N

Contains: AMILORIDE hydrochloride, HYDROCHLOROTHIAZIDE
Other preparations:

Normison
(Wyeth)

A yellow capsule supplied at strengths of 10 mg, 20 mg and used as a sleeping tablet to prevent interrupted sleep, and for short-term treatment of sleeplessness when sedation during the day could present difficulty.

Dose: elderly 10 mg before going to bed; adults usually 10-30 mg but up to 60 mg before going to bed.
Availability: NHS (when prescribed as a generic) and private prescription.
Side effects: drowsiness, confusion, unsteadiness, low blood pressure, rash, changes in vision, changes in libido, retention of urine. Risk of addiction increases with dose and length of treatment. May impair judgement.
Caution: in the elderly, pregnant women, nursing mothers, in women during labour, and in patients suffering from lung disorders, kidney or liver disorders. Avoid long-term use and withdraw gradually.
Not to be used for: children, or for patients suffering from acute lung diseases, some chronic lung diseases, some obsessional and psychotic diseases.
Not to be used with: alcohol, other tranquillizers, anti-convulsants.
Contains: TEMAZEPAM.
Other preparations:

---

nortryptiline *see* Allegron, Aventyl, Motipress, Motival

Norval
(Bencard)

An orange tablet supplied at strengths of 10 mg, 20 mg, 30 mg and used as a TETRACYCLIC anti-depressant to treat depression.

Dose: adults 30-40 mg a day at first increasing gradually after a few days if needed to 30-90 mg or a maximum of 200 mg in divided doses;

elderly up to 30 mg a day.
Availability: NHS and private prescription.
Side effects: drowsiness, bone marrow depression, possible jaundice, hypomania, or convulsions.
Caution: in pregnant women, the elderly or patients suffering from heart attack; discontinue if jaundice, hypomania, or convulsions happen. Your doctor may advise that blood tests should be taken once a month for the first 3 months.
Not to be used for: children, nursing mothers, or for patients suffering from mania or severe liver disease.
Not to be used with: MAOIS, alcohol.
Contains: MIANSERIN hydrochloride.
Other preparations:

Nu-K
(Consolidated)

A blue capsule supplied at a strength of 600 mg and used as a potassium supplement to treat potassium deficiency.

Dose: 1-6 capsules a day in divided doses after food.
Availability: NHS, private prescription, over the counter.
Side effects: ulcers or blockage in the small bowel.
Caution:
Not to be used for: children or patients suffering from advanced kidney disease.
Not to be used with:
Contains: POTASSIUM CHLORIDE.
Other preparations:

Nu-Seals Aspirin
(Eli Lilly)

A red tablet supplied at strengths of 300 mg, 600 mg and used as an analgesic to relieve pain, rheumatism, rheumatoid arthritis.

Dose: adults and children over 12 years 300-900 mg 3-4 times a day to a maximum of 8 g a day.
Availability: NHS and private prescription.
Side effects: stomach upsets, allergy, asthma.
Caution: in pregnant women, the elderly, or in patients with a history

N

of allergy to aspirin, asthma, impaired kidney or liver function, indigestion.

Not to be used for: children under 12 years, nursing mothers, or patients suffering from haemophilia, or ulcers.

Not to be used with: anti-coagulants (blood-thinning drugs), some anti-diabetic drugs, anti-inflammatory agents, METHOTREXATE, SPIRONOLACTONE, steroids, some antacids, some uric acid-lowering drugs.

Contains: ASPIRIN.

Other preparations:

Nuelin SA *see* Theophylline
(3M-Riker)

Nulacin
(Bencard)

A beige tablet used as an antacid to treat dyspepsia, acidity, oesophagitis, hiatus hernia.

Dose: adults 1 or more when required.
Availability: private prescription and over the counter.
Side effects: diarrhoea.
Caution: kidney impairment.
Not to be used for: for children, coeliac disease.
Not to be used with:
Contains: milk solids with dextrins and MALTOSE, MAGNESIUM OXIDE, MAGNESIUM CARBONATE, MAGNESIUM TRISILICATE.
Other preparations:

Numotac
(3M Riker)

A white tablet supplied at a strength of 10 mg and used as a bronchodilator to treat bronchial spasm brought on by bronchial asthma, chronic bronchitis, emphysema.

Dose: 1-2 tablets 3-4 times a day.
Availability: NHS and private prescription.
Side effects: shaking of the hands, rapid or abnormal heart rate,

N

nervous tension, headache, dilation of the blood vessels.
Caution: in patients suffering from diabetes, high blood pressure.
Not to be used for: children or for patients suffering from acute coronary disease, overactive thyroid, cardiac asthma.
Not to be used with: MAOIS, SYMPATHOMIMETICS, TRICYCLICS.
Contains: ISOETHARINE hydrochloride.
Other preparations:

Nutrizym GR
(Merck)

A green/orange capsule used as a source of pancreatic enzymes to treat cystic fibrosis, steatorrhoea, pancreatic disorders.

Dose: 1-2 capsules with meals.
Availability: NHS and private prescription.
Side effects: buccal and perianal irritation.
Caution:
Not to be used for:
Not to be used with:
Contains: PANCREATIN.
Other preparations:

Nystadermal
(Squibb)

A cream used as a steroid and anti-bacterial treatment for thrush, itch, eczema where there is also inflammation.

Dose: apply to the affected area 2-4 times a day.
Availability: NHS and private prescription.
Side effects: fluid retention, suppression of adrenal glands, thinning of the skin may occur.
Caution: use for short periods of time only
Not to be used for: patients suffering from acne or any other skin infections caused by tuberculosis, ringworm, viruses, or fungi, or continuously especially in pregnant women.
Not to be used with:
Contains: NYSTATIN, TRIAMCINOLONE ACETONIDE.
Other preparations:

N

Nystaform
(Bayer)

A cream used as an anti-fungal and anti-bacterial treatment for skin infections or skin conditions where infection may occur.

Dose: apply freely to the affected area 2-3 times a day until 7 days after the wounds have healed.
Availability: NHS and private prescription.
Side effects:
Caution:
Not to be used for:
Not to be used with:
Contains: NYSTATIN, CHLORHEXIDINE.
Other preparations:

Nystaform-HC
(Bayer)

A cream used as a steroid and anti-fungal treatment for skin disorders where there is also infection.

Dose: apply to the affected area 2-3 times a day for 7 days after the condition has healed.
Availability: NHS and private prescription.
Side effects: fluid retention, suppression of adrenal glands, thinning of the skin may occur.
Caution: use for short periods of time only.
Not to be used for: patients suffering from acne or any other skin infections caused by tuberculosis, ringworm, viruses, or fungi, or continuously especially in pregnant women.
Not to be used with:
Contains: NYSTATIN, CHLORHEXIDINE, HYDROCORTISONE.
Other preparations: Nystaform-HC Ointment.

Nystan
(Squibb)

A yellow, diamond-shaped pessary or a brown tablet used as an anti-fungal treatment for vaginal, oral, or intestinal thrush.

N

Dose: vaginal thrush 1-2 pessaries into the vagina for at least 14 nights; children use cream. Other infections 1-2 tablets 4 times a day.
Availability: NHS
Side effects: irritation and burning, nausea, vomiting, diarrhoea in high doses.
Caution:
Not to be used for:
Not to be used with:
Contains: NYSTATIN.
Other preparations: Nystan Vaginal Cream, Nystan Gel, Nystan Oral Tablets, Nystan Triple Pack, NYSTAVESCENT (Squibb).

Nystan Cream
(Squibb)

A cream used as an anti-fungal treatment for thrush of the skin and mucous membranes.

Dose: apply to the affected area 2-4 times a day.
Availability: NHS and private prescription.
Side effects: irritation and burning.
Caution:
Not to be used for:
Not to be used with:
Contains: NYSTATIN.
Other preparations: Nystan Ointment, Nystan Gel, Nystan Powder.

Nystan Oral Suspension
(Squibb)

A supension used as an anti-fungal treatment for thrush.

Dose: hold 1 ml of the supension in contact with the affected area 4 times a day for up to 2 days after the symptoms have abated.
Availability: NHS and private prescription.
Side effects:
Caution:
Not to be used for:
Not to be used with:
Contains: NYSTATIN.
Other preparations: Nystan Granules, Nystan Pastilles.

N

nystatin *see* Gregoderm, Mutilind, Nystadermal, Nystaform, Nystaform-HC, Nystan, Nystan Cream, Nystan Oral Suspension, Timodine, Tinaderm-M, Tri-Adcortyl, Tri-Adcortyl Otic, Tri-Cicatrin, Trimovate

---

Nystavescent *see* Nystan
(Squibb)

---

oat bran meal *see* Lejfibre

Octovit
(S K B)

A maroon, oblong tablet used as a multivitamin treatment for vitamin and mineral deficiencies.

Dose: 1 tablet a day
Availability: private prescription and over the counter.
Side effects:
Caution:
Not to be used for: children.
Not to be used with: TETRACYCLINES, LEVODOPA.
Contains: VITAMIN A, THIAMINE, RIBOFLAVINE, NICOTINAMIDE, PYRIDOXINE, CYANOCOBALAMIN, ASCORBIC ACID, CHOLECALCIFEROL, TOCOPHERYL ACETATE, CALCIUM HYDROGEN PHOSPHATE, FERROUS SULPHATE, MAGNESIUM HYDROXIDE, ZINC.
Other preparations:

Ocusert Pilo
(M & B)

An eye insert used as a cholinergic treatment for glaucoma.

Dose: 1 unit under the eyelid replaced every 7 days.
Availability: NHS and private prescription.
Side effects: irritation, reduced sharpness of vision.

Caution:
Not to be used for: children or for patients suffering from acute eye infection or inflammation.
Not to be used with:
Contains: PILOCARPINE.
Other preparations:

Ocusol *see* **Sulphacetamide**
(Boots)

---

oestradiol *see* **Cyclo-Progynova 1mg, Estraderm, Estra-pak, Hormonin, Progynova, Trisequens**

---

oestriol *see* **Hormonin, Ovestin, Trisequens**

---

oestrone *see* **Hormonin**

Olbetam
(Farmitalia CE)

A red-brown/dark-pink capsule supplied at a strength of 250 mg and used as a lipid-lowering agent to treat elevated lipids.

Dose: 2-3 capsules a day with meals, no more than 1200 mg a day.
Availability: NHS and private prescription.
Side effects: flushes, rash, redness, stomach upset, headache, general feeling of being unwell.
Caution:
Not to be used for: children, pregnant women, nursing mothers, or for patients suffering from peptic ulcer.
Not to be used with:
Contains: ACIPIMOX.
Other preparations:

oleyl alcohol *see* **Polytar Liquid**

---

olive oil *see* **Rowachol, Rowatinex**

---

olsalazine sodium *see* **Dipentum**

---

omeprazole *see* **Losec**

One-Alpha
(Leo)

A white capsule or a brown capsule according to strengths of 0.25 microgram, 1 microgram. and used as a source of vitamin D to treat bone disorders due to kidney disease, rickets, over-or underactive parathyroid glands, low calcium levels in newborn infants, other bone disorders.

Dose: adults and children over 20 kg body weight 1 microgram a day at first adjusting as neded; children under 20 kg 0.05 micrograms per kg a day at first.
Availability: NHS and private prescription.
Side effects:
Caution: in nursing mothers. Your doctor may advise that calcium levels should be checked regularly.
Not to be used for:
Not to be used with: barbiturates, anti-convulsants.
Contains: ALFACALCIDOL.
Other preparations: One-Alpha Solution.

Ophthaine
(Squibb)

Drops used as a local anaesthetic for eye procedures.

Dose: 1-2 drops into the eye as needed.
Availability: NHS and private prescription.
Side effects: irritation, rarely severe sensitivity.
Caution: in patients with a history of allergy, heart disease, or overactive thyroid. Do not use over extended periods.
Not to be used for:
Not to be used with:
Contains: PROXYMETACAINE hydrochloride.
Other preparations:

Opilon
(Parke-Davis)

A yellow, scored tablet supplied at a strength of 40 mg and used as a vasodilator to treat Raynaud's syndrome (a condition caused by spasms of arteries in the hand), chilblains, Ménière's syndrome (dizziness due to ear disease), very cold hands and feet.

Dose: 1 tablet 4 times a day.
Availability: NHS and private prescription.
Side effects: nausea, diarrhoea, vertigo, headache.
Caution: in patients suffering from diabetes, angina, recent heart attack.
Not to be used for: children.
Not to be used with: TRICYCLIC anti-depressants.
Contains: THYMOXAMINE hydrochloride.
Other preparations:

Opticrom
(Fisons)

Drops used as an anti-allergy agent to treat allergic conjunctivitis.

Dose: 1-2 drops into the eyes 4 times a day.
Availability: NHS and private prescription.
Side effects: temporary smarting.
Caution:
Not to be used for: patients who wear soft contact lenses.
Not to be used with:
Contains: SODIUM CROMOGLYCATE.
Other preparations: Opticrom Ointment.

Optimax
(Merck)

A long, yellow scored tablet used as an anti-depressant to treat depression.

Dose: 2 tablets 3 times a day.
Availability: NHS and private prescriptions.
Side effects: nausea, headache.
Caution: in patients suffering from diseased bladder. Patients should be warned of reduced alertness.
Not to be used for: children or when levopoda is also being prescribed.
Not to be used with: MAOIS.
Contains: TRYPTOPHAN, PYRIDOXINE hydrochloride, VITAMIN C.
Other preparations: Optimax Powder, Optimax WV

Optimine
(Kirby-Warrick)

A white, scored tablet supplied at a strength of 1 mg and used as an antihistamine and serotonin antagonist (hormone blocker) to treat bites and stings, itch, allergic rhinitis, urticaria.

Dose: adults 1-2 tablets twice a day; children over 1 year use syrup.
Availability: NHS, private prescription, over the counter.
Side effects: drowsiness, reduced reactions, greater appetite, anorexia, nausea, headache, anti-cholinergic effects.
Caution:
Not to be used for: infants under 1 year or for patients suffering from prostate enlargement, retention of urine, glaucoma, peptic ulcer causing blockage.
Not to be used with: sedatives, MAOIS, alcohol.
Contains: AZATADINE MALEATE.
Other preparations: Optimine Syrup.

Opulets Atropine *see* Atropine
(Alcon)

Opulets Benoxinate
(Alcon)

Drops used as a local anaesthetic for eye procedures.

Dose: 1 drop into the eye as needed.
Availability: NHS and private prescription
Side effects:
Caution:
Not to be used for:
Not to be used with:
Contains: OXYBUPROCAINE hydrochloride.
Other preparations:

Opulets Cyclopentolate
(Alcon)

Drops used as an ANTI-CHOLINERGIC pupil dilator.

Dose: 1-2 drops into the eye as needed.
Availability: NHS and private prescription.
Side effects: temporary smarting, dry mouth, blurrred vision, aversion to light, rapid heart rate, headache, mental and behavioural changes.
Caution:
Not to be used for: for patients suffering from narrow angle glaucoma.
Not to be used with:
Contains: CYCLOPENTOLATE hydrochloride.
Other preparations:

Opulets Pilocarpine
(Alcon)

Drops used as a cholinergic treatment for glaucoma.

Dose: 1 drop into the eye 4-6 times a day.
Availability: NHS and private prescription.
Side effects: reduced sharpness of vision, sensitivity.
Caution:
Not to be used for: patients suffering from acute iritis.

Not to be used with:
Contains: PILOCARPINE hydrochloride.
Other preparations:

Opulets Saline
(Alcon)

Drops used for irrigating the eyes.

Dose: use as needed.
Availability: NHS, private prescription, over the counter.
Side effects:
Caution:
Not to be used for:
Not to be used with:
Contains: SODIUM CHLORIDE.
Other preparations:

Orabase
(Squibb)

An ointment used as a mucoprotectant to protect lesions in the mouth.

Dose: apply to the affected area without rubbing in.
Availability: NHS, private prescription, over the counter.
Side effects:
Caution:
Not to be used for:
Not to be used with:
Contains: CARMELLOSE SODIUM, PECTIN, GELATIN.
Other preparations:

Orabet *see* Glucophage
(Lagap)

Oradexon
(Organon)

A white tablet supplied at strengths of 0.5 mg, 2 mg and used as a corticosteroid treatment for rheumatoid arthritis, allergy, cerebral fluid retention, inflammatory conditions.

Dose: adults 4-8 mg a day at first reducing to 0.5-1.5 mg a day; children 0.01-0.04 mg per kg body weight a day.
Availability: NHS and private prescription.
Side effects: high blood sugar, thin bones, mood changes, ulcers.
Caution: in pregnant women, in patients who have had recent bowel surgery, or who are suffering from inflamed veins, psychiatric disorders, virus infections, some cancers, some kidney diseases, thinning of the bones, ulcers, tuberculosis, other infections, high blood pressure, glaucoma, epilepsy, diabetes, underactive thyroid, liver disease, stress. Withdraw gradually.
Not to be used for: infants under 1 year.
Not to be used with: PHENYTOIN, PHENOBARBITONE, EPHEDRINE, RIFAMPICIN, DIURETICS, ANTI-CHOLINESTERASES, DIGITALIS, anti-diabetic agents, anti-coagulants, NON-STEROID ANTI-INFLAMMATORY DRUGS.
Contains: DEXAMETHASONE.
Other preparations: Oradexon Injection.

Oralcer
(Vitabiotics)

A green pellet used as an anti-bacterial, anti-fungal treatment for mouth ulcers.

Dose: adults allow 6-8 pellets to dissolve slowly near the ulcer on the first day, reducing to 4-6 pellets on the second day; children 3-4 pellets a day.
Availability: NHS, private prescription, over the counter.
Side effects: local irritation.
Caution: do not use for extended periods.
Not to be used for: for patients suffering from kidney or liver disease, overactive thyroid, intolerance to IODINE.
Not to be used with:
Contains: CLIOQUINOL, ASCORBIC ACID.
Other preparations:

Oraldene
(Warner-Lambert)

A solution used as an antiseptic rinse to treat thrush, gingivitis, ulcers, bad breath, stomatitis.

Dose: rinse out the mouth or gargle with 3 5 ml teaspoonsful 2-3 times a day.
Availability: NHS, private prescription, over the counter.
Side effects: local irritation.
Caution:
Not to be used for:
Not to be used with:
Contains: HEXETIDINE.
Other preparations:

Oramorph
(Boehringer Ingelheim)

A solution used as an opiate to control severe pain.

Dose: adults 10-20 mg every 4 hours; children 1-5 years up to 5 mg every 4 hours, 6-12 years up to 5-10 mg every 4 hours.
Availability: controlled drug.
Side effects: tolerance, addiction, constipation, nausea, vomiting, sedation.
Caution: in the elderly, nursing mothers, after surgery, and in patients suffering from underactive thyroid, liver or kidney disease, reduced respiratory reserve, adrenal gland problems, enlarged prostate.
Not to be used for: pregnant women, alcoholics, or for patients suffering from respiratory depression, blocked airways, acute liver disease, head injury, coma, convulsions, or raised intracranial pressure.
Not to be used with: MAOIS, sedatives, alcohol.
Contains: MORPHINE sulphate
Other preparations: Oramorph Concentrated.

Orap
(Janssen)

A white, scored tablet or a green, scored tablet according to strengths of 2 mg, 4 mg, 10 mg and used as a sedative to treat schizophrenia.

Dose: adults 2-20 mg a day; children under 12 years as advised by physician, over 12 years 1-3 mg a day.
Availability: NHS and private prescription.
Side effects: muscle spasms, restlessness, hands shaking, dry mouth, urine retention, palpitations, low blood pressure, weight gain, changes in libido, low body temperature, breast swelling, menstrual changes, jaundice, blood and skin changes, drowsiness, rarely fits.
Caution: care in pregnant women and in patients suffering from endogenous depression, Parkinson's disease, or epilepsy
Not to be used for:
Not to be used with: alcohol, tranquillizers, pain killers, anti-hypertensives, anti-depressants, anti-convulsants, anti-diabetic drugs, LEVODOPA.
Contains: PIMOZIDE.
Other preparations:

Orbenin
(S K B)

An orange/black capsule supplied at strengths of 250 mg, 500 mg and used as a penicillin to treat infections.

Dose: adults 500 mg every 6 hours; children under 2 years ¼ adult dose, over 2 years half adult dose.
Availability: NHS and private prescription.
Side effects: allergy, stomach disturbances.
Caution:
Not to be used for: in patients suffering from penicillin allergy.
Not to be used with:
Contains: CLOXACILLIN.
Other preparations: Orbenin Syrup, Orbenin Injection.

---

orciprenaline sulphate *see* Alupent

Orimeten
(Ciba)

An off-white, scored tablet supplied at a strength of 250 mg and used as a steroid synthesis inhibitor (hormone blocker). to treat breast cancer, prostate cancer, Cushing's syndrome.

Dose: breast or prostate cancer 1 tablet a day increasing by 1 tablet a day every week to 3-4 tablets for prostate or breast cancer; Cushing's syndrome 1 tablet a day increasing to up to 8 a day if needed.
Availability: NHS and private prescription.
Side effects: sedation, stomach disturbances, rash, blood changes, thyroid failure.
Caution: steroids may need to be given. Your doctor may advise regular blood tests.
Not to be used for: children, pregnant women, nursing mothers.
Not to be used with: anti-coagulants, anti-diabetics taken by mouth, artificial glucocorticoids.
Contains: AMINOGLUTETHIMIDE.
Other preparations:

Orovite
(Bencard)

A maroon tablet used as a source of multivitamins to aid recovery from feverish illness, infection, or surgery, and to treat confusion in the elderly, mild alcoholic disorders, or for treatment after intravenous vitamin therapy.

Dose: adults 1 tablet 3 times a day; children use syrup.
Availability: private prescription and over the counter.
Side effects:
Caution:
Not to be used for:
Not to be used with: LEVODOPA.
Contains: THIAMINE, RIBOFLAVINE, PYRIDOXINE, NICOTINAMIDE, ASCORBIC ACID.
Other preparations: Orovite Syrup.

Orovite 7
(Bencard)

Granules in a sachet used as a multivitamin treatment for vitamin deficiencies.

Dose: 1 sachet in water once a day.
Availability: private prescription, over the counter.
Side effects:
Caution:
Not to be used for: for children under 5 years.
Not to be used with: LEVODOPA.
Contains: VITAMIN A PALMITATE, CALCIFEROL, THIAMINE, RIBOFLAVINE, PYRIDOX-
INE, NICOTINAMIDE, ASCORBIC ACID.
Other preparations:

---

orphenadrine *see* Biorphen, Disipal

Ortho Dienoestrol
(Cilag)

A cream with applicator used as an oestrogen treatment for atrophic
inflammation of the vagina, other disease of the vulva or painful intercourse.

Dose: 1-2 applications into the vagina once a day for 1-2 weeks
reducing to half that dose for 1-2 weeks, then 1 application 1-3 times
a week.
Availability: NHS and private prescription.
Side effects: enlarged breasts, bloating and fluid retention, cramps,
leg pains, mood change, reduction in sexual desire, headaches,
nausea, vaginal erosion, discharge, and bleeding, weight gain, skin
changes.
Caution: in patients suffering from high blood pressure, diabetes,
vascular disorders, asthma, depression, kidney disease, multiple
sclerosis, womb diseases. Your doctor may advise you not to smoke,
to have regular examinations. You should stop treatment at the first
sign of serious symptoms such as severe headache or jaundice.
Treatment should be stopped before surgery.
Not to be used for: children, pregnant women, or for patients
suffering from sickle-cell anaemia, history of heart disease or thrombosis, liver disorders, some cancers, undiagnosed vaginal bleeding,
some ear, skin, and kidney disorders.
Not to be used with: diuretics, anti-hypertensives, and drugs that
change liver enzymes.

Contains: DIENOESTROL.
Other preparations:

Ortho-Gynest
(Cilag)

A pessary supplied at a strength of 0.5 mg and used as an oestrogen treatment for atrophic inflammation of the vagina, other disease of the vulva or painful intercourse.

Dose: 1pessary inserted into the vagina each evening at first, then 1 pessary twice a week.
Availability: NHS and private prescription.
Side effects: enlarged breasts, bloating and fluid retention, cramps, leg pains, mood change, reduction in sexual desire, headaches, nausea, vaginal erosion, discharge, and bleeding, weight gain, skin changes.
Caution: in patients suffering from high blood pressure, diabetes, vascular disorders, asthma, depression, kidney disease, multiple sclerosis, womb diseases. Your doctor may advise you not to smoke, to have regular examinations. You should stop treatment at the first sign of serious symptoms such as severe headache or jaundice. Treatment should be stopped before surgery.
Not to be used for: children, pregnant women, or for patients suffering from sickle-cell anaemia, history of heart disease or thrombosis, liver disorders, some cancers, undiagnosed vaginal bleeding, some ear, skin, and kidney disorders.
Not to be used with: diuretics, anti-hypertensives, and drugs that change liver enzymes.
Contains: OESTRIOL.
Other preparations:

Ortho-Novin 1/50
(Cilag)

A white tablet used as an oestrogen, progestogen contraceptive.

Dose: 1 tablet a day for 21 days starting on day 5 of the period.
Availability: NHS and private prescription.
Side effects: enlarged breasts, bloating and fluid retention, cramps,

leg pains, mood change, reduction in sexual desire, headaches, nausea, vaginal erosion, discharge, and bleeding, weight gain, skin changes.

Caution: in patients suffering from high blood pressure, diabetes, vascular disorders, asthma, depression, kidney disease, multiple sclerosis, womb diseases. Your doctor may advise you not to smoke, to have regular examinations. You should stop treatment at the first sign of serious symptoms such as severe headache or jaundice. Treatment should be stopped before surgery.

Not to be used for: pregnant women, or for patients suffering from sickle-cell anaemia, history of heart disease or thrombosis, liver disorders, some cancers, undiagnosed vaginal bleeding, some ear, skin, and kidney disorders.

Not to be used with: RIFAMPICIN, TETRACYCLINES, GRISEOFULVIN, barbiturates, PHENYTOIN, PRIMIDONE, CARBAMAZEPINE, ETHOSUXIMIDE, CHLORAL HYDRATE, DICHLORALPHENAZONE.

Contains: MESTRANOL, NORETHISTERONE.

Other preparations:

Orudis
(M & B)

A green/purple capsule or a pink capsule according to strengths of 50 mg, 100 mg and used as a NON-STEROID ANTI-INFLAMMATORY DRUG to treat rheumatoid arthritis, osteoarthritis, ankylosing spondylitis, acute articular and joint disorders, painful periods.

Dose: 50-100 mg twice a day with food.
Availability: NHS and private prescription.
Side effects: stomach intolerance, rash.
Caution: in pregnant women and in patients suffering from kidney or liver disease.
Not to be used for: children or for patients suffering from severe kidney disease, peptic ulcer or a history of recurring ulcer, asthma, allergy to ASPIRIN/non-steroid anti-inflammatory drugs.
Not to be used with: anti-coagulants, sulphonylureas, hydantoins.
Contains: KETOPROFEN.
Other preparations: ALRHEUMAT (Bayer), ORUVAIL (M & B).

Oruvail *see* **Orudis**
(M & B)

Ossopan 800
(Sanofi)

A buff-coloured tablet supplied at a strength of 830 mg and used as a calcium-phosphorus supplement to treat osteoporosis, rickets, osteomalacia (bone disorders).

Dose: adults 4-8 tablets a day in divided doses before food; children as advised by the physician.
Availability: NHS, private prescription, over the counter.
Side effects:
Caution: in patients suffering from kidney disease, severe loss of movement, or a history of kidney stones.
Not to be used for: patients suffering from elevated blood or urine calcium.
Not to be used with:
Contains: HYDROXYAPATITE compound.
Other preparations: Ossopan Powder

Otosporin
(Calmic)

Drops used as an antibiotic, corticosteroid treatment for bacterial infections and inflammation of the outer ear.

Dose: 3 drops into the ear 3-4 times a day.
Availability: NHS and private prescription.
Side effects: additional infection.
Caution: in infants and in patients suffering from perforated ear drum — do not use over extended periods.
Not to be used for: patients suffering from acne or any other skin infections caused by tuberculosis, ringworm, viruses, or fungi, or continuously especially in pregnant women.
Not to be used with:
Contains: POLYMYXIN B SULPHATE, NEOMYCIN sulphate, HYDROCORTISONE.
Other preparations:

Otrivine
(Ciba)

A spray and drops used as a SYMPATHOMIMETIC preparation to clear blocked nose.

Dose: adults 2-3 drops or 1-2 sprays into each nostril 2-3 times a day; children use paediatric drops.
Availability: NHS (when prescribed as a generic) and private prescription.
Side effects: itching nose, headache, slepplessness, rapid heart rate.
Caution: do not use for extended periods.
Not to be used for:
Not to be used with: MAOIS.
Contains: XYLOMETAZOLINE hydrochloride.
Other preparations: Otrivine Paediatric.

Otrivine-Antistin
(Ciba)

A spray or drops used as a SYMPATHOMIMETIC, antihistamine treatment for hay fever, allergic rhinitis.

Dose: 2-3 drops or 1 spray into each nostril 2-3 times a day.
Availability: private prescription and over the counter.
Side effects: itching nose, headache, rapid heart rate, sleeplessness.
Caution: do not use for extended periods.
Not to be used for: for children.
Not to be used with: MAOIS.
Contains: XYLOMETAZOLINE hydrochloride, ANTAZOLINE sulphate.
Other preparations:

Otrivine-Antistin
(Zyma)

Drops used as a SYMPATHOMIMETIC, antihistamine treatment for allergic conjunctivitis and other eye inflammations.

Dose: adults 1-2 drops into the eye 2-4 times a day; children over 2 years 1 drop 2-4 times a day.

Availability: NHS, private prescription, over the counter.

Side effects: temporary smarting, headache, sleeplessness, drowsiness, rapid heart rate, congestion.

Caution: in patients suffering from high blood pressure, enlarged prostate, coronary disease, diabetes.

Not to be used for: patients suffering from glaucoma or who wear soft contact lenses.

Not to be used with: MAOIS.

Contains: XYLOMETAZOLINE hydrochloride.

Other preparations:

Ovestin
(Organon)

A white tablet supplied at a strength of 0.25 mg and used as an oestrogen treatment for atrophic inflammation of the vagina, itch, as a treatment before vaginal surgery, other diseases of the vulva.

Dose: 1-2 tablets a day.

Availability: NHS and private prescription.

Side effects: enlarged breasts, bloating and fluid retention, cramps, leg pains, mood change, reduction in sexual desire, headaches, nausea, vaginal erosion, discharge, and bleeding, weight gain, skin changes.

Caution: in patients suffering from high blood pressure, diabetes, vascular disorders, asthma, depression, kidney disease, multiple sclerosis, womb diseases. Your doctor may advise you not to smoke, to have regular examinations. You should stop treatment at the first sign of serious symptoms such as severe headache or jaundice. Treatment should be stopped before surgery.

Not to be used for: children, pregnant women, or for patients suffering from sickle-cell anaemia, history of heart disease or thrombosis, liver disorders, some cancers, undiagnosed vaginal bleeding, some ear, skin, and kidney disorders.

Not to be used with: DIURETICS, anti-hypertensives, and drugs that change liver enzymes.

Contains: OESTRIOL.

Other preparations: Ovestin Cream

Ovran
(Wyeth)

A white tablet used as an oestrogen, progestogen contraceptive.

Dose: 1 tablet a day for 21 days starting on day 5 of the period.
Availability: NHS and private prescription.
Side effects: enlarged breasts, bloating and fluid retention, cramps, leg pains, mood change, reduction in sexual desire, headaches, nausea, vaginal erosion, discharge, and bleeding, weight gain, skin changes.
Caution: in patients suffering from high blood pressure, diabetes, vascular disorders, asthma, depression, kidney disease, multiple sclerosis, womb diseases. Your doctor may advise you not to smoke, to have regular examinations. You should stop treatment at the first sign of serious symptoms such as severe headache or jaundice. Treatment should be stopped before surgery.
Not to be used for: pregnant women, or for patients suffering from sickle-cell anaemia, history of heart disease or thrombosis, liver disorders, some cancers, undiagnosed vaginal bleeding, some ear, skin, and kidney disorders.
Not to be used with: RIFAMPICIN, TETRACYCLINES, GRISEOFULVIN, barbiturates, PHENYTOIN, PRIMIDONE, CARBAMAZEPINE, ETHOSUXIMIDE, CHLORAL HYDRATE, DICHLORALPHENAZONE.
Contains: ETHINYLOESTRADIOL, LEVONORGESTREL.
Other preparations: Ovran 30.

Ovranette
(Wyeth)

A white tablet used as an oestrogen, progestogen contraceptive.

Dose: 1 tablet a day for 21 days starting on day 5 of the period.
Availability: NHS and private prescription.
Side effects: enlarged breasts, bloating and fluid retention, cramps, leg pains, mood change, reduction in sexual desire, headaches, nausea, vaginal erosion, discharge, and bleeding, weight gain, skin changes.
Caution: in patients suffering from high blood pressure, diabetes, vascular disorders, asthma, depression, kidney disease, multiple sclerosis, womb diseases. Your doctor may advise you not to smoke, to have regular examinations. You should stop treatment at the first

sign of serious symptoms such as severe headache or jaundice. Treatment should be stopped before surgery.

Not to be used for: pregnant women, or for patients suffering from sickle-cell anaemia, history of heart disease or thrombosis, liver disorders, some cancers, undiagnosed vaginal bleeding, some ear, skin, and kidney disorders.

Not to be used with: RIFAMPICIN, TETRACYCLINES, GRISEOFULVIN, barbiturates, PHENYTOIN, PRIMIDONE, CARBAMAZEPINE, ETHOSUXIMIDE, CHLORAL HYDRATE, DICHLORALPHENAZONE.

Contains: ETHINYLOESTRADIOL, LEVONORGESTREL.

Other preparations:

Ovysmen
(Cilag)

A white tablet used as an oestrogen, progestogen contraceptive.

Dose: 1 tablet a day for 21 days starting on day 5 of the period.
Availability: NHS and private prescription.
Side effects: enlarged breasts, bloating and fluid retention, cramps, leg pains, mood change, reduction in sexual desire, headaches, nausea, vaginal erosion, discharge, and bleeding, weight gain, skin changes.
Caution: in patients suffering from high blood pressure, diabetes, vascular disorders, asthma, depression, kidney disease, multiple sclerosis, womb diseases. Your doctor may advise you not to smoke, to have regular examinations. You should stop treatment at the first sign of serious symptoms such as severe headache or jaundice. Treatment should be stopped before surgery.
Not to be used for: pregnant women, or for patients suffering from sickle-cell anaemia, history of heart disease or thrombosis, liver disorders, some cancers, undiagnosed vaginal bleeding, some ear, skin, and kidney disorders.
Not to be used with: RIFAMPICIN, TETRACYCLINES, GRISEOFULVIN, barbiturates, PHENYTOIN, PRIMIDONE, CARBAMAZEPINE, ETHOSUXIMIDE, CHLORAL HYDRATE, DICHLORALPHENAZONE.
Contains: ETHINYLOESTRADIOL, NORGESTREL.
Other preparations:

Oxanid *see* Oxazepam
(Steinhard)

oxatomide *see* Tinset

oxazepam

A tablet supplied at strengths of 10 mg, 15 mg, 30 mg and used as a sedative to treat anxiety.

Dose: elderly 10-20 mg 3 times a day; adults 15-30 mg a day increasing to 60 mg 3 times a day if needed.
Availability: NHS and private prescription.
Side effects: drowsiness, confusion, unsteadiness, low blood pressure, rash, changes in vision, changes in libido, retention of urine. Risk of addiction increases with dose and length of treatment. May impair judgement.
Caution: in the elderly, pregnant women, nursing mothers, in women during labour, and in patients suffering from lung disorders, kidney or liver disorders. Avoid long-term use and withdraw gradually.
Not to be used for: children, or for patients suffering from acute lung diseases, some chronic lung diseases, some obsessional and psychotic diseases.
Not to be used with: alcohol, other tranquillizers, anti-convulsants.
Contains:
Other preparations: oxazepam capsules, OXANID (Steinhard).

oxerutins *see* Paroven

oxethazaine *see* Mucaine

oxpentifylline *see* Trental

oxprenolol *see* Slow-Trasicor, Trasicor, Trasidrex

oxybuprocaine hydrochloride *see* Opulets Benoxinate

oxymetazoline hydrochloride *see* Afrazine

Oxymycin *see* Tetracycline
(DDSA)

oxypertine *see* Integrin

oxyphenbutazone *see* Tanderil

oxytetracycline hydrochloride *see* Terra-Cortril, Terra-Cortril Spray

p-aminobenzoic acid *see* Labiton

Pacitron
(Rorer)

An oblong orange tablet supplied at a strength of 500 mg and used as an anti-depressant to treat depression.

Dose: 2 tablets 3 times a day.
Availability: NHS and private prescription.
Side effects: nausea, headache.

Caution: in patients suffering from diseased bladder. Patients should be warned of reduced alertness.
Not to be used for: children.
Not to be used with: MAOIS.
Contains: TRYPTOPHAN.
Other preparations:

Paedialyte RS
(Abbott)

A solution used to supply electrolytes in the treatment of dehydration.

Dose: adults dose as required; children equivalent amount to estimate fluid loss in divided doses given over 6-8 hours.
Availability: NHS, private prescription, over the counter.
Side effects:
Caution: in patients suffering from dehydration.
Not to be used for: for patients suffering from kidney disease with kidney failure, blocked intestine, bowel paralysis, severe vomiting, severe dehydration where intravenous fluid treatment is needed.
Not to be used with:
Contains: GLUCOSE, SODIUM CHLORIDE, SODIUM CITRATE, POTASSIUM CITRATE.
Other preparations:

Palaprin Forte
(Nicholas)

An orange, oval, scored tablet supplied at a strength of 600 mg and used as a NON-STEROID ANTI-INFLAMMATORY DRUG to treat rheumatoid arthritis, osteoarthritis, spondylitis.

Dose: 1 tablet per 6.5 kg body weight a day in divided doses dispersed in water, sucked, chewed, or swallowed.
Availability: NHS, private prescription, over the counter.
Side effects: stomach upsets, allergy, asthma.
Caution: in pregnant women, the elderly, or in patients with a history of allergy to aspirin, asthma, impaired kidney or liver function, indigestion.
Not to be used for: children, nursing mothers, or patients suffering from haemophilia, or ulcers.

Not to be used with: anti-coagulants (blood-thinning drugs), some anti-diabetic drugs, anti-inflammatory agents, METHOTREXATE, SPIRONOLAC-TONE, steroids, some antacids, some uric acid-lowering drugs.
Contains: ALOXIPRIN.
Other preparations:

Paldesic *see* Calpol Infant
(RP Drugs)

Palfium
(MCP)

A white, scored tablet or a peach, scored tablet according to strengths of 5 mg, 10 mg and used as an opiate to control severe and prolonged pain.

Dose: adults up to 5 mg and then as advised by physician; children 88 micrograms per kg body weight or as advised by the physician.
Availability: controlled drug.
Side effects: tolerance, addiction, dizziness, sweating, nausea.
Caution: in the elderly, in pregnant women, and in patients suffering from liver disease, underactive thyroid gland.
Not to be used for: women in labour or for patients suffering from respiratory depression or blocked airways.
Not to be used with: MAOIS, sedatives.
Contains: DEXTROMORAMIDE tartrate.
Other preparations: Palfium Injection, Palfium Suppositories.

Paludrine
(ICI)

A white, scored tablet supplied at a strength of 100 mg and used as an anti-malarial drug for the prevention of malaria.

Dose: adults and children over 12 years 1-2 tablets a day after meals; children under 1 year 1/4 tablet, 1-4 years 1/2 tablet, 5-8 years 3/4 tablet, 9-12 years 1 tablet after meals.
Availability: NHS, private prescription, over the counter.

Side effects: stomach upset.
Caution:
Not to be used for:
Not to be used with:
Contains: PROGUANIL hydrochloride.
Other preparations:

Pameton
(Winthrop)

A white tablet used as an analgesic to relieve pain and reduce fever.

Dose: adults 2 tablets up to 4 times a day; children 6-12 years ½ -1 tablet every 4 hours to a maximum of 4 doses a day.
Availability: private prescription only.
Side effects:
Caution: in patients suffering from liver disease.
Not to be used for: children under 6 years.
Not to be used with: LEVODOPA.
Contains: PARACETAMOL, METHIONINE.
Other preparations:

Panadeine
(Winthrop)

A white, scored tablet used as an analgesic to relieve pain and reduce fever.

Dose: adults 2 tablets up to 4 times a day; children 7-12 years ½ -1 tablet up to 4 times a day.
Availability: NHS (when prescribed as a generic), private prescription.
Side effects:
Caution: in patients suffering from liver or kidney disease.
Not to be used for: children under 7 years.
Not to be used with: alcohol and sedatives.
Contains: PARACETAMOL, CODEINE phosphate.
Other preparations: Panadeine Soluble, Panadeine Forte.

Panadol *see* **paracetamol tablets**
(Winthrop)

Panaleve *see* **Calpol Infant**
(Leo)

Pancrease
(Cilag)

A white capsule used as a source of pancreatic enzymes to treat pancreatic exocrine insufficiency as in cystic fibrosis and chronic pancreatitis.

Dose: 1-2 capsules during meals or 1 capsule with a snack
Availability: NHS and private prescription.
Side effects: perianal irritation.
Caution:
Not to be used for:
Not to be used with:
Contains: PANCREATIN.
Other preparations:

pancreatin *see* **Cotazym, Creon, Nutrizym GR, Pancrease, Pancrex V Forte Tablets**

Pancrex V Forte Tablets
(Paines & Byrne)

A white tablet used as a source of pancreatic enzymes to treat cystic fibrosis, steatorrhoea, pancreatic enzyme deficiency states due to pancreatic disease.

Dose: 6-10 tablets 4 times a day before meals.
Availability: NHS and private prescription.
Side effects: buccal and perianal irritation.
Caution:

Not to be used for:
Not to be used with:
Contains: PANCREATIN.
Other preparations: Pancrex V Capsules, Pancrex V Capsules '125', Pancrex V Powder, Pancrex Granules.

Panoxyl
(Stiefel)

A gel used as an anti-bacterial, skin softener to treat acne.

Dose: wash and dry the affected area, then apply once a day.
Availability: NHS, private prescription, over the counter.
Side effects: irritation, peeling.
Caution: keep out of the eyes, nose, mouth.
Not to be used for:
Not to be used with:
Contains: BENZOYL PEROXIDE.
Other preparations: Panoxyl Aquagel, Panoxyl Wash.

panthenol *see* **Lipoflavonoid, Lipotriad**

papaveretum *see* **Aspav**

papaverine *see* **APP, Brovon, Pholcomed-D, Rybarvin**

para-aminosalicylic acid *see* **Cytacon**

paracetamol *see* **Cafadol, Calpol Infant, Co-Codamol, co-dydramol, co-proxamol, Disprol Paed, Femerital, Fortagesic, Lobak, Medised Suspension, Medocodene, Midrid, Migraleve, Pameton, Panadeine, paracetamol tablets,**

Paracodol, Parahypon, Parake, Paramax, Paramol, Pardale, Propain, Salzone, Solpadeine, Syndol, Tylex, Uniflu and Gregovite C

P

paracetamol tablets

A tablet supplied at a strength of 500 mg and used as an analgesic to relieve pain and reduce fever.

Dose: adults 1-2 tablet 4 times a day; children 6-12 years $\frac{1}{2}$ -1 tablet 4 times a day.
Availability: NHS, private prescription, over the counter.
Side effects:
Caution: in patients suffering from kidney or liver disease.
Not to be used for: children under 6 years.
Not to be used with:
Contains:
Other preparations: paracetamol soluble, paracetamol elixir, PANADOL (Winthrop), PANASORB (Winthrop).

Paracodol
(Fisons)

A white, effervescent tablet used as an analgesic to relieve pain.

Dose: adults 1-2 tablets in water every 4-6 hours to a maximum of 8 tablets in 24 hours; children 6-12 years $\frac{1}{2}$ -1 tablet to a maximum of 4 doses in 24 hours.
Availability: NHS (when prescribed as a generic), private presciption, over the counter.
Side effects:
Caution: in patients with kidney or liver disease or who are on a limited consumption of salt.
Not to be used for: children under 6 years.
Not to be used with:
Contains: PARACETAMOL, CODEINE phosphate.
Other preparations:

paradichlorobenzene *see* Cerumol

496

paraffin, liquid *see* **Agarol**

Parahypon
(Calmic)

A pink, scored tablet used as an analgesic to relieve pain.

Dose: adults 1-2 tablets 4 times a day; children 6-12 years half adult dose.
Availability: private presciption and over the counter.
Side effects:
Caution: in patients suffering from kidney or liver disease.
Not to be used for: children under 6 years.
Not to be used with:
Contains: PARACETAMOL, CAFFEINE, CODEINE phosphate.
Other preparations:

Parake
(Galen)

A white tablet used as an analgesic to relieve pain and reduce fever.

Dose: 2 tablets every 4 hours to a maximum of 8 tablets in 24 hours.
Availability: NHS (when prescribed as a generic), private prescription, over the counter.
Side effects:
Caution: in patients suffering from liver or kidney disease.
Not to be used for: children.
Not to be used with: alcohol, sedatives.
Contains: PARACETAMOL, CODEINE phosphate.
Other preparations:

Paramax
(Bencard)

A white, scored tablet used as an analgesic, anti-emetic treatment for migraine.

Dose: adults over 20 years 2 tablets at the beginning of the attack,

then 2 tablets every 4 hours to a maximum of 6 tablets in 24 hours; 15-19 years and with a body weight over 60 kg, 2 tablets at the beginning of the attack to a maximum of 3 tablets in 24 hours; children 12-14 years and body weight over 30 kg 1 tablet at the beginning to a maximum of 3 tablets in 24 hours.
Availability: NHS and private prescription.
Side effects: extrapyramidal reactions (shaking and rigidity).
Caution: in patients suffering from liver or kidney disease.
Not to be used for: children under 12 years.
Not to be used with: ANTI-CHOLINERGICS, sedatives.
Contains: PARACETAMOL, METOCLOPRAMIDE hydrochloride.
Other preparations: Paramax Sachets.

Paramol
(Duncan, Flockhart)

A white tablet used as an opiate, analgesic, antussive (cough medicine) treatment for pain, cough.

Dose: 1 tablet every 4 hours during or after food increasing to 2 tablets 4 times a day if needed.
Availability: NHS (when prescribed as a generic), private prescription.
Side effects: constipation, rarely nausea and headache.
Caution: in the elderly, pregnant women, and in patients suffering from allergies, kidney or liver disease, underactive thyroid.
Not to be used for: children or for patients suffering from respiratory depression or blocked airways.
Not to be used with: alcohol, sedatives.
Contains: PARACETAMOL, DIHYDROCODEINE tartrate.
Other preparations:

Pardale
(Martindale)

A white, scored tablet used as an analgesic to relieve headache, rheumatism, period pain.

Dose: 1-2 tablets 3-4 times a day.
Availability: over the counter and private prescription only.

Side effects:
Caution: in patients suffering from kidney or liver disease.
Not to be used for: children.
Not to be used with:
Contains: PARACETAMOL, CODEINE PHOSPHATE, CAFFEINE hydrate.
Other preparations:

P

Paritane *see* Trasicor
(Berk)

Parlodel
(Sandoz)

A white, scored tablet supplied at strengths of 1 mg, 2.5 mg and used as a hormone blocker to treat Parkinson's disease, inappropriate lactation, infertility, cyclical benign breast disease, elevated prolactin.

Dose: 1-1.25 mg at night with food at first, increasing after 7 days to 2.5 mg at night, then after 14 days to 2.5 mg twice a day with food. Increase if needed every 3-14 days by 2.5 mg a day to 10-80 mg a day in 3 divided doses.
Availability: NHS and private prescription.
Side effects: low blood pressure on standing, brain and stomach disturbances, nausea, vomiting, constipation, headache, drowsiness, poor circulation, movement disorders, dry mouth, leg cramps, lung changes.
Caution: in women, patients suffering from a history of mental disorder, severe cardiovascular disease. Your doctor may advise regular examinations.
Not to be used for: children.
Not to be used with: alcohol.
Contains: BROMOCRIPTINE MESYLATE.
Other preparations: Parlodel Capsules

Parmid *see* Maxolon
(Lagap)

Parnate
(S K B)

A red tablet used as an MAOI anti-depressant to treat depression.

Dose: 1 tablet twice a day at first, increasing after 7 days if necessary to 1 tablet 3 times a day, then usually 1 tablet a day.
Availability: NHS and private prescription.
Side effects: severe high blood pressure reactions with certain foods, sleeplessness, low blood pressure, dizziness, drowsiness, weakness, dry mouth, constipation, stomach upset, blurred vision, urinary difficulties, ankle swelling, rash, jaundice, weight gain, confusion, sexual desire changes.
Caution: in the elderly and in patients suffering from epilepsy.
Not to be used for: children, or for patients suffering from liver disease, blood changes, heart disease, phaeochromocytoma, overactive thyroid, brain artery disease.
Not to be used with: amphetamines or similar SYMPATHOMIMETIC drugs, TRICYCLIC antidepressants, PETHIDINE and other narcotics, some cough mixtures and appetite supressants containing sympathomimetics. Barbiturates, sedatives, alcohol, and anti-diabetics may be enhanced. ANTI-CHOLINERGIC side effects are increased. Cheese, Bovril, Oxo, meat extracts, broad beans, banana, Marmite, yeast extracts, wine, beer, other alcohol, pickled herrings, vegetable proteins. (Up to 14 days after cessation.)
Contains: TRANYLCYPROMINE sulphate.
Other preparations:

Paroven
(Zyma)

A yellow capsule supplied at a strength of 250 mg and used as a vein constrictor to treat ankle swelling, varicose veins.

Dose: 3-4 capsules a day with food at first, then reduce.
Availability: NHS, private prescription, over the counter.
Side effects: stomach disturbances, flushes, headache.
Caution:
Not to be used for: children.
Not to be used with:
Contains: OXERUTINS.
Other preparations:

Parstelin
(S K B)

A green tablet used as an MAOI to treat depression with anxiety.

Dose: 1 tablet twice a day at first, increasing to 1 tablet 3 times a day if needed after 7 days, then usually 1 tablet a day.
Availability: NHS and private prescription.
Side effects: severe high blood pressure reactions with certain foods, low blood pressure, muscle spasms, restlessness, low body temperature, breast swelling, menstrual changes, sleeplessness, low blood pressure, dizziness, drowsiness, weakness, dry mouth, constipation, stomach upset, blurred vision, urinary difficulties, ankle swelling, rash, blood and skin changes, jaundice, weight gain, confusion, sexual desire changes.
Caution: in the elderly, pregnant women, nursing mothers, and in patients suffering from epilepsy. Your doctor may advise regular blood and liver checks.
Not to be used for: children, or for patients suffering from liver disease, blood changes, heart disease, phaeochromocytoma, overactive thyroid, brain artery disease, Parkinson's disease.
Not to be used with: amphetamines or similar SYMPATHOMIMETIC drugs, TRICYCLIC antidepressants, tranquillizers, LEVODOPA, PETHIDINE and other narcotics, some cough mixtures and appetite supressants containing sympathomimetics. Barbiturates, sedatives, alcohol, and anti-diabetics may be enhanced. Anti-cholinergic side effects are increased. Cheese, Bovril, Oxo, meat extracts, broad beans, banana, Marmite, yeast extracts, wine, beer, other alcohol, pickled herrings, vegetable proteins. (Up to 14 days after cessation.)
Contains: TRANYLCYPROMINE sulphate, TRIFLUOPERAZINE.
Other preparations:

Parvolex
(Duncan, Flockhart)

An ampule used to supply amino acid for the treatment of paracetamol overdose.

Dose:
Availability: NHS and private prescription.
Side effects: rash, allergy.
Caution: in patients with a history of asthma. Blood should be

checked regularly.
Not to be used for:
Not to be used with: rubber, metals.
Contains: ACETYLCYSTEINE.
Other preparations:

Pavacol-D
(Boehringer Ingelheim)

A mixture containing opiate and demulcents used to treat cough.

Dose: adults 1-2 5 ml teaspoonsful as needed; children 1-2 years ½ teaspoonful 3-4 times a day,3-5 years 1 teaspoonful 3 times a day, 6-12 years 1 teaspoonful 4-5 times a day.
Availability: NHS, private prescription, over the counter.
Side effects: constipation.
Caution: patients suffering from asthma
Not to be used for: for infants under 1 year or for patients suffering from liver disease.
Not to be used with: MAOIS.
Contains: PHOLCODINE, aromatic oils.
Other preparations:

Paxofen *see* Brufen
(Steinhard)

Paynocil
(S K B)

A white, scored tablet used as an analgesic to relieve pain, reduce fever, and to treat rheumatoid arthritis, and other rheumatic conditions.

Dose: 1 tablet dissolved on the tongue every 4-6 hours. For rheumatic conditions 2-3 tablets three times a day for 2-3 weeks reducing to 1-2 tablets 3 times a day.
Availability: private prescription and over the counter.
Side effects: stomach upsets, allergy, asthma.

Caution: in pregnant women, the elderly, or in patients with a history of allergy to ASPIRIN, asthma, impaired kidney or liver function, indigestion.

Not to be used for: children, nursing mothers, or patients suffering from haemophilia, or ulcers.

Not to be used with: anti-coagulants (blood-thinning drugs), some anti-diabetic drugs, anti-inflammatory agents, METHOTREXATE, SPIRONOLACTONE, steroids, some antacids, some uric acid-lowering drugs.

Contains: ASPIRIN, GLYCINE.

Other preparations:

PC4
(Schering)

A white tablet used as an oestrogen, progestogen contraceptive in an emergency within 72 hours of intercourse where no other precautions have been taken.

Dose: 2 tablets soon after intercourse, then a further 2 tablets 12 hours later.

Availability: NHS and private prescription.

Side effects: vomiting, nausea.

Caution: in patients with a history of depression, diabetes, high blood pressure, epilepsy, porphyria (a rare blood disorder), tetanus, liver and kidney disease, gallstones, cardiovascular disease.

Not to be used for: women whose menstrual bleeding is overdue.

Not to be used with: RIFAMPICIN, TETRACYCLINES, GRISEOFULVIN, barbiturates, PHENYTOIN, PRIMIDONE, CARBAMAZIPINE, MEPROBAMATE, GLUTETHIMIDE, CHORAL HYDRATE, DICHLORALPHENAZONE.

Contains: ETHINYLOESTRADIOL, NORGESTREL.

Other preparations:

pectin *see* **Orabase**

pemoline *see* **Volital**

Penbritin
(S K B)

A black/red capsule supplied at strengths of 250 mg, 500 mg and used as a penicillin to treat respiratory, ear, nose, and throat infections, gonorrhoea, soft tissue infections, urinary infections.

Dose: adults 250 mg-1 g every 6 hours; children 125-250 mg every 6 hours.
Availability: NHS and private prescription.
Side effects: allergy, stomach disturbances.
Caution: in patients suffering from glandular fever.
Not to be used for: patients suffering from penicillin allergy.
Not to be used with:
Contains: AMPICILLIN.
Other preparations:

---

penbutolol *see* Lasipressin

Pendramine
(Degussa)

A white, oblong, scored tablet supplied at strengths of 125 mg, 250 mg and used as an anti-rheumatic drug to treat severe rheumatoid arthritis.

Dose: adults 125-250 mg a day for the first 4-8 weeks, increasing by similar amounts as no less than 4-week intervals to a maximum of 2 g a day; children 15-20 mg per kg body weight a day starting at a lower dose and increasing at 4-week intervals over a period of 3-6 months.
Availability: NHS and private prescription.
Side effects: nausea, anorexia, fever, rash, loss of taste, blood changes, blood or protein in the urine, myasthenia gravis (a muscle disease), systemic lupus erythematosus (a multisystem disorder).
Caution: in patients suffering from kidney disease or who are sensitive to penicillin.
Not to be used for: pregnant women, nursing mothers, or for patients suffering from systemic lupus erythematosus (a multisystem disorder), low platelet levels, agranulocytosis (low white count).
Not to be used with: gold salts, anti-malaria or cytotoxic drugs, PHEN-

YLBUTAZONE.
Contains: PENICILLAMINE.
Other preparations:

penicillamine *see* Distamine, Pendramine

penicillin V potassium *see* Distaquaine V-K, Stabillin V-K, V-Cil-K

pentaerythritol *see* Cardiacap

pentaerythritol tetranitrate *see* Mycardol

pentazocine *see* Fortagesic, Fortral

pentazocine *see* Fortral

penthiazide *see* Trasidrex

Pepcid PM
(Morson)

A brown, square tablet supplied at strengths of 20 mg, 40 mg and used as an H_2 blocker in the prevention and treatment of duodenal and gastric ulcers, Zollinger-Ellison syndrome (high acid production).

Dose: adults prevention 20 mg at night, otherwise 40 mg at night and

up to 480 mg a day.
Availability: NHS and private prescription.
Side effects: headache, dizziness, constipation, diarrhoea, dry mouth, nausea, rash, bowel discomfort, loss of appetite, fatigue.
Caution: in pregnant women, nursing mothers, and in patients suffering from impaired kidney function. Stomach cancer should be excluded as a diagnosis.
Not to be used for: children.
Not to be used with:
Contains: FAMOTIDINE.
Other preparations:

---

peppermint oil *see* **Carbellon, Colpermin, Mintec, Tercoda**

---

pepsin *see* **Muripsin**

Peptard
(3M Riker)

A white tablet supplied at a strength of 0.2 mg and used as an anti-spasm, ANTI-CHOLINERGIC treatment for peptic ulcers, irritable bowel syndrome, excessive sweating.

Dose: children over 10 years 1-2 tablets twice a day, adults 2-3 tablets twice a day.
Availability: NHS and private prescription.
Side effects: blurred vision, confusion, dry mouth.
Caution:
Not to be used for: glaucoma, inflammatory bowel disease, intestinal obstruction, enlarged prostate.
Not to be used with:
Contains: HYOSCYAMINE SULPHATE.
Other preparations:

Percutol
(Rorer)

An ointment used as a NITRATE for the prevention of angina.

Dose: apply every 3-4 hours or as advised.
Availability: NHS and private prescription.
Side effects: headache.
Caution:
Not to be used for: children.
Not to be used with:
Contains: GLYCERYL TRINITRATE.
Other preparations:

Periactin
(MSD)

A white, scored tablet supplied at a strength of 4 mg and used as an antihistamine, serotonin antagonist (hormone blocker) to improve appetite,and to treat allergies, itchy skin conditions.

Dose: adults and children over 7 years 1 tablet 3-4 times a day; children 2-6 years 2 tablets a day or $^1/_2$ tablet 3-4 times a day.
Availability: NHS, private prescription, over the counter.
Side effects: anti-cholinergic effects, reduced reactions, drowsiness, excitement.
Caution: in pregnant women and in patients suffering from bronchial asthma, raised eye pressure, overactive thyroid, cardiovascular disease, high blood pressure.
Not to be used for: for new-born infants, nursing mothers, the elderly, or patients suffering from glaucoma, enlarged prostate, bladder obstruction, retention of urine, stomach blockage, peptic ulcer, or debilitation.
Not to be used with: MAOIS, alcohol, sedatives.
Contains: CYPROHEPTADINE hydrochloride.
Other preparations: Periactin Syrup.

---

pericyazine *see* Neulactil

---

perphenazine *see* Fentazin, Triptafen

Persantin
(Boehringer Ingelheim)

An orange tablet or a white tablet according to strengths of 25 mg, 100 mg and used as an anti-platelet drug in addition to oral anti-coagulants or ASPIRIN in the treatment of thrombosis.

Dose: adults 300-600 mg a day in 3-4 doses before meals; children 5 mg per kg body weight a day in divided doses.
Availability: NHS and private prescription.
Side effects: headache, dizziness, stomach upset, rash.
Caution: care in patients suffering from rapidly worsening agina.
Not to be used for:
Not to be used with: antacids.
Contains: DIPYRIDAMOLE.
Other preparations:

Pertofran
(Geigy)

A pale-pink tablet supplied at a strength of 25 mg and used as an anti-depressant to treat depression.

Dose: adults 1 tablet 3 times a day at first increasing to 2 tablets 3-4 times a day; elderly 1 tablet a day at first.
Availability: NHS and private prescription.
Side effects: dry mouth, constipation, urine retention, blurred vision, palpitations, drowsiness, sleeplessness, dizziness, hands shaking, low blood presure, weight change, skin reactions, jaundice or blood changes, loss of libido may occur.
Caution: in nursing mothers or in patients suffering from heart disease, thyroid disease, epilepsy, diabetes, some other psychiatric conditions. Your doctor may advise regular blood tests.
Not to be used for: children, pregnant women, or for patients suffering from heart attacks, liver disease, heart block.
Not to be used with: alcohol, ANTI-CHOLINERGICS, ADRENALINE, MAOIS, barbiturates, other anti-depressants, anti-hypertensives.
Contains: DESIPRAMINE HYDROCHLORIDE.
Other preparations:

Peru balsam *see* Anugesic-HC, Anusol, Anusol HC

Petrolagar No 1
(Wyeth)

An emulsion supplied in 200 ml and 500 ml bottles and used as a lubricant to treat constipation.

Dose: adults 10 ml night and morning or after meals; children half adult dose.
Availability: private prescription only.
Side effects:
Caution: avoid using for prolonged treatment.
Not to be used for:
Not to be used with:
Contains: liquid PARAFFIN, light liquid paraffin.
Other preparations:

Pevaryl
(Cilag)

A cream used as an anti-fungal treatment for inflammation of the penis, inflammation of the vulva, thrush-like nappy rash, other skin infections such as tinea or nail infections.

Dose: massage gently into the affected area 2-3 times a day.
Availability: NHS, private prescription, over the counter.
Side effects: irritation.
Caution:
Not to be used for:
Not to be used with:
Contains: ECONAZOLE nitrate.
Other preparations: Pevaryl Lotion, Pevaryl Spray, Pevaryl Powder.

---

phaeochromocytoma

a tumour of the adrenal gland which produces excess adrenaline-like hormones.

Phanodorm
(Winthrop)

A white tablet supplied at a strength of 200 mg and used as a barbiturate to treat sleeplessness.

Dose: $^1/_2$ -1 tablet before going to bed.
Availability: controlled drug.
Side effects: drowsiness, hangover, dizziness, allergies, headache, confusion, excitement.
Caution: in patients suffering from kidney or lung disease. Dependence (addiction) may develop.
Not to be used for: children, young adults, pregnant women, nursing mothers, the elderly, patients with a history of drug or alcohol abuse, or suffering from porphyria (a rare blood disorder), or in the management of pain.
Not to be used with: anti-coagulants (blood-thinning drugs), alcohol, other tranquillizers, steroids, the contraceptive pill, GRISEOFULVIN, RIFAMPICIN, PHENYTOIN, METRONIDAZOLE, CHLORAMPHENICOL.
Contains: CYCLOBARBITONE calcium.
Other preparations:

Phasal
(Lagap)

A white tablet supplied at a strength of 300 mg and used as a LITHIUM salt to treat acute manic or hypomanic disorders, prevention of manic depression and recurring depression.

Dose: to maintain blood level in a given range.
Availability: NHS and private prescription.
Side effects: nausea, diarrhoea, hand tremor, muscular weakness, brain and heart changes, weight gain, swelling, under- or overactive thyroid, thirst and excessive urination, kidney changes, skin reactions, intoxication.
Caution: treatment should be started in hospital and a careful check on the functioning of the kidneys and thyroid should be made, as well as ensuring that there is an adequate consumption of salt and fluid. Your doctor may advise blood tests to gauge dose.
Not to be used for: for children, pregnant women, nursing mothers, or for patients suffering from disturbed sodium balance, Addison's disease, kidney or heart disease, or underactive thyroid.
Not to be used with: DIURETICS, NON-STEROID ANTI-INFLAMMATORY DRUGS, CARBAMAZEPINE, FLUPENTHIXOL, METHYLDOPA, PHENYTOIN, HALOPERIDOL, TETRACYCLINES.

Contains: LITHIUM CARBONATE.
Other preparations:

---

phenazocine hydrobromide *see* **Narphen**

---

phenazone *see* **Auralgicin, Auraltone**

---

phenazopyridine hydrochloride *see* **Uromide**

---

phenelzine sulphate *see* **Nardil**

Phenergan
(M & B)

A blue tablet supplied at strengths of10 mg, 25 mg and used as an antihistamine treatment for allergies.

Dose: adults 10-20 mg 2-3 times a day; children 1-5 years 5-15 mg a day, over 5 years 10-25 mg a day.
Availability: NHS, private prescription, over the counter.
Side effects: drowsiness, reduced reactions, dizziness, disorientation, sensitivity to light, convulsions on high doses, extrapyramidal reactions (shaking and rigidity).
Caution:
Not to be used for: infants under 1 year.
Not to be used with: sedatives, MAOIS, alcohol.
Contains: PROMETHAZINE hydrochloride.
Other preparations: Phenergan Elixir, Phenergan Injection.

---

phenethicillin *see* **Broxil**

---

phenindamine tartrate *see* **Thephorin**

phenindione *see* **Dindevan**

pheniramine *see* **Daneral SA**

phenobarbitone *see* **Luminal**

phenol *see* **Chloraseptic**

phenolphthalein *see* **Agarol, Alophen, Kest**

phenoxybenzamine *see* **Dibenyline**

phenoxypropanol *see* **Phytocil**

Phensedyl
(M & B)

A linctus used as an antihistamine, opiate, SYMPATHOMIMETIC treatment for cough.

Dose: adults 1-2 5 ml teaspoonsful 2-3 times a day; children 2-5 years ¹/₂ teaspoonful 2-3 times a day, 6-12 years ¹/₂ -1 teaspoonful 2-3 times a day.
Availability: private prescription and over the counter.
Side effects: constipation, drowsiness, reduced reactions, anxiety, hands shaking, irregular or rapid heart rate, dry mouth, excitement,

rarely skin eruptions.
Caution: in patients suffering from asthma, kidney disease, diabetes.
Not to be used for: children under 2 years or for patients suffering
from liver disease, heart or thyroid isorders.
Not to be used with: MAOIS, alcohol, sedatives, TRICYCLICS.
Contains: PROMETHAZINE hydrochloride, CODEINE phosphate, EPHEDRINE
hydrochloride.
Other preparations:

P

---

phentermine *see* **Duromine, Ionamin**

Phenylephrine
(SNP)

Drops used as a SYMPATHOMIMETIC pupil dilator.

Dose: 1 drop into the eye as needed.
Availability: NHS, private prescription, over the counter.
Side effects:
Caution:
Not to be used for: patients suffering from narrow angle glaucoma,
high blood pressure coronary disease, overactive thyroid.
Not to be used with: ß-BLOCKERS.
Contains: PHENYLEPHRINE.
Other preparations:

---

phenylephrine *see* **Betnovate Rectal, Bronchilator, Dimo-
tapp LA, Duo-Autohaler, Hayphryn, Isopto Frin, Medihaler-
Duo, Neophryn, Phenylephrine, Uniflu and Gregovite C,
Vibrocil**

---

phenylethyl alcohol *see* **Ceanel Concentrate**

---

phenylpropanolamine *see* Dimotapp LA, Eskornade Spansule

P

phenyltoloxamine *see* Pholtex

phenytoin *see* Epanutin

pHiso-Med
(Winthrop)

A solution used as a disinfectant to treat acne, and for disinfecting infants' skin, cleansing and disinfecting skin before surgery.

Dose: use as a liquid soap.
Availability: NHS, private prescription, over the counter.
Side effects:
Caution: in newborn infants dilute 10 times.
Not to be used for:
Not to be used with:
Contains: CHLORHEXIDINE GLUCONATE.
Other preparations:

pholcodine *see* Copholco, Copholcoids, Davenol, Expulin, Galenphol, Pavacol-D, Pholcomed-D, Pholtex

Pholcomed-D
(Medo)

A linctus used as an opiate and bronchial relaxant to treat dry irritating cough.

Dose: adults 2-3 5 ml teaspoonsful 3-4 times a day, children under 2 years ¹/₂ teaspoonful 3-4 times a day, 2-12 years 1 teaspoonful 3-4 times a day.
Availability: NHS, private prescription, over the counter.

Side effects: constipation.
Caution: in patients suffering from asthma
Not to be used for: children under 5 years, or for patients suffering from liver disease.
Not to be used with: MAOIS.
Contains: PHOLCODINE, PAPAVERINE hydrochloride.
Other preparations: Pholcomed Capsules, Pholcomed, Pholcomed Forte, Pholcomed Forte Diabetic, Pholcomed Expectorant.

Pholtex
(3M Riker)

A liquid used as an opiate and antihistamine treatment for dry cough.

Dose: adults 1 5 ml teaspoonful 2-3 times a day; children $\frac{1}{2}$ -1 teaspoonful 2-3 times a day.
Availability: private prescription and over the counter.
Side effects: constipation.
Caution: in patients suffering from asthma.
Not to be used for: children under 5 years, or for patients suffering from liver disease.
Not to be used with: MAOIS.
Contains: PHOLCODINE, PHENYLTOLOXAMINE.
Other preparations:

Phosphate
(Sandoz)

A white, effervescent tablet used as a phosphate supplement to treat elevated calcium levels.

Dose: adults and children over 5 years up to 6 tablets a day; children under 5 years half adult dose.
Availability: NHS, private prescription, over the counter.
Side effects: diarrhoea.
Caution: in patients suffering from kidney disease, congestive heart disease, high blood pressure.
Not to be used for: patients on a low sodium diet.
Not to be used with: antacids.
Contains: SODIUM ACID PHOSPHATE, SODIUM BICARBONATE, POTASSIUM BICARBONATE.

Phospholine-Iodide
(Wyeth)

Drops used as an ANTI-CHOLINESTERASE to treat glaucoma, accommodative esotropia.

Dose: 1 drop into the eye twice a day or as advised by the physician.
Availability: NHS and private prescription.
Side effects: eye irritation at first, heacache, cysts on the iris, rise in pressure, thickening of the conjunctiva, obstruction of the tear duct, poor vision.
Caution: care in patients suffering from low blood pressure or slow heart rate, recent heart attack, epilepsy, Parkinson's disease, peptic ulcer.
Not to be used for: patients suffering from asthma, damaged retina, narrow angle glaucoma, inflamed eye.
Not to be used with: muscle relaxants, anti-cholinesterases.
Contains: ECOTHIOPATE IODIDE.
Other preparations:

phosphorylcolamine *see* Fosfor

Phyllocontin Continus
(Napp)

A pale-yellow tablet supplied at a strength of 225 mg and used as a broncho-dilator to treat left ventricular or congestive heart failure, bronchial spasm associated with asthma, chronic bronchitis, emphysema.

Dose: 1 tablet twice a day for 7 days then 1-2 tablets a day.
Availability: NHS and private prescription.
Side effects: nausea, stomach upset, headache, brain stimulation.
Caution: in pregnant women, nursing mothers, and in patients suffering from other forms of heart disease, liver disease, peptic ulcer.
Not to be used for: children.

Not to be used with: CIMETIDINE, ERYTHROMYCIN, CIPROFLOXACIN, INTER-FERON.
Contains: AMINOPHYLLINE.
Other preparations: Phyllocontin Forte, Phyllocontin Paediatric.

Physeptone
(Calmic)

A white, scored tablet supplied at a strength of 5 mg and used as an opiate to control severe pain.

Dose: 1-2 tablets every 6-8 hours.
Availability: controlled drug.
Side effects: tolerance, addiction, euphoria, dizziness, sedation, nausea.
Caution: in pregnant women and in patients suffering from liver disease or underactive thyroid.
Not to be used for: children, in obstetrics, for ambulant patients, or for patients with respiratory depression or blocked airways.
Not to be used with: MAOIS, sedatives.
Contains: METHADONE hydrochloride.
Other preparations: Physeptone Injection.

Phytex
(Pharmax)

A paint used as an anti-fungal treatment for skin and nail infections.

Dose: paint on to the affected area morning and evening and after bathing for 2-3 weeks after the symptoms have gone.
Availability: NHS, private prescription, over the counter.
Side effects:
Caution:
Not to be used for: children under 5 years or pregnant women.
Not to be used with:
Contains: TANNIC ACID, BORIC ACID, SALICYLIC ACID, METHYL SALICYLATE, ACETIC ACID.
Other preparations:

Phytocil
(Fisons)

A cream used as an anti-fungal treatment for tinea infections.

Dose: apply to the affected area 2-3 times a day.
Availability: NHS, private prescription, over the counter.
Side effects:
Caution:
Not to be used for:
Not to be used with:
Contains: PHENOXYPROPANOL, CHLOROPHENOXYETHANOL, SALICYLIC ACID, MENTHOL.
Other preparations: Phytocil Powder.

Picolax
(Nordic)

Powder supplied in sachets and used as a stimulant and laxative for the evacuation of bowels prior to surgery etc.

Dose: adults 1 sachet dissolved in water before breakfast, repeated 6-8 hours later if required; children 2-4 years 1/2 sachet morning and afternoon, children 4-9 years 1 sachet in morning 1/2 sachet in afternoon, children over 9 years adult dose.
Availability: NHS and private prescription.
Side effects:
Caution: low residue food should be eaten and plenty of water drunk during treatment. Special care should be taken for patients suffering from inflammatory bowel disease.
Not to be used for:
Not to be used with: antibiotics.
Contains: SODIUM PICOSULPHATE, MAGNESIUM CITRATE.
Other preparations:

Pilocarpine
(SNP)

Drops used as a pupil constrictor to treat glaucoma.

Dose: 1 drop into the eye every 5 minutes until constriction is achieved.

Availability: NHS and private prescription.
Side effects:
Caution:
Not to be used for:
Not to be used with:
Contains: PILOCARPINE nitrate.
Other preparations:

---

pilocarpine *see* **Carpine, Ocusert Pilo, Opulets Pilocarpine, Pilocarpine, Sno Pilo**

Pimafucin
(Brocades)

A cream-coloured, pear-shaped vaginal tablet supplied at a strength of 25 mg and used as an anti-fungal treatment for vaginal thrush and trichomonal infections.

Dose: 1 tablet into the vagina at night for 20 days or 1 tablet into the vagina night and morning for 10 days.
Availability: NHS and private prescription.
Side effects: mild burning or irritation
Caution:
Not to be used for: children.
Not to be used with:
Contains: NATAMYCIN.
Other preparations: Pimafucin Cream.

Pimafucin 2¹/₂%
(Brocades)

A suspension used as an antibiotic treatment for lung and respiratory infections.

Dose: inhale 7.5 mg a day in divided doses for 4 weeks, then 5 mg a day until advised by the physician but for not less than 6 weeks in total.
Availability: NHS and private prescription.
Side effects:
Caution:

Pimafucin Cream
(Brocades)

A cream used as an anti-fungal treatment for skin and nail infections.

Dose: apply to the affected area 2-3 times a day.
Availability: NHS and private prescription.
Side effects:
Caution:
Not to be used for:
Not to be used with:
Contains: NATAMYCIN.
Other preparations:

---

pimozide *see* **Orap**

---

pindolol *see* **Viskaldix, Visken**

---

pinene *see* **Rowatinex**

---

pipenzolate bromide *see* **Piptal**

---

piperazine oestrone sulphate *see* **Harmogen**

---

piperazine *see* **Antepar, Pripsin**

Piptal
(MCP)

An orange tablet supplied at a strength of 5 mg and used as an anti-spasm, ANTI-CHOLINERGIC treatment for peptic ulcers, irritable bowel syndrome, excessive sweating.

Dose: 1 tablet 3 times a day and 1-2 tablets at night.
Availability: NHS and private prescription.
Side effects: blurred vision, confusion, dry mouth.
Caution:
Not to be used for: children, or for patients suffering from glaucoma, inflammatory bowel disease, intestinal obstruction, and enlarged prostate.
Not to be used with:
Contains: PIPENZOLATE BROMIDE.
Other preparations: Piptalin (with DIMETHICONE).

Piptalin *see* **Piptal**
(MCP)

---

pirbuterol *see* **Exirel**

---

pirenzepine *see* **Gastrozepin**

---

piretanide *see* **Arelix**

Piriton
(A & H)

A cream-coloured tablet supplied at a strength of 4 mg and used as an antihistamine treatment for allergies.

Dose: adults 1 tablet 3-4 times a day; children 6-12 years $^1/_2$ -1 tablet 3-4 times a day, under 6 years use syrup.
Availability: NHS, private prescription, over the counter.
Side effects: drowsiness, reduced reactions, dizziness, excitation.
Caution: in nursing mothers.

Not to be used for:
Not to be used with: sedatives, MAOIS, alcohol.
Contains: CHLORPHENIRAMINE maleate.
Other preparations: Piriton Syrup, Piriton Spandets, Piriton Injection.

---

piroxicam *see* **Feldene**

---

pivampicillin *see* **Miraxid, Pondocillin**

---

pivmecillinam *see* **Selexid**

---

pizotifen hydrogen malate *see* **Sanomigran**

Plaquenil
(Winthrop)

An orange tablet supplied at a strength of 200 mg and used as an anti-arthritic (anti-malarial) drug to treat rheumatoid arthritis, lupus erythomatosus (a multisystem disease), and for the prevention and treatment of malaria.

Dose: adults 2 tablets a day with food at first, then 1-2 tablets a day or up to 6.5 mg per kg body weight per day for no more than 6 months; children as advised by the physician. Malaria 6 mg per kg body weight a week.
Availability: NHS and private prescription.
Side effects: eye disorders, skin reactions, bleached hair, alopecia, stomach intolerance.
Caution: in pregnant women, nursing mothers, and in patients suffering from porphyria (a rare blood disorder), kidney or liver disease, psoriasis, history of stomach, neurological, or blood disorders. The eyes should be checked regularly.
Not to be used for: patients suffering from maculopathy (eye dis-

ease).
Not to be used with: antacids, aminoglycosides, any drugs likely to cause eye damage.
Contains: HYDROXYCHLOROQUINE sulphate.
Other preparations:

Platet 300
(Nicholas)

A white, effervescent tablet supplied at a strength of 300 mg and used as an anti-platelet drug to reduce risk of heart attack in patients suffering from angina or earlier heart attack.

Dose: 1 tablet a day dissolved in water beginning within 36 hours of surgery.
Availability: NHS and private prescription.
Side effects: bronchospasm, stomach bleeding.
Caution: in patients who are allergic to aspirin or anti-inflammatory drugs, and who are suffering from kidney or liver disease, or a history of bronchospasm.
Not to be used for: nursing mothers or for patients with peptic ulcer or any bleeding conditions.
Not to be used with: oral anti-coagulants, hypoglycaemics, non-steroid anti-inflammatory drugs, uric acid lowering agents, METHOTREXATE, SPIRONOLACTONE, corticosteroids.
Contains: ASPIRIN.
Other preparations: Platet

Plesmet
(Napp)

A syrup used as an iron supplement to treat iron-deficiency anaemia.

Dose: adults 1-2 5 ml teaspoonsful 3 times a day; children $^1/_2$ -1 teaspoonful 2-3 times a day.
Availability: NHS, private prescription, over the counter.
Side effects:
Caution:
Not to be used for:
Not to be used with: TETRACYCLINES.
Contains: FERROUS GLYCINE SULPHATE.

Other preparations:

P

podophyllotoxin *see* **Warticon**

podophyllum resin *see* **Posalfilin**

poldine methylsulphate *see* **Nacton Forte**

Polyalk
(Galen)

A white liquid used as an antacid to treat hyperacidity.

Dose: adults 10-20 ml after meals and at bedtime.
Availability: NHS and private prescription.
Side effects: few; occasionally constipation.
Caution:
Not to be used for: infants.
Not to be used with: TETRACYCLINE antibiotics.
Contains: ALUMINIUM HYDROXIDE AND MAGNESIUM OXIDE.
Other preparations:

Polybactrin
(Calmic)

A powder supplied in an aerosol used as an aminoglycoside antibiotic to treat burns and wounds, and in surgery.

Dose: spray lightly on to the affected area.
Availability: NHS and private prescription.
Side effects: ear damage, kidney damage, allergy.
Caution: in patients with large areas of affected skin.
Not to be used for:
Not to be used with:

Contains: NEOMYCIN sulphate, POLYMYXIN B SULPHATE, BACITRACIN ZINC.
Other preparations:

Polycrol Forte Gel *see* Asilone
(Nicholas)

Polycrol *see* Asilone
(Nicholas)

---

polyethylene glycol *see* Dioctyl Ear Drops, Hypotears

---

polyethylene granules *see* Ionax

Polyfax
(Calmic)

An ointment used as an antibiotic to treat styes, conjunctivitis, other eye inflammations, skin infections.

Dose: apply to the eye at least twice a day or to other areas 2 or more times a day.
Availability: NHS and private prescription.
Side effects: kidney damage, allergy.
Caution: in patients suffering from large open wounds.
Not to be used for:
Not to be used with:
Contains: POLYMYXIN B SULPHATE, BACITRACIN.
Other preparations:

---

polymyxin B sulphate *see* Gregoderm, Maxitrol, Neosporin, Otosporin, Polybactrin, Polyfax, Polytrim, Terra-Cortril, Tribiotic, Uniroid

polynoxylin *see* **Anaflex, Ponoxylan**

polysaccharide-iron complex *see* **Niferex**

Polytar Liquid
(Stiefel)

A liquid used as an anti-psoriatic treatment for psoriasis of the scalp, dandruff, seborrhoea, eczema.

Dose: shampoo once or twice a week.
Availability: NHS, private prescription, over the counter.
Side effects:
Caution:
Not to be used for:
Not to be used with:
Contains: TAR, CADE OIL, COAL TAR, ARACHIS OIL, COAL TAR EXTRACT, OLEYL ALCOHOL.
Other preparations:

polythiazide *see* **Nephril**

Polytrim
(Wellcome)

Drops used as an antibacterial treatment for eye infections.

Dose: 1 drop into the eye 4 times a day until 2 days after the symptoms have gone.
Availability: NHS and private prescription.
Side effects:
Caution:
Not to be used for:
Not to be used with:
Contains: TRIMETHOPRIM, POLYMYXIN B SULPHATE.
Other preparations: Polytrim Ointment

polyvinyl alcohol *see* **Hypotears, Kerecid, Liquifilm Tears, Sno Tears**

Polyvite
(Medo)

A red, oval capsule used as a multivitamin treatment for vitamin deficiency.

Dose: 1-2 capsules a day.
Availability: private prescription and over the counter.
Side effects:
Caution:
Not to be used for:
Not to be used with: LEVODOPA.
Contains: VITAMIN A, CALCIFEROL, THIAMINE, RIBOFLAVINE, PYRIDOXINE, ASCORBIC ACID, CALCIUM PANTOTHENATE, NICOTINAMIDE.
Other preparations:

Ponderax Pacaps
(Servier)

A blue/clear capsule supplied at a strength of 60 mg and used as an appetite suppressant to treat obesity.

Dose: 1-2 capsules a day.
Availability: NHS and private prescription.
Side effects: nervousness, sedation, diarrhoea, dry mouth, frequent urination, depression if the drug is withdrawn suddenly.
Caution: in patients with a history of mental illness.
Not to be used for: children, epileptics, or patients with a history of alcoholism, drug addiction, or depression.
Not to be used with: MAOIS, anti-hypertensives, anti-depressants, diabetic drugs, sedatives, alcohol, other obesity drugs.
Contains: FENFLURAMINE HYDROCHLORIDE.
Other preparations:

Pondocillin
(Leo)

A white, egg-shaped tablet supplied at a strength of 500 mg and used as a penicillin to treat bronchitis, pneumonia, ear, nose, and throat infections, skin, soft tissue infections, urine infections, gonorrhoea.

Dose: adults 1 tablet twice a day with food or drink; children use suspension or sachets.
Availability: NHS and private prescription.
Side effects: allergy, stomach disturbances.
Caution: in patients suffering from kidney disease.
Not to be used for: patients suffering from glandular fever.
Not to be used with:
Contains: PIVAMPICILLIN.
Other preparations: Pondocillin Suspension, Pondocillin Sachets, Pondocillin Plus.

Ponoxylan
(Rorer)

A gel used as an anti-bacterial treatment for infection and inflammation of the skin.

Dose: apply to the affected area as needed.
Availability: NHS, private prescription, over the counter.
Side effects:
Caution:
Not to be used for:
Not to be used with:
Contains: POLYNOXYLIN.
Other preparations:

Ponstan
(Parke-Davis)

An ivory/blue capsule supplied at a strength of 250 mg and used as a NON-STEROID ANTI-INFLAMATORY DRUG to treat pain, headache, period pain, excessively heavy periods.

Dose: 2 tablets 3 times a day.
Availability: NHS and private prescription.
Side effects: diarrhoea, rash, kidney damage, low platelet levels.

Caution: in pregnant women, the elderly, and in patients suffering from bronchial asthma or allergy.
Not to be used for: patients suffering from stomach ulcers, inflammatory bowel disease, kidney or liver disease.
Not to be used with: anti-coagulants, anti-diabetic drugs, anticonvulsants.
Contains: MEFENAMIC ACID.
Other preparations: Ponstan Forte, Ponstan Dispersible, Ponstan Paediatric Suspension.

Ponstan Forte
(Parke-Davis)

A yellow tablet supplied at a strength of 500 mg and used as a NON-STEROID ANTI-INFLAMMATORY DRUG to relieve pain in rheumatoid arthritis including Still's disease, osteoarthritis.

Dose: 1 tablet 3 times a day
Availability: NHS
Side effects: diarrhoea, rash, kidney damage, low platelet levels.
Caution: in the elderly, in pregnant women, and in patients suffering from bronchial asthma, allergy.
Not to be used for: patients suffering from kidney or liver disease, gastro-intestinal ulceration, inflammatory bowel disease.
Not to be used with: anti-coagulants, anti-diabetics, anti-convulsants.
Contains: MEFENAMIC ACID.
Other preparations: Ponstan, Ponstan Dispersible, Ponstan Paediatric Syrup.

Posalfilin
(Norgine)

An ointment used as a skin softener to treat warts.

Dose: protect healthy skin, apply the ointment to the wart, and cover; repeat 2-3 times a week.
Availability: NHS, private prescription, over the counter.
Side effects: pain when the ointment is first applied.

Caution: do not use on healthy skin.
Not to be used for: pregnant women or on warts on the face or anal and genital areas.
Not to be used with:
Contains: SALICYLIC ACID, PODOPHYLLUM RESIN.
Other preparations:

Potaba
(Glenwood)

A powder in a 3 g sachet used as a fibrous tissue dissolver to treat scleroderma (thickened skin), Peyronie's disease.

Dose: 1 sachet with food 4 times a day.
Availability: NHS and private prescription.
Side effects: anorexia, nausea.
Caution: in patients suffering from kidney disease.
Not to be used for: for children.
Not to be used with: sulphonamides.
Contains: POTASSIUM P-AMINOBENZOATE.
Other preparations: Potaba Tablets, Potaba Capsules.

potassium benzoate *see* Kloref

potassium bicarbonate *see* Algicon, Effercitrate, Kloref, Phosphate, Sando-K, Sandocal

potassium chloride *see* Burinex K, Centyl-K, Diarrest, Dioralyte, Diumide-K Continus, Esidrex K, Glandosane, Hygroton K, Kloref, Lasikal, Lasix + K, Leo K, Navidrex-K, Neo-Naclex-K, Nu-K, Rehidrat, Sando-K, Selora, Slow-K

potassium glycerophosphate *see* Verdiviton

potassium hydroxyquinolone sulphate *see* Auralgicin, Quinocort, Quinoderm Cream, Quinoped

---

potassium p-aminobenzoate *see* Potaba

P

---

potassium *see* Metatone

---

povidone-iodine *see* Betadine, Betadine Gargle and Mouthwash, Betadine Ointment, Betadine Scalp and Skin Cleanser, Betadine Spray, Disadine DP, Videne Powder

---

Pragmatar
(Bioglan)

A cream used as an anti-itch, antiseptic, skin softener to treat scaly skin, scalp seborrhoea and similar disorders.

Dose: apply weekly, or daily in severe cases, to wet hair.
Availability: NHS, private prescription, over the counter.
Side effects: irritation.
Caution: dilute the cream first when using for infants.
Not to be used for:
Not to be used with:
Contains: CETYL ALCOHOL/COAL TAR DISTILLATE, SULPHUR, SALICYLIC ACID.
Other preparations:

Pramidex *see* Rastinon
(Berk)

---

pramoxine hydrochloride *see* Anugesic-HC

---

pramoxine *see* Epifoam

Praxilene
(Lipha)

A pink capsule supplied at a strength of 100 mg and used as a blood vessel dilator to treat cerebral and peripheral vascular problems

Dose: 1-2 capsules 3 times a day.
Availability: NHS and private prescription.
Side effects: nausea, stomach pain.
Caution:
Not to be used for: for children.
Not to be used with:
Contains: NAFTIDROFURYL OXALATE.
Other preparations: Praxilene Forte.

---

prazosin *see* Hypovase

Precortysil
(Roussel)

A white tablet or a white, scored tablet according to strengths of 1 mg, 5 mg and used as a corticosteroid treatment for allergies and rheumatic conditions.

Dose: adults 20-40 mg a day at first reducing by 2.5 or 5 mg every 3-4 days to 5-20 mg a day as needed; children 1-7 years quarter to half adult dose, 7-12 years half to three-quarters dose.
Availability: NHS and private prescription.
Side effects: high blood sugar, thin bones, mood changes, ulcers.
Caution: in pregnant women, in patients who have had recent bowel surgery, or who are suffering from inflamed veins, psychiatric disorders, virus infections, some cancers, some kidney diseases, thinning of the bones, ulcers, tuberculosis, other infections, high blood pressure, glaucoma, epilepsy, diabetes, underactive thyroid, liver disease, stress. Withdraw gradually.
Not to be used for: for infants under 1 year

Not to be used with: PHENYTOIN, PHENOBARBITONE, EPHEDRINE, RIFAMPICIN, DIURETICS, ANTI-CHOLINESTERASES, DIGITALIS, anti-diabetic agents, anti-coagulants, NON-STEROID ANTI-INFLAMMATORY DRUGS.
Contains: PREDNISOLONE.
Other preparations: Precortisyl Forte.

Pred Forte
(Allergan)

Drops used as a corticosteroid treatment for inflammation of the eye where no infection is present.

Dose: 1-2 drops into the eye 2-4 times a day or 2 drops every hour for the first two days if needed.
Availability: NHS and private prescription.
Side effects: rise in eye pressure, secondary fungal or viral infections, thinning cornea, cataract.
Caution: in infants and pregnant women.
Not to be used for: patients suffering from glaucoma, viral, fungal, tubercular, or weeping eye infections, dendritic ulcer, or for patients who wear soft contact lenses.
Not to be used with:
Contains: PREDNISOLONE acetate.
Other preparations:

Predenema *see* Predsol
(Pharmax)

Predfoam *see* Predsol

Prednesol
(Glaxo)

A pink, scored tablet supplied at a strength of 5 mg and used as a corticosteroid treatment for allergies, rheumatic and inflammatory conditions.

Dose: adults 2-20 tablets a day in water in divided doses at first reducing to the minimum effective dose; children 1-7 years quarter to half adult dose, 7-12 years half to three-quarters adult dose.
Availability: NHS and private prescription.
Side effects: high blood sugar, thin bones, mood changes, ulcers.
Caution: in pregnant women, in patients who have had recent bowel surgery, or who are suffering from inflamed veins, psychiatric disorders, virus infections, some cancers, some kidney diseases, thinning of the bones, ulcers, tuberculosis, other infections, high blood pressure, glaucoma, epilepsy, diabetes, underactive thyroid, liver disease, stress. Withdraw gradually.
Not to be used for: for infants under 1 year.
Not to be used with: PHENYTOIN, PHENOBARBITONE, EPHEDRINE, RIFAMPICIN, DIURETICS, ANTI-CHOLINESTERASES, DIGITALIS, anti-diabetic agents, anti-coagulants, NON-STEROID ANTI-INFLAMMATORY DRUGS.
Contains: PREDNISOLONE disodium phosphate.
Other preparations:

Prednisolone
(SNP)

Drops used as a corticosteroid treatment for inflammation of the eye where no infection is present.

Dose: 1-2 drops as needed.
Availability: NHS and private prescription.
Side effects: rise in eye pressure, fungal infection, cataract, thinning cornea.
Caution: in pregnant women or infants — do not use for extended periods.
Not to be used for: patients suffering from glaucoma, viral, fungal, tubercular, or acute weeping infections.
Not to be used with:
Contains: PREDNISOLONE sodium phosphate.
Other preparations:

---

prednisolone *see* **Anacal, Deltacortril, Precortysil, Pred Forte, Prednesol, Prednisolone, Predsol, Predsol Drops, Scheriproct, see Sintisone**

prednisone *see* **Decortisyl**

Predsol
(Glaxo)

An enema supplied at a strength of 20 mg and used as a steroid treatment for ulcerative colitis.

Dose: 1 at night for 2-4 weeks.
Availability: NHS and private prescription.
Side effects: systemic corticosteroid effects.
Caution: in pregnant women. Do not use for prolonged periods.
Not to be used for: children.
Not to be used with:
Contains: PREDNISOLONE.
Other preparations: Predsol Suppositories, predsol drops, Predsol-N. PREDFOAM (Pharmax), PREDENEMA (Pharmax).

Predsol Drops
(Glaxo)

Drops used as a corticosteroid treatment for inflammation of the ear or eye where no infection is present.

Dose: 2-3 drops into the ear every 2-3 hours or 1-2 drops into the eye every 1-2 hours.
Availability: NHS and private prescription.
Side effects: allergy, resistance to neomycin rise in eye pressure, thinning cornea, cataract.
Caution: do not use unless necessary, and avoid use over extended periods for infants or pregnant women.
Not to be used for: patients suffering from viral, fungal, tubercular, or weeping infections, dendritic ulcer, glaucoma or for patients who wear soft contact lenses.
Not to be used with:
Contains: PREDNISOLONE sodium phosphate.
Other preparations: Predsol-N (contains NEOMYCIN).

Prefil
(Norgine)

Brown granules used as a bulking agent to treat obesity.

P

Dose: 2 5 ml spoonsful swallowed with water $\frac{1}{2}$-1 hour before eating.
Availability: NHS, private prescription, over the counter.
Side effects:
Caution:
Not to be used for: patients suffering from a blocked intestine.
Not to be used with:
Contains: STERCULIA.
Other preparations:

Pregaday
(Duncan, Flockhart)

A brownish-red tablet used as an iron and folic acid supplement
prevention of iron and folic acid deficiency in pregnancy.

Dose: 1 tablet a day.
Availability: NHS, private prescription, over the counter.
Side effects: stomach upset, allergy.
Caution: in patients with a history of peptic ulcer or who are in the first
three months of pregnancy.
Not to be used for: patients suffering from vitamin B_{12} deficiency.
Not to be used with: TETRACYCLINES, antacids, anti-convulsant drugs,
CO-TRIMOXAZOLE.
Contains: FERROUS FUMARATE, FOLIC ACID.
Other preparations:

Pregnavite Forte F
(Bencard)

A lilac-coloured tablet used as an iron, folic acid, and vitamin supplement to treat iron and vitamin deficiencies.

Dose: 1 tablet 3 times a day after meals starting at least 1 month
before conception and continuing at least until the second missed
period date.
Availability: NHS, private prescription, over the counter.

Side effects: stomach upset.
Caution:
Not to be used for: children or for patients suffering from megaloblastic anaemia.
Not to be used with: TETRACYCLINES, LEVODOPA.
Contains: ferrous sulphate, FOLIC ACID, CALCIFEROL, THIAMINE hydrochloride, RIBOFLAVINE, PYRIDOXINE hydrochloride, NICOTINAMIDE, ASCORBIC ACID, CALCIUM PHOSPHATE.
Other preparations:

Premarin
(Wyeth)

A maroon, oval tablet, yellow, oval tablet, or purple, oval tablet according to strengths of 0.625 mg, 1.25 mg, 2.5 mg and used as an oestrogen for hormone replacement during and after the menopause, and to treat atrophic inflammation of the vagina, inflammation of the urethra, prostate cancer, certain kinds of breast cancer.

Dose: menopause 0.625 mg a day for 21 days starting on the fifth day of the period if present, then 7 days without tablets. Other, as advised by the physician.
Availability: NHS and private prescription.
Side effects: enlarged breasts, bloating and fluid retention, cramps, leg pains, mood change, reduction in sexual desire, headaches, nausea, vaginal erosion, discharge, and bleeding, weight gain, skin changes.
Caution: in patients suffering from high blood pressure, diabetes, vascular disorders, asthma, depression, kidney disease, multiple sclerosis, womb diseases. Your doctor may advise you not to smoke, to have regular examinations. You should stop treatment at the first sign of serious symptoms such as severe headache or jaundice. Treatment should be stopped before surgery.
Not to be used for: children, pregnant women, or for patients suffering from sickle-cell anaemia, history of heart disease or thrombosis, liver disorders, some cancers, undiagnosed vaginal bleeding, some ear, skin, and kidney disorders.
Not to be used with: DIURETICS, anti-hypertensives, and drugs that change liver enzymes.
Contains: conjugated oestrogens.
Other preparations: Premarin Vaginal Cream.

Prempak-C
(Wyeth)

A maroon, oval tablet or yellow, oval tablet according to strengths of 0.625 mg, 1.25 mg plus a brown tablet 0.15 mg and used as an oestrogen, progestogen for hormone replacement during and after the menopause, and treatment of post-menopausal osteoporosis, atrophic inflammation of the vagina, inflammation of the urethra.

Dose: beginning on the first day of the period if present,1 maroon or yellow tablet a day for 16 days then 1 maroon or yellow tablet plus 1 brown tablet a day for 12 days.
Availability: NHS and private prescription.
Side effects: enlarged breasts, bloating and fluid retention, cramps, leg pains, mood change, reduction in sexual desire, headaches, nausea, vaginal erosion, discharge, and bleeding, weight gain, skin changes.
Caution: in patients suffering from high blood pressure, diabetes, vascular disorders, asthma, depression, kidney disease, multiple sclerosis, womb diseases. Your doctor may advise you not to smoke, to have regular examinations. You should stop treatment at the first sign of serious symptoms such as severe headache or jaundice. Treatment should be stopped before surgery.
Not to be used for: children, pregnant women, or for patients suffering from sickle-cell anaemia, history of heart disease or thrombosis, liver disorders, some cancers, undiagnosed vaginal bleeding, some ear, skin, and kidney disorders.
Not to be used with: DIURETICS, anti-hypertensives, and drugs that change liver enzymes.
Contains: conjugated oestrogens plus NORGESTREL.
Other preparations:

Prepulsid
(Janssen)

A white tablet supplied at a strength of 10 mg and used as a a stomach-emptying drug to treat gastric reflux and to encourage emptying of the stomach in conditions where the nerve supply is impaired.

Dose: 1-4 tablets a day for 6-12 weeks.
Availability: NHS and private prescription.
Side effects: stomach rumbling, diarrhoea, occasionally headaches

and convulsions.

Caution: in the elderly, nursing mothers, and in patients suffering from kidney or liver impairment.

Not to be used for: pregnant women or for patients suffering from stomach block, perforation, or bleeding.

Not to be used with: sedatives, H$_2$ ANTAGONISTS, anti-coagulants, ANTI-CHOLINERGICS.

Contains: cisapride.

Other preparations:

Prescal
(Ciba)

A yellow scored tablet supplied at a strength of 2.5 mg and used as a calcium antagonist to treat high blood pressure.

Dose: adults 1 tablet morning and evening, increasing after 3-4 weeks to 2 tablets twice a day if needed, up to a maximum of 4 tablets twice a day.

Availability: private prescription, over the counter.

Side effects: weight gain, palpitations, rapid heart rate, swelling, headache, flushing, dizziness, tiredness, abdominal pain, skin rash, liver enzyme changes, rise in liver enzymes.

Caution: pregnant women, nursing mothers, and in patients suffering from some rare heart conditions.

Not to be used for: children.

Not to be used with: anti-convulsants.

Contains: ISRADIPINE.

Other preparations:

Prestim
(Leo)

A white, scored tablet used as a ß-BLOCKER/THIAZIDE DIURETIC combination to treat high blood pressure.

Dose: 1-4 tablets a day.

Availability: NHS and private prescription.

Side effects: cold hands and feet, sleep disturbance, slow heart rate, tiredness, wheezing, heart failure, stomach upset.

Caution: in pregnant women, nursing mothers, and in patients suffering from diabetes, kidney or liver disorders, asthma. May need to be withdrawn before surgery. Withdraw gradually. Your doctor may advise additional treatment with diuretics or digitalis.

Not to be used for: children, or for patients suffering from heart block or failure.

Not to be used with: VERAPAMIL, CLONIDINE withdrawal, some anti-arrhythmic drugs and anaesthetics, RESERPINE, some anti-hypertensives, ergot alkaloids, CIMETIDINE, sedatives, SYMPATHOMIMETICS, INDOMETHACIN.

Contains: TIMOLOL MALEATE, BENDROFLUAZIDE.

Other preparations: Prestim Forte

Priadel
(Delandale)

A white, scored tablet supplied at strengths of 200 mg, 400 mg and used as a lithium salt to treat mania, manic depression, recurring depression, agression, and self-injuring behaviour.

Dose: to keep blood levels in a given range.

Availability: NHS and private prescription.

Side effects: nausea, diarrhoea, hand tremor, muscular weakness, brain and heart disturbances, weight gain, fluid retention, under- or overactive thyroid, thirst and excessive urination, skin reactions. Your doctor may advise blood tests to gauge dose.

Caution: treatment should start in hospital. Kidney heart, and thyroid function should be checked regularly. Salt and fluid consumption should be maintained.

Not to be used for: children, pregnant women, nursing mothers, or for patients suffering from Addison's disease, weak kidneys or heart, underactive thyroid, disturbed sodium balance.

Not to be used with: DIURETICS, NON-STEROID ANTI-INFLAMMATORY DRUGS, PHENYTOIN, CARBAMAZEPIDE, FLUPENTHIXOL, HALOPERIDOL, DIAZEPAM, METHYLDOPA, TETRACYCLINES.

Contains: LITHIUM CARBONATE.

Other preparations:

Primalan
(M & B)

A white tablet supplied at a strength of 5 mg and used as an antihistamine treatment for allergy, itch, hay fever, rhinitis.

Dose: 1 tablet twice a day.
Availability: NHS and private prescription.
Side effects: drowsiness, reduced reactions, anti-cholinergic effects, convulsions at high doses, extrapyramidal reactions (shaking and rigidity).
Caution:
Not to be used for: children, pregnant women, or for patients suffering from epilepsy, enlarged prostate, liver disease.
Not to be used with: sedatives, MAOIS, SYMPATHOMIMETICS, alcohol.
Contains: MEQUITAZINE.
Other preparations:

---

primidone *see* **Mysoline**

Primolut N
(Schering)

A white tablet supplied at a strength of 5 mg and used as a progestogen treatment for postponing menstruation, and for other menstrual and womb disorders.

Dose: usually 1 tablet 3 times a day.
Availability: NHS and private prescription.
Side effects: liver disturbances, masculinization.
Caution: in patients suffering from epilepsy or migraine.
Not to be used for: children, pregnant women, or patients suffering from severe liver disease, a history of itch or idiopathic jaundice Dubin-Johnson and Rotor syndromes during pregnancy.
Not to be used with:
Contains: NORETHISTERONE.
Other preparations:

Primperan *see* **Maxolon**
(Berk)

Prioderm
(Napp Consumer)

A lotion used as a pediculicide, scabicide to treat scabies, lice of the head and pubic areas.

Dose: rub in and shampoo after 2-12 hours; repeat after 7-9 days.
Availability: NHS, private prescription, over the counter.
Side effects:
Caution: keep out of the eyes.
Not to be used for:
Not to be used with:
Contains: MALATHION.
Other preparations: Prioderm Cream Shampoo.

Pripsen
(Reckitt & Colman)

A sachet used to treat worms.

Dose: adults and children over 6 years 1 sachet and then a second dose of 1 sachet after 14 days; infants 3 months-1 year $1/3$ sachet then a second dose after 14 days; children 1-6 years $2/3$ sachet then a secon dose after 14 days.
Availability: NHS, private prescription, over the counter.
Side effects: rarely sight disorders, vertigo.
Caution: care in nursing mothers and in patients suffering from nervous disorders.
Not to be used for: patients suffering from epilepsy, liver or kidney disease.
Not to be used with:
Contains: PIPERAZINE phosphate, SENNOSIDE.
Other preparations:

Pro-Actidil
(Wellcome)

A white tablet supplied at a strength of 10 mg and used as an antihis-tamine treatment for allergies.

Dose: 1 tablet a day 5-6 hours before going to bed.

Availability: NHS, private prescription, over the counter.
Side effects: drowsiness, reduced reactions, rarely skin eruptions.
Caution: in nursing mothers and in patients suffering from liver or kidney disease.
Not to be used for: children.
Not to be used with: sedatives, MAOIS, alcohol.
Contains: TRIPROLIDINE hydrochloride.
Other preparations:

Pro-banthine
(Gold Cross)

A pink tablet supplied at a strength of 15 mg and used as an anti-spasm, ANTI-CHOLINERGIC treatment for ulcers, irritable bowel syndrome, bed wetting.

Dose: adults up to 8 daily individual doses.
Availability: NHS and private prescription.
Side effects: blurred vision, confusion, dry mouth.
Caution: in the elderly and in patients suffering from ulcerative colitis, heart disease, autonomic neuropathy, kidney and liver disease.
Not to be used for: children or for patients suffering from glaucoma, obstructive bowel disease, obstructive disease of the urinary tract.
Not to be used with: DIGOXIN.
Contains: PROPANTHELINE bromide.
Other preparations:

Pro-Vent *see* Theophylline
(Wellcome)

Pro-Viron
(Schering)

A white, scored tablet supplied at a strength of 25 mg and used as an androgen to treat low androgen levels, infertility in men.

Dose: 1 tablet 3-4 times a day for several months, then 2-3 tablets a day.
Availability: NHS and private prescription.

Side effects: fluid retention, weight gain, raised calcium levels, increased bone growth, erect penis, premature closure of epiphyses (bone ends), reduced fertility in males, masculinization of women, inflammation of the prostate in the elderly.

Caution: in patients suffering from heart, kidney, or liver impairment, high blood pressure, epilepsy, migraine.

Not to be used for: children, or for patients suffering from prostate or breast cancer, kidney damage, raised calcium levels, heart disease, untreated heart failure.

Not to be used with: liver-enzyme inducing drugs.

Contains: MESTEROLONE.

Other preparations:

---

probenecid *see* **Benemid**

---

probucol *see* **Lurselle**

Procainamide Durules
(Astra)

A pale yellow tablet supplied at a strength of 500 mg and used as a heart rhythm regulator to treat abnormal heart rhythm, some muscle disorders.

Dose: 1 tablet 2-3 times a day.

Availability: NHS and private prescription.

Side effects: SLE, stomach and brain disturbance, blood changes.

Caution: in patients suffering from kidney, liver, or heart failure. Your doctor may advise regular blood tests.

Not to be used for: for children or for patients suffering from heart block, SLE (a multisystem disorder), myasthenia gravis (a muscle disorder).

Not to be used with:

Contains: PROCAINAMIDE hydrochloride.

Other preparations:

---

procainamide *see* **Procainamide Durules, Pronestyl**

prochlorperazine *see* **Buccastem, Stemetil**

P

Proctofibe
(Roussel)

A beige tablet used as a bulking agent to treat diverticular disease, irritable colon, constipation because of a diet low in fibre.

Dose: adults and children over 3 years 4-12 tablets a day in divided doses.
Availability: private prescription only.
Side effects:
Caution:
Not to be used for: infants or for patients suffering from intestinal obstruction.
Not to be used with:
Contains: GRAIN FIBRE, CITRUS FIBRE.
Other preparations:

Proctofoam HC
(Stafford-Miller)

Foam supplied in an aerosol with an applicator and used as a steroid, local anaesthetic treatment for haemorrhoids, bowel inflammation, fissures.

Dose: in the rectum 1 application 2-3 times a day and after passing motions; around the anus apply as required.
Availability: NHS and private prescription.
Side effects: systemic corticosteroid effects.
Caution: in pregnant women; do not use for prolonged periods.
Not to be used for: children or for patients suffering from tuberculous, fungal and viral infections.
Not to be used with:
Contains: HYDROCORTISONE acetate, PROXAMINE hydrochloride.
Other preparations:

Proctosedyl
(Roussel)

Suppositories used as a steroid, local anaesthetic treatment for haemorrhoids, anal fissure, inflammation, itch.

Dose: 1 suppository night and morning and after passing motions.
Availability: NHS and private prescription.
Side effects: systemic corticosteroid effects.
Caution: in pregnant women; do not use for prolonged periods.
Not to be used for: patients suffering from tuberculous, fungal or viral infections.
Not to be used with:
Contains: HYDROCORTISONE, CINCHOCAINE hydrochloride.
Other preparations: Proctosedyl ointment.

---

procyclidine *see* Arpicolin, Kemadrin

Progesic *see* Fenopron
(Eli Lilly)

---

progesterone *see* Cyclogest

---

proguanil hydrochloride *see* Paludrine

Progynova
(Schering)

A beige tablet or a blue tablet according to strengths of 1 mg, 2 mg and used as an oestrogen for the short-term treatment of the menopause.

Dose: 1 mg a day for 21 days then 7 or more days without tablets.
Availability: NHS and private prescription.
Side effects: enlarged breasts, bloating and fluid retention, cramps,

leg pains, mood change, reduction in sexual desire, headaches, nausea, vaginal erosion, discharge, and bleeding, weight gain, skin changes.

Caution: in patients suffering from high blood pressure, diabetes, vascular disorders, asthma, depression, kidney disease, multiple sclerosis, womb diseases. Your doctor may advise you not to smoke, to have regular examinations. You should stop treatment at the first sign of serious symptoms such as severe headache or jaundice. Treatment should be stopped before surgery.

Not to be used for: pregnant women, or for patients suffering from sickle-cell anaemia, history of heart disease or thrombosis, liver disorders, some cancers, undiagnosed vaginal bleeding, some ear, skin, and kidney disorders.

Not to be used with: DIURETICS, anti-hypertensives, and drugs that change liver enzymes.

Contains: OESTRADIOL valerate.

Other preparations:

---

prolintane *see* **Villescon**

---

promazine embonate *see* **Sparine**

---

promethazine *see* **Avomine, Medised Suspension, Phenergan, Phensedyl, Sominex**

Prominal
(Winthrop)

A white tablet supplied at strengths of 30 mg, 60 mg, 200 mg and used as a barbiturate to treat epilepsy.

Dose: adults 100-600 mg a day; children 5-15 mg per kg body weight a day.

Availability: controlled drug.

Side effects: drowsiness, hangover, dizziness, allergies, headache, confusion, excitement.

Caution: in patients suffering from kidney or lung disease. Dependence (addiction) may develop.
Not to be used for: children, young adults, pregnant women, nursing mothers, the elderly, patients with a history of drug or alcohol abuse, or suffering from porphyria (a rare blood disorder), or in the management of pain.
Not to be used with: anti-coagulants (blood-thinning drugs), alcohol, other tranquillizers, steroids, the contraceptive pill, GRISEOFULVIN, RIFAMPICIN, PHENYTOIN, METRONIDAZOLE, CHLORAMPHENICOL.
Contains: METHYLPHENOBARBITONE.
Other preparations:

Prondol
(Wyeth)

A yellow tablet supplied at strengths of 15 mg, 30 mg and used as an anti-depressant to treat depression.

Dose: adults 15-30 mg 3 times a day at first, to a maximum of 60 mg 3 times a day; elderly 15 mg 3 times a day at first.
Availability: NHS and private prescription.
Side effects: dry mouth, constipation, urine retention, blurred vision, palpitations, drowsiness, sleeplessness, dizziness, hands shaking, low blood pressure, weight change, skin reactions, jaundice or blood changes, loss of libido may occur.
Caution: in nursing mothers or in patients suffering from heart disease, thyroid disease, epilepsy, diabetes, some other psychiatric conditions. Your doctor may advise regular blood tests.
Not to be used for: children under 6 years, pregnant women, or for patients suffering from heart attacks, liver disease, heart block.
Not to be used with: alcohol, anti-cholinergics, ADRENALINE, MAOIS, barbiturates, other anti-depressants, anti-hypertensives.
Contains: IPRINDOLE hydrochloride.
Other preparations:

Pronestyl
(Squibb)

A white, scored tablet supplied at a strength of 250 mg and used as an anti-arryhthmic drug to treat abnormal heart rhythm.

Dose: 50 mg per kg body weight a day in divided doses every 3-6 hours.
Availability: NHS and private prescription.
Side effects: SLE (a multi-system disorder), stomach and brain disturbance, blood changes.
Caution: in patients suffering from kidney, liver, or heart failure. Your doctor may advise regular blood tests.
Not to be used for: for children or for patients suffering from heart block, SLE, myasthenia gravis (a muscle disorder).
Not to be used with:
Contains: PROCAINAMIDE hydrochloride.
Other preparations: Pronestyl Injection

Propaderm
(A & H)

A cream used as a steroid treatment for skin disorders.

Dose: rub in a small quantity to the affected area twice a day.
Availability: NHS and private prescription.
Side effects: fluid retention, suppression of adrenal glands, thinning of the skin may occur.
Caution: use for short periods of time only.
Not to be used for: patients suffering from acne or any other skin infections caused by tuberculosis, ringworm, viruses, or fungi, or continuously especially in pregnant women.
Not to be used with:
Contains: BECLOMETHASONE diproprionate.
Other preparations: Propaderm Ointment, Propaderm-A

---

propaferone *see* **Arhythmol**

Propain
(Panpharma)

A yellow, scored tablet used as an analgesic, antihistamine treatment for headache, migraine, muscle pain, period pain.

Dose: 1-2 tablets every 4 hours to a maximum of 10 tablets in 24 hours.
Availability: private prescription and over the counter.
Side effects: drowsiness.
Caution: in patients suffering from kidney or liver disease.
Not to be used for: children.
Not to be used with: alcohol, sedatives.
Contains: CODEINE PHOSPHATE, DIPHENHYDRAMINE HYDROCHLORIDE, PARACETAMOL, CAFFEINE.
Other preparations:

---

propanolol hydrochloride *see* Inderal, Inderal LA, Inderetic

---

propantheline bromide *see* Pro-banthine

Propine
(Allergan)

Drops used as a SYMPATHOMIMETIC treatment for glaucoma, hypertension of the eye.

Dose: 1 drop into the eye every 12 hours.
Availability: NHS and private prescription.
Side effects: temporary smarting, redness, allergy, rarely raised blood pressure.
Caution: in patients suffering from narrow-angle glaucoma, absence of the lens.
Not to be used for: children or for patients suffering from closed angle glaucoma or who wear soft contact lenses.
Not to be used with:
Contains: DIPIVEFRIN HYDROCHLORIDE.
Other preparations:

---

propyl salicylate *see* Monphytol

propyl undecoanate *see* **Monphytol**

---

propylene glycol *see* **Aserbine, Malatex**

Prostigimin
(Roche)

A white, scored tablet supplied at a strength of 15 mg and used as an anti-cholinesterase to treat distension, urinary retention following surgery, bowel paralysis, myasthenia gravis (a muscle disorder).

Dose: adults bowel paralysis 1-2 tablets as required; children $\frac{1}{6}$-1 tablet as required. Adults myasthenia gravis 5-20 tablets a day in divided doses; infants 1-5 mg every 4 hours, children 15-90 mg a day in divided doses; after surgery 2.5-15 mg as needed.
Availability: NHS and private prescription.
Side effects: nausea, diarrhoea, colic, salivation.
Caution: in patients suffering from bronchial asthma, heart disease, epilepsy, Parkinson's disease.
Not to be used for: patients suffering from intestinal or urinary obstruction.
Not to be used with: muscle relaxants, CYCLOPROPANE, HALOTHANE.
Contains: NEOSTIGMINE bromide.
Other preparations: Prostigimin Injection.

Prothiaden
(Boots)

A red/brown capsule supplied at a strength of 25 mg and used as an anti-depressant to treat depression, anxiety.

Dose: 3-6 capsules a day.
Availability: NHS and private prescription.
Side effects: dry mouth, constipation, urine retention, blurred vision, palpitations, drowsiness, sleeplessness, dizziness, hands shaking, low blood presure, weight change, skin reactions, jaundice or blood changes, loss of libido may occur.
Caution: in nursing mothers or in patients suffering from heart

disease, thyroid disease, epilepsy, diabetes, some other psychiatric conditions. Your doctor may advise regular blood tests.
Not to be used for: children under 6 years, pregnant women, or for patients suffering from heart attacks, liver disease, heart block.
Not to be used with: alcohol, anti-cholinergics, ADRENALINE, MAOIS, barbiturates, other anti-depressants, anti-hypertensives.
Contains: DOTHIEPIN hydrochloride.
Other preparations: Prothiaden tablets

---

protryptiline *see* Concordin

Provera
(Upjohn)

A white, scored tablet supplied at strengths of 5 mg, 100 mg, 200 mg, 400 mg and used as a progestogen treatment for abnormal bleeding of the uterus, secondary absence of periods, hormone-dependent disorders such as breast cancer.

Dose: abnormal bleeding 2.5-20 mg a day for 5-10 days, repeated on 2-3 menstrual consecutive cycles; breast cancer 400-800 mg a day; other cancers 200-400 mg a day.
Availability: NHS and private prescription.
Side effects: nausea; on high doses breast pain, lactation, abnormal menstrual bleeding, corticoid symptoms.
Caution: in patients with a history of depression, diabetes, epilepsy, migraine, asthma, heart or kidney failure.
Not to be used for: children, pregnant women, or patients suffering from cancer of the genitals or breast, liver disease, abnormal vaginal bleeding, or a history of thromboembolic disorders, thrombophlebitis, history of, or presence of, raised calcium levels.
Not to be used with:
Contains: MEDROXYPROGESTERONE.
Other preparations: Provera Suspension.

---

proxamine *see* Proctofoam HC

---

proxymetacaine hydrochloride *see* **Ophthaine**

Prozac
(Dista)

A green/off-white capsule supplied at a strength of 20 mg and used as an anti-depressant to treat depression.

Dose: adults 1 capsule a day up to a maximum of 4 capsules; elderly no more than 3 capsules a day.
Availability: NHS and private prescription.
Side effects: nausea, headache, anxiety, sleeplessness, dizziness, rash, weakness, reduced judgement and abilities; rarely convulsions, hypomania, mania.
Caution: in pregnant women and in patients suffering from unstable epilepsy, liver failure, moderate kidney failure, heart disease.
Not to be used for: children, nursing mothers, or for patients suffering from severe kidney failure or allergy to FLUOXETINE.
Not to be used with: MAOIS, tryptophan (this is in many health foods), LITHIUM.
Contains: FLUOXETINE.
Other preparations:

---

pseudoephedrine *see* **Actifed Compound, Congesteze, Dimotane Expectorant, Dimotane Plus, Expulin, Galpseud, Sudafed, Sudafed Plus**

Psoradrate
(Norwich Eaton)

A cream used as an anti-psoriatic, drying agent to treat psoriasis.

Dose: wash and dry the area, then apply the cream twice a day.
Availability: NHS, private prescription, over the counter.
Side effects: irritation, hypersensitivity.
Caution:
Not to be used for: patients suffering from pustular psoriasis.
Not to be used with:
Contains: DITHRANOL, UREA.

Psoriderm
(Dermal)

An emulsion used as an anti-psoriatic to treat psoriasis.

Dose: add 30 ml of the emulsion to the bath water, soak for 15 minutes, dry, then apply the cream to the affected area.
Availability: NHS, private prescription, over the counter.
Side effects: irritation, sensitivity to light.
Caution:
Not to be used for: patients suffering from acute psoriasis.
Not to be used with:
Contains: COAL TAR.
Other preparations: Psoriderm Cream, Psoriderm Scalp Lotion.

Psorigel
(Alcon)

A gel used as an anti-psoriatic treatment for psoriasis, eczema, dermatoses.

Dose: rub into the affected area and allow to dry 1-2 times a day.
Availability: NHS, private prescription, over the counter.
Side effects: irritation, sensitivity to light.
Caution:
Not to be used for: patients suffering from acute psoriasis.
Not to be used with:
Contains: COAL TAR solution.
Other preparations:

Psorin
(Thames)

An ointment used as an anti-psoriatic, skin softener to treat psoriasis, eczema.

Dose: apply to the affected areas twice a day.

Availability: NHS, private prescription, over the counter.
Side effects:
Caution: keep out of the eyes, and avoid direct sunlight.
Not to be used for: patients suffering from unstable psoriasis.
Not to be used with:
Contains: COAL TAR, DITHRANOL, SALICYLIC ACID.
Other preparations:

Pulmadil
(3M Riker)

An aerosol supplied at a strength of 0.2 mg and used as a broncho-dilator to treat bronchial spasm brought on by chronic bronchitis, bronchial asthma.

Dose: 1-3 sprays and again after 30 minutes if needed, up to a maximum of 24 sprays in 24 hours.
Availability: NHS and private prescription.
Side effects: headache, dilation of the blood vessels.
Caution: in pregnant women and in patients suffering from abnormal heart rhythms, high blood pressure, overactive thyroid, heart muscle disorders, angina.
Not to be used for:
Not to be used with: SYMPATHOMIMETICS.
Contains: RIMITEROL HYDROBROMIDE.
Other preparations: Pulmadil Auto.

Pulmicort
(Astra)

An aerosol supplied at a strength of 200 micrograms and used as a corticosteroid to treat bronchial asthma.

Dose: 1 spray twice a day up to a maximum of 6 sprays a day if needed.
Availability: NHS and private prescription.
Side effects: hoarseness, thrush of the mouth and throat.
Caution: in pregnant women, in patients suffering from tuberculosis of the lungs, and in those transferring from systemic steroids.
Not to be used for: children.
Not to be used with:

Contains: BUDESONIDE.
Other preparations: Pulmicort LS.

P

pumilio pine oil *see* Tercoda

Pyralvex
(Norgine)

A liquid used as an anti-inflammatory treatment for mouth inflammations.

Dose: apply to the affected area 3-4 times a day.
Availability: NHS, private prescription, over the counter.
Side effects: local irritation.
Caution:
Not to be used for:
Not to be used with:
Contains: ANTHRAQUINONE GLYCOSIDES, SALICYLIC ACID.
Other preparations:

pyrantel *see* Combantrin

pyrazinamide *see* Rifater, Zinamide

pyridostigmine *see* Mestinon

pyridoxine *see* Abidec, Allbee with C, Apisate, BC 500, BC 500 with Iron, Becosym, Calcimax, Complement Continus, Fefol-Vit Spansule, Fesovit Spansule, Fesovit Z Spansule, Galfervit, Givitol, Ketovite, Lipoflavonoid, Lipotriad, Octovit, Optimax, Orovite, Orovite 7, Polyvite, Pregnavite Forte F, Surbex T, Tonivitan B, Verdiviton, Villescon

pyrimethamine *see* **Daraprim, Fansidar, Maloprim**

Pyrogastrone *see* **Biogastrone**
(Sterling Research Laboratories)

Q

Quellada
(Stafford-Miller)

A lotion used as a scabicide to treat scabies.

Dose: apply as directed.
Availability: NHS, private prescription, over the counter.
Side effects:
Caution: keep out of the eyes.
Not to be used for: infants under 1 month.
Not to be used with:
Contains: LINDANE.
Other preparations: Quellada Application PC.

Questran
(Bristol-Myers)

A powder in a sachet used as a lipid-lowering agent to treat elevated lipids.

Dose: adults 12-24 g a day in divided doses to a maximum of 36 g a day; children over 6 years in proportion to dose for 70 kg adult.
Availability: NHS and private prescription.
Side effects: constipation.
Caution: in pregnant women, nursing mothers, and patients on long-term treatment should take Vitamin A, D, K supplements.
Not to be used for: children under 6 years or for patients suffering from complete biliary blockage.
Not to be used with: DIGITALIS, antibiotics, DIURETICS; allow 1 hour between treatment and any other drugs.
Contains: CHOLESTYRAMINE.
Other preparations:

quinalbarbitone *see* **Seconal Sodium, Tuinal**

---

quinidine *see* **Kinidin Durules**

Q

Quinocort
(Quinoderm)

A cream used as a steroid, anti-fungal, anti-bacterial treatment for skin disorders where there is also infection.

Dose: massage into the affected area 2-3 times a day.
Availability: NHS and private prescription
Side effects: fluid retention, suppression of adrenal glands, thinning of the skin may occur.
Caution: use for short periods of time only.
Not to be used for: patients suffering from acne or any other skin infections caused by tuberculosis, ringworm, viruses, or fungi, or continuously especially in pregnant women.
Not to be used with:
Contains: POTASSIUM HYDROXYQUINOLONE SULPHATE, HYDROCORTISONE.
Other preparations:

Quinoderm Cream
(Quinoderm)

A cream used as an anti-bacterial, skin softener to treat acne, acne-like eruptions, inflammation of the follicles.

Dose: massage into the affected area 1-3 times a day.
Availability: NHS, private prescription, over the counter.
Side effects: irritation, peeling.
Caution: keep out of the eyes, nose, mouth.
Not to be used for:
Not to be used with:
Contains: POTASSIUM HYDROXYQUINOLONE SULPHATE, BENZOYL PEROXIDE.
Other preparations: Quinoderm Cream 5, Quinoderm Lotio-Gel, Quinoderm Lotio-Gel 5%, Quinoderm with Hydrocortisone.

Quinoped
(Quinoderm)

A cream used as an anti-fungal treatment for athlete's foot and similar infections.

Dose: rub lightly into the affected area night and morning.
Availability: NHS, private prescription, over the counter.
Side effects:
Caution:
Not to be used for:
Not to be used with:
Contains: BENZOYL PEROXIDE, POTASSIUM HYDROXYQUINOLONE SULPHATE.
Other preparations:

Rabro *see* Caved-S
(Sinclair)

---

ranitidine *see* Zantac

Rastinon
(Hoechst)

A white, scored tablet supplied at a strength of 500 mg and used as an anti-diabetic treatment for diabetes.

Dose: 2 tablets a day at first adjust to 1-3 tablets a day as needed.
Availability: NHS and private prescription.
Side effects: allergy including skin rash.
Caution: in the elderly and in patients suffering from kidney failure.
Not to be used for: children, pregnant women, nursing mothers, during surgery, or for patients suffering from juvenile diabetes, liver or kidney disorders, stress, infections.
Not to be used with: ß-BLOCKERS, MAOIS, steroids, DIURETICS, alcohol, anti-coagulants, lipid-lowering agents, ASPIRIN, some antibiotics (RIFAMPICIN, sulphonamides, CHLORAMPHENICOL), GLUCAGON, CYCLOPHOSPHAMIDE.
Contains: TOLBUTAMIDE.
Other preparations: PRAMIDEX (Berk).

Redoxon
(Roche)

A white tablet supplied at strengths of 25 mg, 50 mg, 200 mg and used as a vitamin C treatment for scurvy, and as an additional treatment for wounds and infections.

Dose: adults 500 mg-1 g 2-3 times a day; children under 4 years quarter adult dose, 4-12 years half adult dose, 12-14 years three-quarters adult dose.
Availability: NHS (when prescribed as a generic), private prescription, over the counter.
Side effects: diarrhoea.
Caution:
Not to be used for:
Not to be used with:
Contains: ASCORBIC ACID.
Other preparations: Redoxon Effervescent

Refolinon
(Farmitalia CE)

A light-yellow, scored tablet supplied at a strength of 15 mg and used as a folinic acid treatment for megaloblastic anaemia.

Dose: 1 tablet a day.
Availability: NHS and private prescription.
Side effects:
Caution:
Not to be used for: patients suffering from vitamin B_{12} deficiency anaemia.
Not to be used with:
Contains: CALCIUM FOLINATE.
Other preparations:

Regulan
(Gold Cross)

An effervescent powder supplied in sachets of 3.6 g and used as a bulking agent to treat constipation owing to lack of fibre in the diet.

Dose: adults1 sachet in water 1-3 times a day; children over 6 years
$^1/_2$ -1 5 ml spoonful 3 times a day.
Availability: NHS and private prescription.
Side effects:
Caution:
Not to be used for: children under 6 years and patients suffering from
intestinal obstruction.
Not to be used with:
Contains: ISPAGHULA husk.
Other preparations:

Rehibin
(Serono)

A white, scored tablet supplied at a strength of 100 mg and used as
an a anti-oestrogen treatment for infertility due to failure of ovulation
caused by impaired hypothalamic-pituitary function.

Dose: 2 tablets morning and evening for 10 days beginning on the
third day of the period; continue the treatment for at least 3 cycles.
Availability: NHS and private prescription.
Side effects: hot flushes, nausea, uncomfortable abdomen, jaun-
dice.
Caution:
Not to be used for: pregnant women or for patients suffering from
liver disease, endometrial (womb) cancer, or bleeding from the uterus.
Not to be used with:
Contains: CYCLOFENIL.
Other preparations:

Rehidrat
(Searle)

A lemon and lime, and orange-flavoured powder used to provide
electrolytes in fluid and electrolyte loss.

Dose: adults and children drink until thirst is quenched; infants
substitute for feeds or after breast feeding.
Availability: NHS, private prescription, over the counter.
Side effects:

Caution:
Not to be used for: care in patients suffering from kidney disease, blocked intestine, bowel paralysis.
Not to be used with:
Contains: SODIUM CHLORIDE, POTASSIUM CHLORIDE, SODIUM BICARBONATE, CITRIC ACID, GLUCOSE, SUCROSE, LAEVULOSE.
Other preparations:

Relaxit
(Pharmacia)

A micro-enema used as a faecal softener to treat constipation.

Dose: 1 enema.
Availability: NHS and private prescription.
Side effects:
Caution:
Not to be used for:
Not to be used with:
Contains: SODIUM CITRATE, SODIUM LAURYL SULPHATE, SORBIC ACID, GLYCEROL, SORBITOL solution.
Other preparations:

Relifex
(Bencard)

A red tablet supplied at a strength of 500 mg and used as a NON-STEROID ANTI-INFLAMMATORY DRUG to treat rheumatoid arthritis, osteoarthritis.

Dose: adults 2 tablets at bed time and, if needed, 1-2 tablets in the morning; elderly 1-2 tablets a day.
Availability: NHS and private prescription.
Side effects: diarrhoea, dyspepsia, nausea, constipation, stomach pain, wind, headache, dizziness, rash, sedation.
Caution: in patients suffering from kidney disease or with a history of peptic ulcer.
Not to be used for: children, or patients suffering from peptic ulcer or allergy to aspirin/non-steroid anti-inflammatory drugs.
Not to be used with: anti-coagulants taken by mouth, HYDANTOIN, anti-convulsants, anti-diabetics.

Contains: nabumetone.
Other preparations:

Remnos *see* **Mogadon**
(DDSA)

---

reproterol *see* **Bronchodil**

Rescufolin
(Nordic)

A cream-coloured, scored tablet supplied at a strength of 15 mg and used as a folinic acid treatment for megaloblastic anaemia.

Dose: 1 tablet a day.
Availability: NHS and private prescription.
Side effects:
Caution:
Not to be used for: patients suffering from vitamin B_{12} anaemia.
Not to be used with:
Contains: CALCIUM FOLINATE.
Other preparations:

---

reserpine *see* **Serpasil, Serpasil Esidrex**

Resonium-A
(Winthrop)

A powder used for ion-exchange to lower potassium levels.

Dose: 15 g 3-4 times a day.
Availability: NHS, private prescription, over the counter.
Side effects:
Caution: potassium and sodium levels should be checked regularly.

Not to be used for:
Not to be used with:
Contains: SODIUM POLYSTYRENE SULPHONATE.
Other preparations:

---

resorcinol *see* Anugesic-HC, Anusol HC, Dome-Acne, Eskamel

Restandol
(Organon)

A brown, oval capsule supplied at a strength of 40 mg and used as an androgen to treat hypogonadism and osteoporosis in men caused by low androgen levels.

Dose: 3-4 tablets a day for 3 weeks, then 1-3 tablets a day as needed.
Availability: NHS and private prescription.
Side effects: fluid retention, weight gain, raised calcium levels, increased bone growth, erect penis, premature closure of epiphyses (bone ends), reduced fertility in males, masculinization of women, inflammation of the prostate in the elderly.
Caution: in patients suffering from heart, kidney, or liver impairment, high blood pressure, epilepsy, migraine.
Not to be used for: children, or for patients suffering from prostate or breast cancer, kidney damage, raised calcium levels, heart disease, untreated heart failure.
Not to be used with: liver-enzyme inducing drugs.
Contains: TESTOSTERONE UNDECANOATE.
Other preparations:

Retcin *see* Erythrocin
(DDSA)

Retin-A
(Cilag)

A lotion used as a VITAMIN A derivative to treat acne where there are comedones, papules, and pustules.

Dose: apply to the affected area 1-2 times a day for at least 8 weeks.
Availability: NHS and private prescription.
Side effects: redness, irritation, loss or gain of skin pigment.
Caution: in pregnant women; avoid direct sunlight or ultra-violet lamps, and keep the lotion away from the eyes, nose, and mouth etc.
Not to be used for: patients suffering from eczema, cuts, abrasion,
Not to be used with: skin softener.
Contains: TRETINOIN.
Other preparations: Retin-A Gel, Retin-A Cream.

R

Retrovir
(Wellcome)

A white capsule or blue/white capsule according to strengths of 100 mg, 250 mg and used as an anti-viral treatment for serious HIV infections in patients suffering from AIDS, or to delay the onset of AIDS in HIV positive people.

Dose: 200-300 mg every 4 hours including during the night.
Availability: NHS and private prescription.
Side effects: anaemia, white cell changes, headache, nausea, rash, stomach pain, fever, pins and needles, anorexia, myalgia, sleeplessness.
Caution: in the elderly, pregnant women, and in patients suffering from kidney or liver disease. Regular blood tests should be carried out.
Not to be used for: nursing mothers or for patients suffering from low white cell counts.
Not to be used with: analgesics, especially PARACETAMOL, drugs inducing liver enzymes, cytotoxic drugs, PROBENECID.
Contains: ZIDOVUDINE.
Other preparations:

Rheumox
(Robins)

A light/dark orange capsule supplied at a strength of 300 mg and used as a NON-STEROID ANTI-INFLAMMATORY DRUG to treat rheumatoid arthritis, osteoarthritis, ankylosing spondylitis, acute gout.

Dose: adults 4 capsules a day in 2 or 4 divided doses; acute gout 8 capsules in divided doses for 24 hours then 6 capsules a day reducing to 4 capsules a day until symptoms are relieved. Elderly 1 capsule morning and night increasing to 3 capsules a day if the kidneys function normally.

Availability: NHS and private prescription.

Side effects: sensitivity to light, fluid retention, stomach bleeding, alveolitis, positive Coombs test.

Caution: in pregnant women and in patients with a history of peptic ulcer. Patients on long-term treatment should be checked regularly.

Not to be used for: children or for patients suffering from peptic ulcer, history of blood changes, or kidney disease.

Not to be used with: PHENYTOIN, anti-coagulants, anti-diabetics, sulphonamides.

Contains: AZAPROPAZONE.

Other preparations: Rheumox Tablets.

Rhinocort
(Astra)

An aerosol supplied at a strength of 50 micrograms and used as a corticosteroid treatment for rhinitis.

Dose: 2 sprays into each nostril twice a day at first, then 1 spray into each nostril twice a day.

Availability: NHS and private prescription.

Side effects: sneezing.

Caution: in pregnant women and in patients suffering from fungal, viral, or tubercular infections of the nose.

Not to be used for: children for prolonged treatment.

Not to be used with:

Contains: BUDESONIDE.

Other preparations:

Rhumalgan *see* Voltarol
(Lagap)

---

riboflavine *see* **Abidec, Allbee with C, Apisate, BC 500, BC**

500 with Iron, Becosym, Calcimax, Concavit, Fefol-Vit Spansule, Fesovit Spansule, Fesovit Z Spansule, Galfervit, Givitol, Ketovite, Lipoflavonoid, Octovit, Orovite, Orovite 7, Polyvite, Pregnavite Forte F, Surbex T, Tonivitan B, Verdiviton, Villescon

---

Ridaura
(Bridge)

A pale-yellow, square tablet supplied at a strength of 3 mg and used as an oral gold salt to treat progressive rheumatoid arthritis which cannot be controlled effectively by NON-STEROID ANTI-INFLAMMATORY DRUGS.

Dose: 1 tablet in the morning and 1 tablet in the evening for the first 3-6 months, then increase to 3 tablets a day if needed for no longer than a further 3 months when the treatment should be discontinued.
Availability: NHS and private prescription.
Side effects: diarrhoea, nausea, stomach pain, ulcerative enterocolitis, rash, itch, mouth inflammation, alopecia, conjunctivitis, disturbance of taste, blood changes, liver effects, lung fibrosis.
Caution: in patients suffering from kidney or liver disease, inflammatory bowel disease, rash, history of bone marrow depression. Your doctor may advise that blood counts should be checked regularly. Women should take contraceptive measures.
Not to be used for: children, pregnant women, nursing mothers, or for patients suffering from severe kidney or liver disease, SLE (a multisystem disorder), history of necrotizing enterocolitis, lung fibrosis, exfoliative dermatitis, bone marrow aplasia, severe blood changes.
Not to be used with:
Contains: AURANOFIN.
Other preparations:

Rifadin
(Merrell Dow)

A red/blue capsule or a red capsule according to strengths of 150 mg, 300 mg and used as an antibiotic in the additional treatment for tuberculosis, and other infections.

Dose: adults 600 mg twice a day for 2 days; children 3 months-1 year

5 mg per kg body weight twice a day for 2 days, 1-12 years 10 mg per kg body weight twice a day for 2 days. Tuberculosis 450-600 mg as a single dose.
Availability: NHS and private prescription.
Side effects: symptoms similar to influenza, rash, stomach disturbances, orange-coloured urine and faeces.
Caution: in the elderly, underfed or very young infants, and in patients suffering from liver disease.
Not to be used for: pregnant women or for patients suffering from jaundice.
Not to be used with: anti-coagulants, DIGITALIS, anti-diabetics, contraceptive pill, corticosteroids.
Contains: RIFAMPCIN.
Other preparations: Rifadin Syrup, RIMACTANE (Ciba).

---

rifampcin *see* Rifadin, Rifinah, Rimactane

Rifater
(Merrell Dow)

A pink/beige tablet used as an antibiotic combination to treat tuberculosis of the lungs.

Dose: adults under 40 kg body weight 3 tablets a day, 40-49 kg 4 tablets a day, 50-64 kg 5 tablets a day, over 65 kg 6 tablets a day; children as advised by the physician.
Availability: NHS and private prescription.
Side effects: flu-like symptoms, skin reactions, stomach disturbances, change in urine colour.
Caution: care in the elderly and in patients suffering from liver disease, gout, or coughing blood.
Not to be used for: pregnant women, nursing mothers, or for patients suffering from jaundice.
Not to be used with: anti-convulsants, anti-coagulants, DIGITALIS, QUINIDINE, corticosteroids, the contraceptive pill, DAPSONE, narcotics, analgesics, anti-diabetics taken by mouth.
Contains: ISONIAZID, PYRAZINAMIDE, RIFAMPCIN.
Other preparations:

Rifinah
(Merrell Dow)

A pink tablet or an orange, oval-shaped tablet according to strength and used as an antibiotic combination to treat tuberculosis.

Dose: under 50 kg body weight 3 pink tablets once a day before breakfast; over 50 kg body weight 2 orange tablets once a day before breakfast.
Availability: NHS and private prescription.
Side effects: sleeplessness, muscle twitching, flu-like symptoms, skin reactions, stomach and liver disturbances, orange urine and faeces.
Caution: in children under 2 years, nursing mothers, the elderly, and patients suffering from kidney or liver disease, chronic alcoholism, or with a history of epilepsy.
Not to be used for: pregnant women or patients suffering from jaundice.
Not to be used with: anti-coagulants, digitalis, corticosteroids, the contraceptive pill, anti-diabetics.
Contains: RIFAMPCIN, ISONIAZID.
Other preparations: RIMACTAZID (Ciba)

Rimactane
(Ciba)

A red capsule or a brown/red capsule according to strengths of 150 mg, 300 mg and used as an antibiotic in the additional treatment for tuberculosis and other similar infections.

Dose: adults 450-600 mg a day in a single dose $\frac{1}{2}$ hour before breakfast; children up to 20 mg per kg a day to a maximum of 600 mg in a single dose.
Availability: NHS and private prescription.
Side effects: sleeplessness, muscle twitching, flu-like symptoms, skin reactions, stomach and liver disturbances, orange urine and faeces.
Caution: in the elderly or in very young undernourished patients, and in patients suffering from liver disease.
Not to be used for: pregnant women, nursing mothers, and in patients suffering from jaundice.
Not to be used with: anti-coagulants, contraceptive pill, corticosteroids,

DIGITALIS, anti-diabetics.
Contains: RIFAMPCIN.
Other preparations: Rimactane Syrup, Rimactane Infusion.

Rimactane *see* **Rifadin**
(Ciba)

R

Rimactazid *see* **Rifinah**
(Ciba)

---

rimiterol hydrobromide *see* **pulmadil**

---

ritodrine hydrochloride *see* **Yutopar**

Rivotril
(Roche)

A beige tablet or white tablet according to strengths of 0.5 mg, 2 mg and used as an anti-convulsant to treat epilepsy.

Dose: adults 1 mg a day at first, up to 4-8 mg a day; children and the elderly reduced doses.
Availability: NHS and private prescription.
Side effects: drowsiness, confusion, unsteadiness, low blood pressure, rash, changes in vision, changes in libido, retention of urine. Risk of addiction increases with dose and length of treatment. May impair judgement.
Caution: in children, the elderly, pregnant women, nursing mothers, in women during labour, and in patients suffering from lung disorders, kidney or liver disorders. Avoid long-term use and withdraw gradually.
Not to be used for: patients suffering from acute lung diseases, some chronic lung diseases, some obsessional and psychotic diseases.
Not to be used with: alcohol, other tranquillizers, anti-convulsants.

Contains: CLONAZEPAM.
Other preparations: Rivotril Injection.

Ro-A-Vit
(Roche)

A white tablet used as a source of VITAMIN A to treat vitamin A deficiency.

Dose: adults 1-6 tablets a day; children up to 1 tablet a day.
Availability: NHS and private prescription.
Side effects: vitamin A poisoning.
Caution:
Not to be used for: pregnant women.
Not to be used with:
Contains: vitamin A.
Other preparations: Ro-A-Vit Injection.

Roaccutane
(Roche)

A white/red capsule used as a VITAMIN A derivative to treat severe acne.

Dose: 0.5 mg per kg body weight a day with food for the first 4 weeks, then adjust according to response for another 8-12 weeks.
Availability: NHS (hospitals only).
Side effects: dryness, erosion of mucous membranes, alopecia, rise in liver enzymes and serum lipids, nausea, headache, sweating, moodiness, seizures, irregular periods, rarely loss of hearing, blood changes, blood vessel inflammation.
Caution: women of child-bearing age must take contraceptive precautions before, during, and after treatment. Your doctor may advise that liver and blood should be checked regularly.
Not to be used for: children, pregnant women, nursing mothers, or for patients suffering from liver or kidney disease.
Not to be used with: vitamin A.
Contains: ISOTRETINOIN.
Other preparations:

Robaxin
(Robins)

A white, oblong, scored tablet supplied at a strength of 750 mg and used as a muscle relaxant to treat skeletal muscle spasm.

Dose: adults 2 tablets 4 times a day; elderly 1 tablet 4 times a day.
Availability: NHS and private prescription.
Side effects: drowsiness, allergy.
Caution: in pregnant women, nursing mothers, and in patients suffering from kidney or liver disease.
Not to be used for: children or for patients in a coma or suffering from brain damage, epilepsy, myasthenia gravis (a muscle disorder).
Not to be used with: alcohol, sedatives and stimulants, ANTI-CHOLINERGICS.
Contains: METHOCARBAMOL.
Other preparations: Robaxin Injectable.

Robaxisal Forte
(Robins)

A pink/white, two-layered, scored tablet used as a muscle relaxant and analgesic to treat skeletal muscle spasm.

Dose: adults 2 tablets 4 times a day; elderly 1 tablet 4 times a day.
Availability: private prescription only.
Side effects: drowsiness, allergy, stomach bleeding.
Caution: in pregnant women, nursing mothers, and in patients suffering from kidney or liver disease, allergy to anti-inflammatory drugs, or a history of bronchospasm.
Not to be used for: children or for patients suffering from coma, brain damage, epilepsy, myasthenia gravis (a muscle disorder), peptic ulcer, haemophilia.
Not to be used with: alcohol, sedatives and stimulants, ANTI-CHOLINERGICS, anti-coagulants, anti-diabetics, hydantoins.
Contains: METHOCARBAMOL, ASPIRIN.
Other preparations:

Rocaltrol
(Roche)

A white/red capsule or a red capsule according to strengths of 0.25 micrograms, 0.5 micrograms and used as a source of VITAMIN D for correcting calcium and phosphate metabolism in patients suffering from kidney osteodystrophy (bone disease due to kidney disorder).

Dose: 1-2 micrograms a day increasing if needed by 0.25-0.5 micrograms at a time to no more than 2-3 micrograms a day.
Availability: NHS and private prescription.
Side effects: increased blood and urine calcium levels.
Caution: in pregnant women. Do not take any other vitamin D preparations. Your doctor may advise that calcium levels should be checked regularly.
Not to be used for: patients suffering from metastatic calcification (laying down of calcium), raised calcium levels.
Not to be used with:
Contains: CALCITRIOL.
Other preparations:

Roccal
(Winthrop)

A solution used as a disinfectant for cleansing and disinfecting the skin before surgery.

Dose: dilute the solution and use as needed.
Availability: NHS, private prescription, over the counter.
Side effects:
Caution:
Not to be used for:
Not to be used with:
Contains: BENZALKONIUM CHLORIDE.
Other preparations:

Rohypnol
(Roche)

A purple, diamond-shaped, scored tablet supplied at a strength of 1 mg and used as a sedative for the short-term treatment of sleeplessness or to bring on sleep at other times.

Dose: elderly ¹/₂ tablet before going to bed; adults ¹/₂ -1 tablet before going to bed.
Availability: private prescription only.
Side effects: drowsiness, confusion, unsteadiness, low blood pressure, rash, changes in vision, changes in libido, retention of urine. Risk of addiction increases with dose and length of treatment. May impair judgement.
Caution: in the elderly, pregnant women, nursing mothers, in women during labour, and in patients suffering from lung disorders, kidney or liver disorders. Avoid long-term use and withdraw gradually.
Not to be used for: children, or for patients suffering from acute lung diseases, some chronic lung diseases, some obsessional and psychotic diseases.
Not to be used with: alcohol, other tranquillizers, anti-convulsants.
Contains: FLUNITRAZEPAM.
Other preparations:

Ronicol
(Roche)

A white, scored tablet supplied at a strength of 25 mg and used as a vaso-dilator to treat poor circulation, spasm of blood vessels, Ménière's syndrome (dizziness and deafness)

Dose: 1-2 tablets 4 times a day.
Availability: NHS and private prescription.
Side effects: flushes.
Caution: care in long-term treatment of diabetics.
Not to be used for: children.
Not to be used with:
Contains: NICOTINYL ALCOHOL TARTRATE.
Other preparations: Ronicol Timespan.

Rose Bengal
(SNP)

Drops used as a dye to stain the eye for finding degenerated cells in dry eye syndrome.

Dose: 1-2 drops into the eye as needed.

Availability: NHS, private prescription, over the counter.
Side effects: severe smarting.
Caution:
Not to be used for: children.
Not to be used with:
Contains: ROSE BENGAL.
Other preparations:

Roter
(Roterpharma)

A pink tablet used as an antacid and antibulking agent to treat peptic ulcers, gastritis.

Dose: adults 1-2 tablets 3 times a day.
Availability: private prescription and over the counter.
Side effects: constipation, nerve damage.
Caution:
Not to be used for: for infants.
Not to be used with: TETRACYCLINE antibiotics.
Contains: MAGNESIUM CARBONATE, BISMUTH SUBNITRATE, SODIUM BICARBONATE, FRANGULA.
Other preparations:

Rotersept
(Roterpharma)

An aerosol used as a disinfectant for the prevention of mastitis, and to treat cracked nipples.

Dose: spray on to the breast before and after feeding.
Availability: NHS, private prescription, over the counter.
Side effects:
Caution:
Not to be used for: children.
Not to be used with:
Contains: CHLORHEXIDINE GLUCONATE.
Other preparations:

Rowachol
(Tillotts)

A solution containing essential oils used to treat cholelithiasis (gall stones), biliary and liver disorders.

Dose: adults 3-5 drops 4-5 times a day.
Availability: NHS and private prescription.
Side effects:
Caution:
Not to be used for: for children.
Not to be used with:
Contains: MENTHOL, MENTHONE, ALPHA-BETA-PINENES, CAMPHENE, CINEOLE, BORNEOL, OLIVE OIL.
Other preparations: Rowachol Capsules.

R

Rowatinex
(Tillotts)

Volatile oils used to treat urinary stones, kidney disorders, prevention of urinary stones

Dose: 3-5 drops 4-5 times a day before food.
Availability: NHS, private prescription, over the counter.
Side effects:
Caution:
Not to be used for: children.
Not to be used with:
Contains: PINENE, CAMPHENE, BORNEOL, ANETHOL, FENCHONE, CINEOLE, OLIVE OIL.
Other preparations: Rowatinex Capsules.

Rybarvin
(Rybar)

A solution used as an anti-asthmatic drug to treat asthma

Dose: adults inhale for 1-2 minutes 3 times a day and during an attack if needed; children inhale for 30 seconds-1 minute twice a day.
Availability: NHS, private prescription, over the counter.
Side effects: nervousness, restlessness, sleeplessness, shaking, abnormal heart rhythms, anti-cholinergic effects.

Caution: care in patients suffering from glaucoma, enlarged prostate, diabetes.
Not to be used for: patients suffering from overactive thyroid, high blood pressure, coronary disease, cardiac asthma.
Not to be used with: MAOIS, TRICYCLICS, SYMPATHOMIMETICS.
Contains: ATROPINE methonitrate, ADRENALINE, PAPAVERINE hydrochloride, BENZOCAINE.
Other preparations:

Rynacrom Spray
(Fisons)

A spray used as an anti-allergy treatment for allergic rhinitis.

Dose: 1 spray into each nostril 4-6 times a day.
Availability: NHS, private prescription, over the counter.
Side effects: temporary itching nose, rarely bronchial spasm.
Caution:
Not to be used for:
Not to be used with:
Contains: SODIUM CROMOGLYCATE.
Other preparations: Rynacrom Nasal Drops, Rynacrom Cartridges, Rynacrom Compound.

Rythmodan
(Roussel)

A yellow/green capsule or a white capsule according to strengths of 100 mg, 150 mg and used as an anti-arrhythmic treatment for abnormal heart rhythm

Dose: 300-800 mg a day in divided doses.
Availability: NHS and private prescription.
Side effects: anti-cholinergic effects, rarely jaundice, mood changes, low blood sugar.
Caution: in pregnant women, and in patients suffering from heart conduction block, heart, liver, and kidney failure, enlarged prostate, glaucoma, urine retention, low potassium levels.
Not to be used for: for patients suffering from severe heart conduction block, heart failure.
Not to be used with: ß-BLOCKERS, DIURETICS, ANTI-CHOLINERGICS, other

anti-arrhythmics.
Contains: DISOPYRAMIDE.
Other preparations: Rythmodan Retard, Rythmodan Injection.

Sabidal SR *see* Theophylline
(Zyma)

Salactol
(Dermal)

A paint used as a skin softener to treat warts.

Dose: apply to the wart once a day and rub down with a pumice stone between treatments.
Availability: NHS, private prescription, over the counter.
Side effects:
Caution: do not apply to healthy skin.
Not to be used for: warts on the face or anal and genital areas.
Not to be used with:
Contains: SALICYLIC ACID, LACTIC ACID.
Other preparations:

Salazopyrin
(Pharmacia)

An orange, scored tablet supplied at a strength of 500 mg and used as a salicylate-sulphonamide treatment for ulcerative colitis, Crohn's disease.

Dose: adults 2-4 tablets 4 times a day for 2-3 weeks; children over 2 years 40-60 mg/kg body weight a day.
Availability: NHS and private prescription.
Side effects: nausea, headache, rash, high temperature, loss of appetite.
Caution: in patients with liver or kidney disease. Your doctor may advise regular blood tests.
Not to be used for: children under 2 years.
Not to be used with: DIGOXIN.
Contains: SULPHASALAZINE.

Other preparations: Salazopyrin EN-Tabs, Salazopyrin suspension, enema, suppositories.

Salazopyrin EN-tablets
(Pharmacia)

An orange, oval tablet supplied at a strength of 500 mg and used as a salicylate-sulphonamide. treatment for rheumatoid arthritis which is not responding to NON-STEROID ANTI-INFLAMMATORY DRUGS.

Dose: 1 tablet a day for the first 7 days increasing by 1 tablet a day each subsequent 7 days to a maximum of 6 tablets a day in divided doses.
Availability: NHS and private prescription.
Side effects: nausea, headache, rash, fever, loss of appetite.
Caution: in patients suffering from liver or kidney disease. Your doctor may advise that blood should be checked regularly and any other analgesics taken at the same time should only be withdrawn after response has been monitored.
Not to be used for: children.
Not to be used with: DIGOXIN.
Contains: SULPHASALAZINE.
Other preparations:

Salbulin
(3M Riker)

A white tablet or a pink tablet according to strengths of 2 mg, 4 mg and used as a broncho-dilator to treat bronchial spasm brought on by bronchitis, bronchial asthma, emphysema.

Dose: adults 2-4 mg 3-4 times a day; children 2-6 years 1-2 mg 3-4 times a day, 6-12 years 2 mg 3-4 times a day.
Availability: NHS and private prescription.
Side effects: hands shaking, nervous tension, headache, dilation of the blood vessels.
Caution: in pregnant women and in patients suffering from overactive thyroid, heart muscle disease, angina, abnormal heart rhythms, high blood pressure.
Not to be used for:
Not to be used with: SYMPATHOMIMETICS.

Contains: SALBUTAMOL sulphate.
Other preparations: Salbulin Inhaler.

---

salbutamol *see* **Cobutolin, Salbulin, Ventide, Ventodisks, Ventolin**

---

salicylamide *see* **Intralgin**

---

salicylic acid *see* **Aserbine, Cuplex, Diprosalic, Dithrolan, Duofilm, Gelcosal, Ional T, Keralyt, Malatex, Monphytol, Movelat, Phytex, Phytocil, Posafilin, Pragmatar, Psorin, Pyralvex, Salactol, Verrugon**

Salonair
(Salonpas)

An aerosol used as an analgesic rub to relieve muscular and rheumatic pain.

Dose: spray on to the affected area 1-2 times a day.
Availability: NHS, private prescription , over the counter.
Side effects: may be irritant.
Caution:
Not to be used for: areas such as near the eyes, on broken or inflamed skin, or on membranes (such as the mouth).
Not to be used with:
Contains: GLYCOL SALICYLATE, MENTHOL, CAMPHOR, SQUALANE, BENZYL NICOTINATE.
Other preparations:

---

salsalate *see* **Disalcid**

Saluric
(MSD)

A white, scored tablet supplied at a strength of 500 mg and used as a DIURETIC to treat fluid retention, high blood pressure.

Dose: adults fluid retention 1-2 tablets a day or from time to time, high blood pressure 1-2 a day up to 4 a day if needed; children under 2 years 125-375 mg a day in two doses, 2-12 years 375-1 g a day in two doses.
Availability: NHS and private prescription.
Side effects: low potassium level, rash, sensitivity to light, blood changes, gout, tiredness.
Caution: in pregnant women and in patients suffering from diabetes, kidney or liver disease, gout. Potassium supplements may be needed.
Not to be used for: nursing mothers or for patients suffering from severe kidney failure.
Not to be used with: DIGITALIS, LITHIUM, anti-hypertensives.
Contains: CHLOROTHIAZIDE.
Other preparations:

S

Salzone
(Wallace)

A syrup supplied at a strength of 120 mg/5 ml teaspoonful and used as an analgesic to relieve pain and reduce fever.

Dose: children 1/2-2 5 ml teaspoonsful every 4 hours according to age.
Availability: NHS, private prescription, over the counter.
Side effects:
Caution: in children suffering from kidney or liver disease.
Not to be used for:
Not to be used with:
Contains: PARACETAMOL.
Other preparations:

Sando-K
(Sandoz)

A white, effervescent tablet used as a potassium supplement to treat potassium deficiency.

Dose: 2-4 tablets a day dissolved in water.
Availability: NHS, private prescription, over the counter.
Side effects: stomach upset.
Caution: in patients suffering from kidney disease.
Not to be used for: children.
Not to be used with:
Contains: POTASSIUM BICARBONATE, POTASSIUM CHLORIDE.
Other preparations:

Sandocal
(Sandoz)

An orange, effervescent tablet used as a calcium supplement in additional treatment for osteoporosis, osteomalacia, rickets, pregnancy, lactation, undernourishment, and after gastric surgery when absorption is poor.

Dose: adults 3-4 tablets a day dissolved in water; children 1-2 tablets a day dissolved in water.
Availability: NHS, private prescription, over the counter.
Side effects: diarrhoea, nausea, flushes.
Caution: in patients suffering from kidney disease, unbalanced electrolyte levels, congestive heart failure. Your doctor may advise that calcium levels should be checked regularly.
Not to be used for: for patients suffering from raised calcium levels in the blood or urine, severe kidney failure, kidney stones, galactosaemia.
Not to be used with: THIAZIDES, TETRACYCLINES.
Contains: CALCIUM LACTATE GLUCONATE, SODIUM BICARBONATE, POTASSIUM BICARBONATE.
Other preparations: Calcium Sandoz Syrup, Calcium Sandoz Injection.

Sanomigran
(Sandoz)

An ivory, scored tablet supplied at strengths of 0.5 mg, 1.5 mg and used as a blood vessel stabilizer to treat migraine or headache.

Dose: adults 1.5 mg a day as a single dose at night or in 3 divided doses to a maximum of 6 mg a day in divided doses; children up to 1.5

mg a day in divided doses, or 1 mg at night.
Availability: NHS and private prescription.
Side effects: drowsiness, weight gain.
Caution: in patients suffering from glaucoma or retention of urine.
Not to be used for:
Not to be used with:
Contains: PIZOTIFEN HYDROGEN MALATE.
Other preparations: Sanomigran Eleixir.

Saventrine
(Pharmax)

A white, mottled tablet supplied at a strength of 30 mg and used as a circulatory stimulant to treat shock, Stokes-Adams attacks, low blood pressure.

Dose: as advised by physician.
Availability: NHS and private prescription.
Side effects: palpitations, tremor, sweating, headache, diarrhoea.
Caution: in patients suffering from high blood pressure and diabetes.
Not to be used for: patients suffering from some heart diseases and overactive thyroid.
Not to be used with:
Contains: ISOPRENALINE hydrochloride
Other preparations: Saventrine I.V.

Savloclens
(ICI)

A solution in a sachet used as a disinfectant for cleansing and disinfecting wounds and burns.

Dose: use neat as needed.
Availability: NHS, private prescription, over the counter.
Side effects:
Caution:
Not to be used for:
Not to be used with:
Contains: CHLORHEXIDINE gluconate, CETRIMIDE.
Other preparations:

Savlodil
(ICI)

A solution in a sachet used as a disinfectant for cleansing and disinfecting wounds and burns.

Dose: use neat as needed.
Availability: NHS, private prescription, over the counter.
Side effects:
Caution:
Not to be used for:
Not to be used with:
Contains: CHLORHEXIDINE gluconate, CETRIMIDE.
Other preparations:

Savlon Hospital Concentrate
(ICI)

A solution used as a disinfectant and general antiseptic.

Dose: adequate amounts.
Availability: NHS, private prescription, over the counter.
Side effects:
Caution:
Not to be used for:
Not to be used with:
Contains: CHLORHEXIDINE gluconate, CETRIMIDE.
Other preparations:

Scheriproct
(Schering)

An ointment used as a steroid, local anaesthetic, antihistamine treatment for haemorrhoids, anal fissure, itch, bowel inflammation.

Dose: apply 2-4 times a day.
Availability: NHS and private prescription.
Side effects: systemic corticosteroid effects.
Caution: in pregnant women; do not use for prolonged periods.
Not to be used for: patients suffering from tuberculous, fungal, or viral infections
Not to be used with:

Contains: PREDNISOLONE hexanoate, CINCHOCAINE hydrochloride
Other preparations: Scheriproct suppositories.

Scopoderm
(Ciba)

A pink, self-adhesive patch used as a ANTI-CHOLINERGIC to prevent travel sickness.

Dose: 1 patch applied to clean dry skin behind the ear 5-6 hours before a journey, replacing after 3 days if needed. Remove after journey is completed.
Availability: NHS and private prescription.
Side effects: local skin irritation, rash, dry mouth, drowsiness, dizziness, rention of urine.
Caution: care in pregnant women, nursing mothers, and in patients suffering from blocked bladder outflow, bowel obstruction, kidney or liver disease.
Not to be used for: children under 10 years or for patients suffering from glaucoma.
Not to be used with: sedatives, anti-cholinergics.
Contains: HYOSCINE.
Other preparations:

Secadrex
(M & B)

A white tablet supplied at a strength of 400 mg and used as a ß-BLOCKER/THIAZIDE DIURETIC combination to treat high blood pressure.

Dose: 1-2 tablets a day.
Availability: NHS and private prescription.
Side effects: cold hands and feet, sleep disturbance, slow heart rate, tiredness, wheezing, heart failure, stomach upset.
Caution: in pregnant women, nursing mothers, and in patients suffering from diabetes, kidney or liver disorders, asthma. May need to be withdrawn before surgery. Withdraw gradually. Your doctor may advise additional treatment with diuretics or digitalis.
Not to be used for: children, or for patients suffering from heart block or failure.
Not to be used with: VERAPAMIL, CLONIDINE withdrawal, some anti-

arrhythmic drugs and anaesthetics, RESERPINE, some anti-hypertensives, ergot alkaloids, CIMETIDINE, sedatives, SYMPATHOMIMETICS, INDOMETHACIN.
Contains: ACEBUTOLOL hydrochloride, HYDROCHLOROTHIAZIDE.
Other preparations:

Seconal Sodium
(Eli Lilly)

An orange capsule supplied at strengths of 60 mg, 200 mg and used as a barbiturate to treat sleeplessness.

Dose: 50-100 mg at night.
Availability: controlled drug.
Side effects: drowsiness, hangover, dizziness, allergies, headache, confusion, excitement.
Caution: in patients suffering from kidney or lung disease. Dependence (addiction) may develop.
Not to be used for: children, young adults, pregnant women, nursing mothers, the elderly, patients with a history of drug or alcohol abuse, or suffering from porphyria (a rare blood disorder), or in the management of pain.
Not to be used with: anti-coagulants (blood-thinning drugs), alcohol, other tranquillizers, steroids, the contraceptive pill, GRISEOFULVIN, RIFAMPICIN, PHENYTOIN, METRONIDAZOLE, CHLORAMPHENICOL.
Contains: QUINALBARBITONE sodium.
Other preparations:

Sectral
(M. & B.)

A buff/white capsule or a buff/pink capsule according to strengths of 100 mg, 200 mg, or a white tablet supplied at a strength of 400 mg and used as a ß-BLOCKER to treat angina, abnormal heart rhythm, or high blood pressure.

Dose: 100-200 mg 2-3 times a day; high blood pressure up to 800 mg a day.
Availability: NHS and private prescription.
Side effects: cold hands and feet, sleep disturbance, slow heart rate,

tiredness, wheezing, heart failure, stomach upset.

Caution: in pregnant women, nursing mothers, and in patients suffering from diabetes, kidney or liver disorders, asthma. May need to be withdrawn before surgery. Withdraw gradually. Your doctor may advise additional treatment with diuretics or digitalis.

Not to be used for: children or for patients suffering from heart block or failure.

Not to be used with: VERAPAMIL, CLONIDINE withdrawal, some anti-arrhythmic drugs and anaesthetics, RESERPINE, some anti-hypertensives, ergot alkaloids, CIMETIDINE, sedatives, SYMPATHOMIMETICS, IN-DOMETHACIN.

Contains: ACEBUTOLOL hydrochloride.

Other preparations:

Securon
(Knoll)

A white tablet or a white, scored tablet according to strengths of 40 mg, 80 mg, 120 mg, 160 mg and used as a calcium blocker to treat angina.

Dose: 120 mg 3 times a day.

Availability: NHS and private prescription.

Side effects: constipation, flushes; occasionally headache, nausea, allergies.

Caution: in pregnant women and in patients suffering from slow heart rate, heart failure, liver damage, some heart rhythm disturbances.

Not to be used for: children or for patients suffering from severe shock or heart block, heart failure, heart attacks.

Not to be used with: ß-BLOCKERS, DIGOXIN, anti-arrhythmics.

Contains: VERAPAMIL hydrochloride.

Other preparations:

Securon SR
(Knoll)

A green, scored, oblong tablet supplied at a strength of 240 mg and used as a calcium blocker to treat high blood pressure.

Dose: ¹/₂ tablet at first, the usually 1 tablet a day to a maximum of 2 tablets a day if needed.

Availability: NHS and private prescription.
Side effects: constipation, flushes, rarely headaches, nausea, allergies.
Caution: in pregnant women and in patients suffering from slow heart rate, heart failure, liver damage, some heart rhythm disturbances.
Not to be used for: children or for patients suffering from severe shock or heart block, heart failure, heart attacks.
Not to be used with: ß-BLOCKERS, DIGOXIN, anti-arrhythmics.
Contains: VERAPAMIL hydrochloride.
Other preparations: Securon.

---

selegiline *see* Eldepryl

---

selenium sulphide *see* Lenium, Selsun

Selexid
(Leo)

A white tablet supplied at a strength of 200 mg and used as a penicillin to treat urinary system and other infections.

Dose: 2 tablets immediately followed by 1 tablets 3 times a day.
Availability: NHS and private prescription.
Side effects: allergy, stomach disturbances.
Caution: in patients suffering from kidney disease.
Not to be used for:
Not to be used with:
Contains: PIVMECILLINAM hydrochloride.
Other preparations: Selexid Suspension.

Selora
(Winthrop)

Fine white granules used as a common salt substitute for patients on low-sodium diets.

Dose: normal salt use.
Availability: private prescription and over the counter.
Side effects:
Caution:
Not to be used for: patients suffering from kidney disease.
Not to be used with:
Contains: POTASSIUM CHLORIDE.
Other preparations:

Selsun
(Abbott)

A suspension used as an anti-dandruff treatment for dandruff, tinea versicolor (a scalp condition).

Dose: shampoo twice a week for 2 weeks, then once a week for 2 weeks, or apply to lesions and leave overnight.
Availability: NHS, private prescription, over the counter.
Side effects:
Caution: keep out of the eyes or broken skin; do not use within 48 hours of using waving or colouring substances.
Not to be used for:
Not to be used with:
Contains: SELENIUM SULPHIDE.
Other preparations:

Semprex
(Calmic)

A white capsule supplied at a strength of 8 mg and used as an anti-histamine treatment for allergic rhinitis, other allergies.

Dose: 1 capsule 3 times a day.
Availability: NHS and private prescription
Side effects: rarely drowsiness.
Caution: in nursing mothers and in patients suffering from liver or kidney disease.
Not to be used for: children, the elderly, or for patients suffering from kidney failure.
Not to be used with: sedatives, alcohol.
Contains: ACRIVASTINE.

senna tablets

A tablet supplied at a strength of 7.5 mg and used as a stimulant laxative to treat constipation.

Dose: adults 2-4 tablets at bedtime; children 6-12 years half adult dose.
Availability: NHS and private prescription.
Side effects:
Caution:
Not to be used for: pregnant women, children under 6 years.
Not to be used with:
Contains: SENNOSIDES.
Other preparations:

sennoside B *see* Senokot

sennosides *see* Manevac, Pripsin, senna tablets

Senokot
(Reckitt & Colman)

A brown tablet supplied at a strength of 7.5 mg and used as a stimulant to treat constipation.

Dose: adults 2-4 tablets at bedtime; children 2-6 years 2.5-5 ml syrup (see below) in morning; children over 6 years half adult dose in morning.
Availability: NHS (when prescribed as a generic) and private prescription.
Side effects:
Caution:
Not to be used for: infants under 2 years.
Not to be used with:

Contains: SENNOSIDE B.
Other preparations: Senokot granules, Sennokott syrup.

Sential
(Pharmacia)

A cream used as a steroid, wetting agent to treat dry eczema.

Dose: apply lightly to the affected area twice a day.
Availability: NHS and private prescription.
Side effects: fluid retention, suppression of adrenal glands, thinning of the skin may occur.
Caution: use for short periods of time only.
Not to be used for: patients suffering from acne or any other skin infections caused by tuberculosis, ringworm, viruses, or fungi, or continuously especially in pregnant women.
Not to be used with:
Contains: HYDROCORTISONE, UREA, SODIUM CHLORIDE.
Other preparations:

Septrin
(Wellcome)

A white tablet or an orange, dispersible tablet used as an antibiotic to treat respiratory, stomach, and skin infections.

Dose: adults 1-3 tablets twice a day; children under 6 years use paediatric syrup, 6-12 years 1 tablet twice a day.
Availability: NHS and private prescription.
Side effects: nausea, vomiting, tongue inflammation, rash, blood changes, folate (vitamin) deficiency, rarely skin changes.
Caution: in nursing mothers and in patients suffering from kidney disease. Your doctor may advise that patients undergoing prolonged treatment should have regular blood tests.
Not to be used for: pregnant women, new-born infants, or for patients suffering from severe kidney or liver disease, or blood changes.
Not to be used with: folate inhibitors, anti-coagulants, anti-convulsants, anti-diabetics.
Contains: TRIMETHOPRIM, SULPHAMETHOXAZOLE.
Other preparations: Septrin Adults Suspension, Septrin Forte, Septrin Paediatric Tablets, Septrin Paediatric Suspension, Septrin IM Injec-

tion, Septrin for Infusion. BACTRIM (Roche), CHEMOTRIM PAEDIATRIC (RP Drugs), COMOX (Norton).

Serc
(Duphar)

A white tablet supplied at a strength of 8 mg and used as a histamine-type drug to treat vertigo, tinnitus, and hearing loss caused by Ménière's disease.

Dose: 2 tablets 3 times a day at first then 3-6 tablets a day.
Availability: NHS and private prescription.
Side effects: stomach upset.
Caution: in patients suffering from bronchial asthma, peptic ulcer.
Not to be used for: children or patients suffering from phaeochromocytoma (a disease of the adrenal glands).
Not to be used with:
Contains: BETAHISTINE dihydrochloride.
Other preparations:

Serenace
(Searle)

A green/pale-green capsule supplied at a strength of 0.5 mg and used as a sedative for an additional treatment in the short-term management of anxiety.

Dose: 1 capsule twice a day.
Availability: NHS and private prescription.
Side effects: muscle spasms, restlessness, hands shaking, dry mouth, urine retention, palpitations, low blood pressure, weight gain, changes in libido, low body temperature, breast swelling, menstrual changes, jaundice, blood and skin changes, drowsiness, rarely fits.
Caution: in pregnant women or in patients suffering from hperthyroidism, liver or kidney failure, severe cardiovascular disease, tardive dyskinesia (a movement disorder), epilepsy
Not to be used for: nursing mothers, unconscious patients, or for patients suffering from Parkinson's disease.
Not to be used with: alcohol, tranquillizers, pain killers, anti-hypertensives, anti-depressants, anti-convulsants, anti-diabetic drugs, LEVODOPA.

Contains: HALOPERIDOL.
Other preparations: Serenace Liquid, Serenace Tablets, Serenace Injection.

Serophene
(Serono)

A white, scored tablet supplied at a strength of 50 mg and used as a anti-oestrogen treatment for infertility due to failure of ovulation caused by impaired hypothalamic-pituitary function.

Dose: 1 tablet a day for 5 days beginning within 5 days of the start of the period.
Availability: NHS and private prescription.
Side effects: enlargement of the ovaries, hot flushes, uncomfortable abdomen, blurred vision.
Caution:
Not to be used for: children, pregnant women, or patients suffering from liver disease, large ovarian cyst, endometrial cancer, bleeding from the uterus.
Not to be used with:
Contains: CLOMIPHENE citrate.
Other preparations:

Serpasil
(Ciba)

A blue tablet or a blue, scored tablet according to strengths of 0.1 mg, 0.25 mg and used as an anti-hypertensive drug to treat high blood pressure.

Dose: up to 1 mg a day at first, then up to 0.5 mg a day.
Availability: NHS and private prescription.
Side effects: blocked nose, lethargy, diarrhoea, depression, rash, peptic ulcer, low blood pressure, failure to ejaculate, Parkinson-like problems.
Caution: in pregnant women, nursing mothers, and in patients suffering from abnormal heart rhythm, bronchitis, asthma, heart attack.

Not to be used for: children or for patients with a history of depression, active peptic ulcer, ulcerative colitis.
Not to be used with: DIGITALIS, QUINIDINE.
Contains: RESERPINE.
Other preparations:

Serpasil Esidrex
(Ciba)

A white, scored tablet used as an anti-hypertensive combination to treat high blood pressure.

Dose: 2-3 tablets a day.
Availability: NHS and private prescription.
Side effects: anorexia, blocked nose, lethargy, diarrhoea, rash, depression, blood changes, peptic ulcer, low blood pressure, failure to ejaculate, Parkinson-like problems.
Caution: pregnant women, nursing mothers, and in patients suffering from diabetes, gout, liver disease, bronchitis, asthma. Potassium supplements may be needed.
Not to be used for: children or for patients with a history of depression, active peptic ulcer, ulcerative colitis, severe kidney failure.
Not to be used with: LITHIUM, DIGITALIS.
Contains: RESERPINE, HYDROCHLOROTHIAZIDE.
Other preparations:

Siloxyl *see* Asilone
(Martindale)

---

silver sulphadiazine *see* Flamazine

Simeco *see* Asilone
(Wyeth)

Simplene
(SNP)

Drops used as a SYMPATHOMIMETIC treatment for primary open angle or secondary glaucoma.

Dose: 1 drop into the eye 1-2 times a day.
Availability: NHS and private prescription.
Side effects: pain in the eye, headache, redness, skin reactions, melanosis, rarely systemic effects.
Caution:
Not to be used for: patients suffering from narrow angle glaucoma, absence of the lens.
Not to be used with:
Contains: ADRENALINE.
Other preparations:

---

simvastatin *see* Zocor

Sinemet
(MSD)

A blue, scored, oval tablet or a yellow, scored tablet according to strengths of LS 50/12.5 mg, 110 110/10 mg, Plus 100/25 mg, 275 250/25 mg and used as an anti-parkinsonian preparation to treat Parkinson's disease.

Dose: 1 'plus' 3 times a day at first, increasing gradually to a maximum of 8 'plus' a day, then 1 '275' 3-4 times a day if needed.
Availability: NHS and private prescription.
Side effects: nausea, vomiting, anorexia, low blood pressure on standing, involuntary movements, heart and brain disturbances, discoloration of urine.
Caution: in pregnant women and in patients suffering from cardiovascular, liver, kidney, lung, or endocrine disease, peptic ulcer, or glaucoma. Your doctor may advise that blood, liver, kidney, and cardiovascular system should be checked regularly.
Not to be used for: patients under 18 years, nursing mothers, or for patients suffering from severe mental disorders or glaucoma.
Not to be used with: drugs affecting brain peptides, MAOIS, anti-hypertensives, and SYMPATHOMIMETICS.

Contains: LEVODOPA, CARBIDOPA monohydrate.
Other preparations:

Sinequan
(Pfizer)

An orange capsule or a blue/orange capsule accodring to strengths of 10 mg, 25 mg and used as an anti-depressant to treat depression.

Dose: 10-100 mg a day.
Availability: NHS and private prescription.
Side effects: dry mouth, constipation, urine retention, blurred vision, palpitations, drowsiness, sleeplessness, dizziness, hands shaking, low blood presure, weight change, skin reactions, jaundice or blood changes. Loss of sexual desire may occur.
Caution: in nursing mothers or in patients suffering from heart disease, thyroid disease, epilepsy, diabetes, some other psychiatric conditions. Your doctor may advise regular blood tests.
Not to be used for: children under 6 years, pregnant women, or for patients suffering from heart attacks, liver disease, heart block.
Not to be used with: alcohol, ANTI-CHOLINERGICS, ADRENALINE, MAOIS, barbiturates, other anti-depressants, anti-hypertensives.
Contains: DOXEPIN hydrochloride
Other preparations:

Sinthrome
(Geigy)

A pink tablet or a white, quarter-scored tablet according to strengths of 1 mg, 4 mg and used as an anti-coagulant drug to treat thrombotic disorders.

Dose: 8-12 mg on the first day, 4-8 mg second day, and then adjust as required.
Availability: NHS and private prescription.
Side effects: bleeding, allergies, liver damage, reversible alopecia, rarely nausea, anorexia, headache, skin necrosis.
Caution: in nursing mothers, the elderly, and in patients suffering from high blood pressure, reduced protein binding, severe heart failure, liver dysfunction, gastro-intestinal disorders.

Not to be used for: children, pregnant women, the unco-operative, and in patients suffering from bleeding conditions, blood changes, damaged kidney or liver function, inflammation of the heart or lungs, or within 24 hours of surgery.
Not to be used with: NON-STEROID ANTI-INFLAMMATORY DRUGS, oral anti-diabetics, sulphonamides, QUINIDINE, antibiotics, PHENFORMIN, CIMETID-INE, corticosteroids, drugs affecting liver chemistry.
Contains: NICOUMALONE.
Other preparations:

Sintisone
(Farmatalia CE)

A white, scored tablet supplied at a strength of 5 mg and used as a corticosteroid treatment for bronchial asthma, rheumatoid arthritis, rheumatic fever, allergies, inflammatory skin problems.

Dose: adults 2-4 tablets twice a day at first, reducing to 1-3 tablets a day; children 0.6-2 mg per kg body weight a day at first adjusting to 1 mg per kg a day.
Availability: NHS and private prescription.
Side effects: high blood pressure, thin bones, mood changes, ulcers.
Caution: in pregnant women, in patients who have had recent bowel surgery, or who are suffering from inflamed veins, psychiatric disorders, virus infections, some cancers, some kidney diseases, thinning of the bones, ulcers, tuberculosis, other infections, high blood pressure, glaucoma, epilepsy, diabetes, underactive thyroid, liver disease, stress. Withdraw gradually.
Not to be used for: infants under 1 year.
Not to be used with: PHENYTOIN, PHENOBARBITONE, EPHEDRINE, RIFAMPICIN, DIURETICS, ANTI-CHOLINESTERASES, DIGITALIS, anti-diabetic agents, anti-coagulants, NON-STEROID ANTI-INFLAMMATORY DRUGS.
Contains: PREDNISOLONE steaglate.
Other preparations:

Slo-Phyllin *see* Theophylline
(Lipha)

Slow Sodium
(Ciba)

A white tablet supplied at a strength of 600 mg and used as a salt supplement to treat salt deficiency.

Dose: adults 4-20 tablets a day, children in proportion to dose for 70 kg adult.
Availability: NHS, private prescription, over the counter.
Side effects:
Caution:
Not to be used for: patients suffering from fluid retention, heart disease, heart failure.
Not to be used with: DIURETICS, LITHIUM.
Contains: SODIUM CHLORIDE.
Other preparations:

Slow-Fe
(Ciba)

An off-white tablet supplied at a strength of 160 mg and used as a iron supplement. to treat iron-deficiency anaemia.

Dose: adults 1-2 tablets a day; children 6-12 years 1 tablet a day.
Availability: NHS, private prescription, over the counter.
Side effects: nausea, constipation.
Caution:
Not to be used for: children under 6 years.
Not to be used with: TETRACYCLINES.
Contains: FERROUS SULPHATE.
Other preparations:

Slow-Fe Folic
(Ciba)

A cream-coloured tablet used as an iron and folic acid supplement for the prevention of iron and folic acid deficiencies in pregnancy.

Dose: 1-2 tablets a day.
Availability: NHS and private prescription.
Side effects: nausea, constipation.

Caution:
Not to be used for: for children.
Not to be used with: TETRACYCLINES.
Contains: FERROUS SULPHATE, FOLIC ACID.
Other preparations:

Slow-K
(Ciba)

An orange tablet supplied at a strength of 600 mg and used as a potassium supplement to treat potassium deficiency.

Dose: adults 2-6 tablets a day or every other day after food; children as advised by the physician.
Availability: NHS, private prescription, over the counter.
Side effects: blocked or ulcerated small bowel.
Caution: in patients suffering from kidney disease or peptic ulcer.
Not to be used for: patients suffering from advanced kidney disease.
Not to be used with:
Contains: POTASSIUM CHLORIDE.
Other preparations:

Slow-Pren *see* Slow Trasicor
(Norton)

Slow-Trasicor
(Ciba)

A white tablet supplied at a strength of 160 mg and used as a ß-BLOCKER to treat high blood pressure.

Dose: 1 tablet a day in the morning at first, then increase to 2-3 tablets a day if needed.
Availability: NHS and private prescription.
Side effects: cold hands and feet, sleep disturbance, slow heart rate, tiredness, wheezing, heart failure, stomach upset.
Caution: in pregnant women, nursing mothers, and in patients suffering from diabetes, kidney or liver disorders, asthma. May need to be withdrawn before surgery. Withdraw gradually. Your doctor may

advise additional treatment with DIURETICS or digitalis.
Not to be used for: children or for patients suffering from heart block or failure.
Not to be used with: VERAPAMIL, CLONIDINE withdrawal, some anti-arrhythmic drugs and anaesthetics, RESERPINE, some anti-hypertensives, ergot alkaloids, CIMETIDINE, sedatives, SYMPATHOMIMETICS, INDOMETHACIN.
Contains: OXPRENOLOL hydrochloride.
Other preparations: SLOW-PREN (Norton).

Sno Phenicol *see* Chlormoycetin
(SNP)

Sno Pilo
(SNP)

Drops used as a cholinergic treatment for glaucoma.

Dose: 1-2 drops into the eye 4 times a day.
Availability: NHS and private prescription.
Side effects: temporary reduction of visual sharpness.
Caution:
Not to be used for: patients suffering from acute iritis or who wear soft contact lenses.
Not to be used with:
Contains: PILOCARPINE.
Other preparations:

Sno Tears
(SNP)

Drops used to lubricate the eyes.

Dose: 1 or more drops into the eye as needed.
Availability: NHS, private prescription, over the counter.
Side effects:
Caution:
Not to be used for: patients who wear soft contact lenses.
Not to be used with:

Contains: POLYVINYL ALCOHOL.
Other preparations:

---

sodium acid phosphate (anhydrous) *see* **Carbalax, Fletcher's Phosphate, Phosphate**

---

sodium alginate *see* **Gaviscon**

---

sodium alkylsulphoacetate *see* **Micralax**

Sodium Amytal
(Eli Lilly)

A blue capsule supplied at strengths of 60 mg, 200 mg and used as a barbiturate to treat sleeplessness, status epilepticus (severe epilepsy).

Dose: 60-200 mg at night.
Availability: controlled drug.
Side effects: drowsiness, hangover, dizziness, allergies, headache, confusion, excitement.
Caution: in patients suffering from kidney or lung disease. Dependence (addiction) may develop.
Not to be used for: children, young adults, pregnant women, nursing mothers, the elderly, patients with a history of drug or alcohol abuse, or suffering from porphyria (a rare blood disorder), or in the management of pain.
Not to be used with: anti-coagulants (blood-thinning drugs), alcohol, other tranquillizers, steroids, the contraceptive pill, GRISEOFULVIN, RIFAMPICIN, PHENYTOIN, METRONIDAZOLE, CHLORAMPHENICOL.
Contains: AMYLOBARBITONE sodium.
Other preparations: Sodium Amytal Tablets, Sodium Amytal Vials.

---

sodium bicarbonate *see* **Carbalax, Caved-S, Dioralyte,**

Gastrocote, Gastron, Gaviscon, Mictral, Phosphate, Rehidrat, Roter, Sandocal

---

sodium cellulose *see* Calcisorb

---

sodium chloride *see* Diarrest, Dioralyte, Glandosane, Minims Saline, Normasol, Opulets Saline, Rehidrat, Sential, Slow Sodium, Topiclens

---

S

sodium citrate *see* Benylin Expectorant, Diarrest, Guanor, Histalix, Micolette, Micralax, Mictral, Relaxit, Urisal

---

sodium cromoglycate *see* Intal, Intal Compound, Nalcrom, Opticrom, Rynacrom Spray

---

sodium docusate *see* Molcer, Soliwax

---

sodium fluorescein *see* Lignocaine and Fluorescein

---

sodium fusidate *see* Fucidin, Fucidin H

---

sodium glycerophosphate *see* Verdiviton

---

sodium hydrogen tartrate *see* Bocasan

---

sodium hypochlorite *see* Chlorasol

---

sodium iron edetate *see* Sytron

---

sodium lauryl sulphate *see* Relaxit

---

sodium lauryl sulphoacetate *see* Micolette

---

sodium nedocromil *see* Tilade

---

sodium oleate *see* Alcos-Anal

---

sodium perborate *see* Bocasan

---

sodium phenolate *see* Chloraseptic

---

sodium phosphate *see* Fletcher's Phosphate

---

sodium picosulphate *see also* Laxoberal, Picolax

A stimulant laxative used to treat constipation.

Dose: adults 5-15 ml at night; children 0-5 years 2.5 ml at night; children 5-10 years 5 ml at night.
Availability: NHS and private prescription.
Side effects:

Caution: in patients suffering from inflammatory bowel disease.
Not to be used for:
Not to be used with: antibiotics.
Contains:
Other preparations:

---

sodium polystyrene sulphonate *see* **Resonium-A**

---

sodium *see* **Metatone**

S

---

sodium sulphacetamide *see* **Cortucid, Sulphacetamide**

---

sodium sulphosuccinated undecylenic monoalkylolamide
see **Genisol, Synogist**

---

sodium thyroxine *see* **Eltroxin**

---

sodium valproate *see* **Epilim**

Sofradex
(Roussel)

Drops used as a antibiotic, corticosteroid treatment for inflammation of the outer ear.

Dose: 2-3 drops into the ear 3-4 times a day.
Availability: NHS and private prescription.
Side effects: additional infection.
Caution: in pregnant women and infants — do not use over extended periods.

Not to be used for: patients suffering from perforated ear drum.
Not to be used with:
Contains: FRAMYCETIN sulphate, DEXAMETHASONE, GRAMICIDIN.
Other preparations: SOFRADEX OINTMENT.

Sofradex Ointment
(Roussel)

An ointment used as a corticosteroid, aminoglycoside antibiotic treatment for eyelid inflammation, infected eczema.

Dose: apply to the eye 2-3 times a day and at night.
Availability: NHS and private prescription.
Side effects: rise in eye pressure, fungal infection, thinning cornea, cataract.
Caution: in pregnant women and infants — do not use for extended periods.
Not to be used for: patients suffering from glaucoma, viral, fungal, tubercular, or weeping infections.
Not to be used with:
Contains: DEXAMETHASONE, FRAMYCETIN sulphate, GRAMICIDIN.
Other preparations: SOFRADEX.

Soframycin
(Roussel)

A white, scored tablet supplied at a strength of 250 mg and used as an aminoglycoside antibiotic for the prevention of infections before and after stomach surgery, and to treat stomach infections.

Dose: adults prior to surgery 1 tablet 4 times a day for 2-3 days, infections 4-6 tablets a day; children infections $1/2$ -1 tablet a day.
Availability: NHS and private prescription.
Side effects: ear and kidney damage.
Caution: in patients suffering from myasthenia gravis (a muscle disorder), Parkinson's disease. Your doctor may advise that blood levels and dose should be carefully controlled especially if the patient is suffering from kidney disease.
Not to be used for: pregnant women.
Not to be used with: neuromuscular blockers, anaesthetics, ETH-ACRYNIC ACID, FRUSEMIDE.

Contains: FRAMYCETIN sulphate.
Other preparations: SOFRAMYCIN DROPS, SOFRAMYCIN OINTMENT.

Soframycin Cream
(Roussel)

A cream used as a aminoglycoside antibiotic treatment for infective dermatitis, boils, sycosis barbae (infected beard), impetigo, inflammation of the follicles, nail infections.

Dose: apply to the affected area up to 3 times a day if needed.
Availability: NHS and private prescription.
Side effects: ear damage, sensitization.
Caution: in patients with large areas of affected skin.
Not to be used for:
Not to be used with:
Contains: FRAMYCETIN sulphate.
Other preparations: SOFRAMYCIN OINTMENT.

Soframycin Drops
(Roussel)

Drops used as an aminoglycoside antibiotic treatment for conjunctivitis, styes, eyelid inflammation

Dose: 1-2 drops into the eye 3-4 times a day.
Availability: NHS and private prescription.
Side effects:
Caution:
Not to be used for:
Not to be used with:
Contains: FRAMYCETIN sulphate.
Other preparations: SOFRAMYCIN OINTMENT.

Solis *see* Valium
(Galen)

Soliwax
(Martindale)

A red capsule used as a wax softener to soften and remove hardened ear wax and to clean the canal.

Dose: insert the contents of 1 capsule into the ear, plug, and leave overnight then syringing if necessary.
Availability: NHS, private prescription,over the counter.
Side effects:
Caution:
Not to be used for: patients suffering from perforated ear drum.
Not to be used with:
Contains: SODIUM DOCUSATE.
Other preparations:

Solpadeine
(Sterling Research Laboratories)

A white, effervescent tablet used as an analgesic to relieve rheumatic, muscle, bone pain, headache, sinusitis, influenza.

Dose: adults 2 tablets in water 3-4 times a day; children 7-12 years $\frac{1}{2}$ -1 tablet 3-4 times a day.
Availability: private prescription and over the counter.
Side effects: constipation.
Caution: in patients with liver or kidney disease, or who have a restricted salt consumption.
Not to be used for: children under 7 years.
Not to be used with:
Contains: PARACETAMOL, CODEINE PHOSPHATE, CAFFEINE.
Other preparations:

Solprin
(Reckitt & Colman)

A white, soluble tablet supplied at a strength of 300 mg and used as an analgesic for the relief of pain, and to treat rheumatic conditions.

Dose: 1-3 tablets in water every 4 hours to a maximum of 12 tablets in 24 hours; higher doses for rheumatoid arthritis.
Availability: NHS (when prescribed as a generic), private prescrip-

tion, over the counter.
Side effects:
Caution:
Not to be used for: children.
Not to be used with:
Contains: ASPIRIN.
Other preparations: Solprin 75 mg.

Solvazinc
(Thames)

An off-white, effervescent tablet supplied at a strength of 200 mg and used as a zinc supplement to treat zinc deficiency.

Dose: adults and children over 30 kg body weight 1 tablet dissolved in water 1-3 times a day after food; children under 10 kg body weight $^1/_2$ tablet in water once a day after food, 10-30 kg half adult dose.
Availability: NHS, private prescription, over the counter.
Side effects: stomach upset.
Caution: in patients suffering from kidney failure.
Not to be used for:
Not to be used with: TETRACYCLINES.
Contains: ZINC SULPHATE.
Other preparations:

Sominex
(S K B)

A white, scored tablet supplied at a strength of 20 mg and used as an antihistamine treatment for occasional sleeplessness.

Dose: 1 tablet immediately before or up to 1 hour after going to bed.
Availability: NHS and private prescription.
Side effects: anti-cholinergic effects, brain and stomach upsets, allergies, blood disorders.
Caution: in patients suffering from glaucoma, enlarged prostate, epilepsy, liver disease. Patients should be warned of drowsiness and should not drive or carry out any functions requiring alertness.
Not to be used for: children under 16 years.
Not to be used with: alcohol, sedatives, ANTI-CHOLINERGICS.
Contains: PROMETHAZINE hydrochloride.

Somnite *see* Mogadon
(Norgine)

Soneryl
(M & B)

A pink, scored tablet supplied at a strength of 100 mg and used as a barbiturate to treat sleeplessness.

Dose: 1-2 tablets before going to bed.
Availability: NHS and private prescription.
Side effects: drowsiness, hangover, dizziness, allergies, headache, confusion, excitement.
Caution: patients suffering from kidney or lung disease. Dependence (addiction) may develop.
Not to be used for: children, young adults, pregnant women, nursing mothers, the elderly, patients with a history of drug or alcohol abuse, or suffering from porphyria (a rare blood disorder), or in the management of pain.
Not to be used with: anti-coagulants (blood-thinning drugs), alcohol, other tranquillizers, steroids, the contraceptive pill, GRISEOFULVIN, RIFAMPICIN, PHENYTOIN, METRONIDAZOLE, CHLORAMPHENICOL.
Contains: BUTOBARBITONE.
Other preparations:

Soni-Slo
(Lipha)

A pink, clear capsule or a red/clear capsule according to strengths of 20 mg, 40 mg, and containing off-white pellets used as a NITRATE for the prevention of angina.

Dose: 40-120 mg a day in 2-3 divided doses.
Availability: NHS and private prescription.
Side effects: flushes, headache, dizziness.
Caution:
Not to be used for: children.

Not to be used with:
Contains: ISOSORBIDE DINITRATE.
Other preparations:

---

sorbic acid *see* Micralax, Relaxit

Sorbichew
(Stuart)

A green, scored tablet supplied at a strength of 5 mg and used as a NITRATE to treat acute angina attacks.

Dose: 1-2 tablets chewed thoroughly.
Availability: NHS and private prescription.
Side effects: flushes, headache, dizziness.
Caution:
Not to be used for: children.
Not to be used with:
Contains: ISOSORBIDE DINITRATE.
Other preparations:

Sorbid SA
(Stuart)

A red/yellow capsule or a red/clear capsule according to strengths of 20 mg, 40 mg and used as a NITRATE for the prevention of angina.

Dose: 20-80 mg twice a day.
Availability: NHS and private prescription.
Side effects: flushes, headache, nausea.
Caution:
Not to be used for: children.
Not to be used with:
Contains: ISOSORBIDE DINITRATE.
Other preparations:

---

sorbitol *see* Glandosane, Relaxit

Sorbitrate
(Stuart)

A yellow, oval, scored tablet or a blue, oval scored tablet according to strengths of 10 mg, 20 mg and used as a NITRATE for the prevention of angina.

Dose: 10-40 mg 3-4 times a day.
Availability: NHS and private prescription.
Side effects: flushes, headache, dizziness.
Caution:
Not to be used for: children.
Not to be used with:
Contains: ISOSORBIDE DINITRATE.
Other preparations:

S

Sotacor
(Bristol-Meyers)

A pink tablet or a blue tablet according to strengths of 80 mg, 160 mg and used as a ß-BLOCKER to treat angina, abnormal heart rhythm, and for the prevention of heart attacks.

Dose: angina 160 mg a day in single or divided doses; for other uses higher doses.
Availability: NHS and private prescription.
Side effects: cold hands and feet, sleep disturbance, slow heart rate, tiredness, wheezing, heart failure, stomach upset.
Caution: in pregnant women, nursing mothers, and in patients suffering from diabetes, kidney or liver disorders, asthma. May need to be withdrawn before surgery. Withdraw gradually. Your doctor may advise additional treatment with diuretics or digitalis.
Not to be used for: children, or for patients suffering from heart block or failure.
Not to be used with: VERAPAMIL, CLONIDINE withdrawal, some anti-arrhythmic drugs and anaesthetics, RESERPINE, some anti-hypertensives, ergot alkaloids, CIMETIDINE, sedatives, SYMPATHOMIMETICS, INDOMETHACIN.
Contains: SOTALOL hydrochloride.
Other preparations: Sotacor Injection.

sotalol *see* Beta-Cardone, Sotacor, Sotazide, Tolerzide

Sotazide
(Bristol-Myers)

A blue, oblong, scored tablet used as a ß-BLOCKER to treat high blood pressure.

Dose: 1 tablet a day at first increasing to 2 tablets a day if needed.
Availability: NHS and private prescription.
Side effects: cold hands and feet, sleep disturbance, slow heart rate, tiredness, wheezing, heart failure, stomach upset.
Caution: in pregnant women, nursing mothers, and in patients suffering from diabetes, kidney or liver disorders, asthma. May need to be withdrawn before surgery. Withdraw gradually. Your doctor may advise additional treatment with DIURETICS or DIGITALIS.
Not to be used for: children or for patients suffering from heart block or failure.
Not to be used with: VERAPAMIL, CLONIDINE withdrawal, some anti-arrhythmic drugs and anaesthetics, reserpine, some anti-hyperten-sives, ergot alkaloids, CIMETIDINE, sedatives, SYMPATHOMIMETICS, IN-DOMETHACIN.
Contains: SOTALOL hydrochloride, HYDROCHLOROTHIAZIDE.
Other preparations:

---

soya oil *see* Balneum with Tar

Sparine
(Wyeth)

A suspension used as a sedative to treat agitation or restlessness in the elderly, additional short-term treatment for psychomotor agitation.

Dose: adults 2-4 5 ml spoonsful 4 times a day; elderly half adult dose or $^1/_2$ -1 5 ml spoonful for restlessness.
Availability: NHS and private prescription.
Side effects: muscle spasms, restlessness, hands shaking, dry mouth, urine retention, palpitations, low blood pressure, weight gain, changes in libido, low body temperature, breast swelling, menstrual

changes, jaundice, blood and skin changes, drowsiness, rarely fits.
Caution: in pregnant women, nursing mothers, and in patients suffering from liver disease, Parkinson's disease, or cardiovascular disease.
Not to be used for: children or for patients suffering from bone marrow depression or in an unconscious state
Not to be used with: alcohol, tranquillizers, pain killers, anti-hypertensives, anti-depressants, anti-convulsants, anti-diabetic drugs, LEVODOPA.
Contains: PROMAZINE embonate.
Other preparations: Sparine Injection.

Spasmonal
(Norgine)

A blue/grey capsule supplied at a strength of 60 mg and used as an anti-spasmodic treatment for irritable bowel syndrome.

Dose: adults 1-2 tablets 1-3 times a day.
Availability: NHS, private prescription, over the counter.
Side effects: blurred vision, confusion, dry mouth.
Caution:
Not to be used for: children, or for patients suffering from glaucoma, inflammatory bowel disease, intestinal obstruction, enlarged prostate.
Not to be used with:
Contains: ALVERINE CITRATE.
Other preparations:

Spiretic *see* Aldactone
(DDSA)

Spiroctan
(MCP)

A blue tablet or a green tablet according to strengths of 25 mg, 50 mg and used as a potassium-sparing DIURETIC to treat congestive heart failure, liver cirrhosis, fluid retention, kidney and adrenal gland disorders.

Dose: adults 50-200 mg a day to a maxium of 600 mg a day; children 1.5-3 mg per kg of bodyweight a day.
Availability: NHS and private prescription.
Side effects: heart enlargement, stomach upset, drowsiness, headache, confusion, rash.
Caution: in pregnant women , young patients, and in patients suffering from kidney or liver disease.
Not to be used for: nursing mothers and for patients suffering from severe or progressive kidney failure, raised potassium levels, Addison's disease.
Not to be used with: potassium supplements, potassium-sparing diuretics, CARBENOXOLONE, anti-hypertensives, ACE INHIBITORS.
Contains: SPIRONOLACTONE.
Other preparations: Spiroctan Capsules, Spiroctan-M

Spirolone *see* Aldactone
(Berk)

spironolactone *see* Aldactide 50, Aldactone, Diatensic, Lasilactone, Spiroctan

Sporanox
(Janssen)

A blue/pink capsule supplied at a strength of 100 mg and used as an anti-fungal treatment for skin or vaginal infections.

Dose: 1-2 tablets a day for 1-30 days.
Availability: NHS and private prescription.
Side effects: headache, indigestion, nausea, stomach pain.
Caution: in patients suffering from liver disease.
Not to be used for: pregnant women, nursing mothers.
Not to be used with: RIFAMPCIN, CYCLOSPORIN, H_2-ANTAGONISTS, antacids.
Contains: ITRACONAZOLE.
Other preparations:

squalane *see* **Salonair**

Stabillin V-K
(Boots)

A tablet supplied at a strength of 250 mg and used as a penicillin treatment for infections.

Dose: adults 2-6 tablets a day in divided doses; children under 1 year 62.5 mg every 6 hours, 1-5 years 125 mg every 6 hours, 6-12 years 250 mg every 6 hours.
Availability: NHS and private prescription.
Side effects: allergy, stomach upset.
Caution: in patients suffering from kidney disease.
Not to be used for:
Not to be used with:
Contains: PENICILLIN V-POTASSIUM.
Other preparations: Stabillin V-K Elixir.

Stafoxil
(Brocades)

A brown/cream capsule supplied at strengths of 250 mg, 500 mg and used as a penicillin treatment for infections.

Dose: adults 250 mg 4 times a day 1 hour before food; children over 2 years half adult dose.
Availability: NHS and private prescription.
Side effects: allergy, stomach upset.
Caution:
Not to be used for: children under 2 years.
Not to be used with:
Contains: FLUCLOXACILLIN sodium.
Other preparations:

---

stanozolol *see* **Stromba**

Staphlipen
(Lederle)

A brown capsule supplied at strengths of 250 mg, 500 mg and used as a penicillin treatment for infections.

Dose: adults 250 mg 4 times a day; children under 2 years quarter adult dose, over 2 years half adult dose.
Availability: NHS and private prescription.
Side effects: allergy, stomach upset.
Caution: in pregnant women and in patients suffering from kidney disease.
Not to be used for:
Not to be used with:
Contains: FLUCLOXACILLIN.
Other preparations: Staphlipen Injection.

---

starch *see* Arobon

Stelazine
(S K B)

A blue tablet supplied at strengths of 1 mg, 5 mg and used as a sedative to treat anxiety, depression, agitation, schizophrenia, mental disorders, severe agitation, dangerous impulsive behaviour, nausea, vomiting.

Dose: anxiety etc, adults 2-4 mg up to a maximum of 6 mg a day in divided doses; children 3-5 years up to 1 mg a day, 6-12 up to 4 mg a day.For schizophrenia etc, adults 5 mg twice a day increasing after 7 days to 15 mg; children up to 5 mg a day. For nausea and vomiting adults 2-6 mg a day; children 3-5 years up to 1 mg a day, 6-12 up to 4 mg a day.
Availability: NHS and private prescription.
Side effects: brain disturbances, dry mouth, blurred vision, ECG and hormone changes, allergies, impaired judgement and ability, rarely extrapyramidal symptoms (shaking and rigidity).
Caution: in the elderly, pregnant women, nursing mothers, and in patients suffering from undiagnosed vomiting, epilepsy, cardiovascular disease or Parkinson's disease. Your doctor may advise you to watch for loss of dexterity.

Not to be used for: patients in an unconscious state or patients suffering from depression, liver disease, bone marrow depression.
Not to be used with: sedatives, alcohol, analgesics, blood pressure-lowering drugs.
Contains: TRIFLUOPERAZINE hydrochloride.
Other preparations: Stelazine Syrup, Stelazine Spansule Stelazine Concentrate, Stelazine Injection.

Stemetil
(M & B)

A cream tablet or a cream, scored tablet according to strengths of 5 mg, 25 mg and used as a anti-sickness medication for minor mental and emotional problems, schizophrenia and other mental disorders, vertigo caused by Ménière's disease, severe nausea, vomiting.

Dose: 15-20 mg a day in divided doses up to a maximum of 40 mg a day for minor problems, 75-100 mg a day for schizophrenia.
Availability: NHS and private prescription.
Side effects: brain disturbances, anti-cholinergic effects, ECG and hormone changes, allergies, reduced judgement and abilities, rarely extrapyramidal effects.
Caution: in pregnant women, nursing mothers, and in patients suffering from cardiovascular disease, Parkinson's disease, undiagnosed or prolonged vomiting.
Not to be used for: patients in an unconscious state or patients suffering from bone marrow depression or liver disease.
Not to be used with: sedatives, alcohol, analgesics, blood pressure-lowering drugs, anti-depressants, anti-convulsants, anti-diabetics.
Contains: PROCHLORPERAZINE maleate.
Other preparations: Stemetil Syrup, Stemetil EFF, Stemetil Suppositories, Stemetil Injection.

Ster-Zac Bath Concentrate
(Hough, Hoseason)

A liquid used as an anti-bacterial treatment for skin infections.

Dose: add 28.5 ml to the bath water.
Availability: NHS, private prescription, over the counter.
Side effects:

Caution: keep out of the eyes.
Not to be used for:
Not to be used with:
Contains: TRICLOSAN.
Other preparations:

Ster-Zac DC
(Hough, Hoseason)

A cream used as a disinfectant for cleansing and disinfecting the hands before surgery.

Dose: use as a liquid soap.
Availability: NHS and private prescription.
Side effects:
Caution: in children under 2 years.
Not to be used for:
Not to be used with:
Contains: HEXACHLOROPHANE.
Other preparations:

Ster-Zac Powder
(Hough, Hoseason.)

A powder used as a disinfectant for the prevention of infections in new-born infants, and to treat recurring skin infections.

Dose: adults apply to the affected area once a day; infants dust the affected area at each change of nappy.
Availability: NHS, private prescription, over the counter.
Side effects:
Caution: in patients where the skin is broken.
Not to be used for:
Not to be used with:
Contains: HEXACHLOROPHANE.
Other preparations:

---

sterculia *see* Normacol

sterculia *see* **Prefil**

Stesolid *see* **Valium**
(CP Pharmaceuticals)

Stiedex
(Stiefel)

An oily cream used as a steroid treatment for skin disorders.

Dose: massage a small quantity into the affected area 2-3 times a day.
Availability: NHS and private prescription.
Side effects: fluid retention, suppression of adrenal glands, thinning of the skin may occur.
Caution: use for short periods of time only.
Not to be used for: patients suffering from acne or any other skin infections caused by tuberculosis, ringworm, viruses, or fungi, or continuously especially in pregnant women.
Not to be used with:
Contains: DESOXYMETHASONE.
Other preparations: Stiedex LP, Stiedex LPN.

Stiemycin
(Stiefel)

A solution used as an antibiotic treatment for acne.

Dose: wash and dry the affected area and apply twice a day.
Availability: NHS and private prescription.
Side effects: irritation, dryness.
Caution:
Not to be used for:
Not to be used with:
Contains: ERYTHROMYCIN.
Other preparations:

---

stilboesterol *see* **Tampovagan**

Stromba
(Sterling Research Laboratories)

A white, quarter-scored tablet supplied at a strength of 5 mg and used as an anabolic steroid to treat vascular disorders.

Dose: adults vascular complications 1 tablet twice a day, angio-oedema $^1/_2$-2 tablets a day at first reducing as appropriate.
Availability: NHS and private prescription.
Side effects: masculinization, liver poisoning, fluid retention, dyspepsia, cramp, headache.
Caution: in patients suffering from heart or kidney disease. Your doctor may advise blood tests for liver function.
Not to be used for: for pregnant women or for patients suffering from prostate cancer, liver disease, porphyria (a rare blood disorder).
Not to be used with: anti-coagulants taken by mouth.
Contains: STANOZOLOL.
Other preparations:

Stugeron
(Janssen)

A white, scored tablet supplied at a strength of 15 mg and used as an antihistamine treatment for vestibular disorders, travel sickness.

Dose: vestibular disorders adults, 2 tablets 3 times a day; travel sickness 1 tablet 2 hours before journey, then 1 every 8 hours during the journey. Children 5-12 years half adult dose.
Availability: NHS, private prescription, over the counter.
Side effects: drowsiness, reduced reactions, rarely skin eruptions.
Caution: in patients suffering from liver or kidney disease.
Not to be used for: children under 5 years.
Not to be used with: alcohol, sedatives, some anti-depressants (MAOIS).
Contains: CINNARIZINE.
Other preparations:

Stugeron Forte
(Janssen)

An orange/cream capsule supplied at a strength of 75 mg and used as an anti-histamine treatment for peripheral vascular disease including intermittent claudication and Raynaud's syndrome (a disease of the arteries of the hands).

Dose: 1 capsule 3 times a day.
Availability: NHS and private prescription.
Side effects: drowsiness, rash.
Caution: in patients suffering from high blood pressure.
Not to be used for: children.
Not to be used with: alcohol, sedatives.
Contains: CINNARIZINE.
Other preparations:

---

sucralfate *see* **Antepsin**

---

sucrose *see* **Rehidrat**

Sudafed
(Calmic)

A red tablet supplied at a strength of 60 mg and used as a SYMPATH-OMIMETIC treatment to relieve congestion of the nose, sinuses, and upper respiratory tract.

Dose: adults 1 tablet 3 times a day; children use elixir.
Availability: NHS, private prescription, over the counter.
Side effects: anxiety, tremor, rapid or abnormal heart rate, dry mouth, brain stimulation.
Caution: in patients suffering from diabetes.
Not to be used for: patients suffering from cardivascular disorders, overactive thyroid.
Not to be used with: MAOIS, TRICYCLICS.
Contains: PSEUDOEPHEDRINE.
Other preparations: Sudafed Elixir, Sudafed SA, Sudafed-Co, Sudafed Expectorant.

Sudafed Plus

(Calmic)

A white, scored tablet used as an antihistamine, SYMPATHOMIMETIC treatment for allergic rhinitis.

Dose: adults 1 tablet 3 times a day; children over 2 years use syrup.
Availability: NHS, private prescription, over the counter.
Side effects: drowsiness, rash, disturbed sleep, rarely hallucinations.
Caution: in patients suffering from raised eye pressure, enlarged prostate.
Not to be used for: infants under 2 years or for patients suffering from severe high blood pressure, coronary artery disease, overactive thyroid.
Not to be used with: MAOIS, SYMPATHOMIMETICS, FURAZOLIDONE, alcohol.
Contains: TRIPROLIDINE hydrochloride, PSEUDOEPHEDRINE hydrochloride.
Other preparations: Sudafed Plus Syrup.

---

sulconazole *see* Exelderm

Suleo-C
(International)

A lotion used as a pediculicide to treat head lice.

Dose: rub into the scalp as directed.
Availability: NHS, private prescription, over the counter.
Side effects:
Caution: keep out of the eyes.
Not to be used for:
Not to be used with:
Contains: CARBARYL.
Other preparations: Suleo-C Shampoo.

Suleo-M
(International)

A lotion used as a pediculicide to treat head lice.

Dose: rub into the scalp as directed.
Availability: NHS, private prescription, over the counter.

Side effects:
Caution: keep out of the eyes.
Not to be used for:
Not to be used with:
Contains: MALATHION.
Other preparations:

---

sulfadoxine *see* **Fansidar**

---

sulfametopyrazine *see* **Kelfizine W**

S

---

sulindac *see* **Clinoril**

---

sulphabenzamide *see* **Sultrin**

---

sulphacarbamide *see* **Uromide**

Sulphacetamide
(SNP)

Drops used as a sulphonamide treatment for eye infections.

Dose: 1 drop into the eye every 2 hours.
Availability: NHS and private prescription.
Side effects:
Caution:
Not to be used for:
Not to be used with:
Contains: SODIUM SULPHACETAMIDE.
Other preparations: OCUSOL (Boots).

---

sulphacetamide, sodium *see* **Albucid, Ocusol, Sultrin, Sulphacetamide**

---

sulphamethoxazole *see* **Septrin**

---

sulphasalazine *see* **Salazopyrin, Salazopyrin EN-tablets**

---

sulphathiazole *see* **Sultrin**

---

sulphinpyrazone *see* **Anturan**

---

sulphur *see* **Actinac, Dome-Acne, Eskamel, Medrone Lotion, Neo-Medrone Lotion, Pragmatar**

---

sulpiride *see* **Dolmatil, Sulpitil**

Sulpitil
(Tillotts)

A white, scored tablet supplied at a strength of 200 mg and used as a sedative to treat schizophrenia.

Dose: elderly $^1/_4$ -$^1/_2$ a tablet twice a day at first increasing to adult dose; adults over 14 years 1-2 tablets twice a day up to a maximum of 9 tablets a day.
Availability: NHS and private prescription.
Side effects: muscle spasms, restlessness, hands shaking, dry mouth, urine retention, palpitations, low blood pressure, weight gain, changes in libido, low body temperature, breast swelling, menstrual changes, jaundice, blood and skin changes, drowsiness, rarely fits.

Caution: in pregnant women and in patients suffering from hypertension, kidney disease, hypomania, or epilepsy
Not to be used for: children under 14 years or for patients suffering from phaeochromocytoma (a disease of the adrenal glands).
Not to be used with: alcohol, tranquillizers, pain killers, anti-hypertensives, anti-depressants, anti-convulsants, anti-diabetic drugs, LEVODOPA.
Contains: SULPIRIDE.
Other preparations:

Sultrin
(Cilag)

A white, lozenge-shaped vaginal tablet used as a sulphonamide antibacterial treatment for bacterial inflammation of the vagina or cervix, and for care after surgery.

Dose: 1 tablet into the vagina twice a day for 10 days.
Availability: NHS and private prescription.
Side effects: sensitivity
Caution:
Not to be used for: children or patients suffering from kidney disease.
Not to be used with:
Contains: SULPHATHIAZOLE, SULPHACETAMIDE, SULPHABENZAMIDE.
Other preparations: Sultrin Cream.

Suprefact
(Hoechst)

A nasal spray used as a hormone treatment for prostate cancer.

Dose: 1 spray into each nostril 6 times a day.
Availability: NHS and private prescription.
Side effects: hot flushes, loss of sex drive, temporary irritation of the nose.
Caution:
Not to be used for: tumours which are not sensitive to hormones, or following removal of a testicle.
Not to be used with:
Contains: BUSERELIN.
Other preparations: Suprefact Injection.

Surbex T
(Abbott)

An orange, oval tablet used as a multivitamin treatment for vitamin B and VITAMIN C deficiencies.

Dose: adults 1 or more tablets a day; children 6-12 years 1 tablet a day.
Availability: private prescription, over the counter.
Side effects:
Caution:
Not to be used for: children under 6 years.
Not to be used with: LEVODOPA.
Contains: THIAMINE, RIBOFLAVINE, NICOTINAMIDE, PYRIDOXINE, ASCORBIC ACID.
Other preparations:

Surem *see* Mogadon
(Galen)

Surgam SA
(Roussel)

A maroon/pink capsule supplied at a strength of 300 mg and used as a NON-STEROID ANTI-INFLAMMATORY DRUG rheumatoid arthritis, osteoarthritis, ankylosing spondylitis, lumbago, acute bone or muscular problems.

Dose: 2 capsules once a day.
Availability: NHS and private prescription.
Side effects: stomach upset, headache, drowsiness, rash.
Caution: in pregnant women, nursing mothers, and in patients suffering from severe kidney or liver disease, asthma, allergy to aspirin/non-steroid anti-inflammatory drugs.
Not to be used for: children or for patients suffering from peptic ulcer or a history of peptic ulcer.
Not to be used with: anti-coagulants, anti-diabetics, hydantoins, sulphonamides.
Contains: TIAPROFENIC ACID.
Other preparations: Surgam Tablets, Surgam Sachets.

Surmontil
(M & B)

A white tablet supplied at strengths of 10 mg, 25 mg and used as an anti-depressant to treat depression, anxiety, sleep disturbance, agitation.

Dose: 50-75 mg 2 hours before going to bed for at least 3 weeks.
Availability: NHS and private prescription.
Side effects: dry mouth, constipation, urine retention, blurred vision, palpitations, drowsiness, sleeplessness, dizziness, hands shaking, low blood presure, weight change, skin reactions, jaundice or blood changes. Loss of sexual desire may occur.
Caution: in nursing mothers or in patients suffering from heart disease, thyroid disease, epilepsy, diabetes, some other psychiatric conditions. Your doctor may advise regular blood tests.
Not to be used for: children, pregnant women, or for patients suffering from heart attacks, liver disease, heart block.
Not to be used with: alcohol, ANTI-CHOLINERGICS, ADRENALINE, MAOIS, barbiturates, other anti-depressants, anti-hypertensives.
Contains: TRIMIPRAMINE maleate.
Other preparations: Surmontil Capsules.

Suscard Buccal
(Pharmax)

A white tablet supplied at strengths of 1 mg, 2 mg, 3 mg, 5 mg and used as a NITRATE to treat angina, acute heart failure, congestive heart failure.

Dose: 5 mg 3 times a day at first or repeated until symptoms are relieved, allowing tablet to dissolve between upper lip and gum. For angina 1 mg as required or 1 mg 3 times a day increasing strength and frequency as needed.
Availability: NHS and private prescription.
Side effects: headache, flushes.
Caution:
Not to be used for: for children.
Not to be used with:
Contains: GLYCERYL TRINITRATE.
Other preparations:

Sustac
(Pharmax)

A pink, mottled tablet supplied at strengths of 2.6 mg, 6.4 mg, 10 mg and used as a NITRATE for the prevention of angina.

Dose: 2.6-12.8 mg 2-3 times a day.
Availability: NHS and private prescription.
Side effects: headache, flushes.
Caution:
Not to be used for: children.
Not to be used with:
Contains: GLYCERYL TRINITRATE.
Other preparations:

Sustamycin *see* Tetracycline
(MCP)

Symmetrel
(Geigy)

A brownish-red capsule supplied at a strength of 100 mg and used as an anti-parkinsonian/anti-viral drug to treat Parkinson's disease, virus infections.

Dose: for Parkinson's disease 1 tablet a day for 7 days then 1 tablet twice a day; virus infections twice the above dose.
Availability: NHS and private prescription.
Side effects: skin changes, fluid retention, rash, sight, brain and stomach disturbances.
Caution: in pregnant women, confused patients, and in patients suffering from liver disease or congestive heart failure.
Not to be used for: patients suffering from severe kidney disease or with a history of convulsions or gastric ulcers.
Not to be used with: ANTI-CHOLINERGIC DRUGS, LEVODOPA, sedatives.
Contains: AMANTADINE hydrochloride.
Other preparations: Symmetrel Syrup.

sympathomimetic

a drug which functions like ADRENALINE and causes narrowing of the blood vessels but which may open other organs, such as the bronchial tubes. Example EPHEDRINE *see* Phensedyl.

Synalar
(ICI)

An ointment used as a steroid treatment for skin disorders.

Dose: apply to the affected area 2-3 times a day.
Availability: NHS and private prescription.
Side effects: fluid retention, suppression of adrenal glands, thinning of the skin may occur.
Caution: use for short periods of time only.
Not to be used for: patients suffering from acne or any other skin infections caused by tuberculosis, ringworm, viruses, or fungi, or continuously especially in pregnant women.
Not to be used with:
Contains: FLUOCINOLONE ACETONIDE.
Other preparations: Synalar Cream, Synalar 1:4, Synalar Cream 1:10, Synalar C, Synalar N, Synalar Gel.

Syndol
(Merrell Dow)

A yellow, scored tablet used as an analgesic, antihistamine treatment for tension headache after dental or other surgery.

Dose: 1-2 tablets every 4-6 hours up to a maximum of 8 tablets in 24 hours.
Availability: over the counter and private prescription only.
Side effects: drowsiness, constipation.
Caution: in patients suffering from liver or kidney disease.
Not to be used for: children.
Not to be used with: alcohol, sedatives.
Contains: PARACETAMOL, CODEINE PHOSPHATE, DOXYLAMINE SUCCINATE, CAFFEINE.
Other preparations:

Synflex
(Syntex)

An orange tablet supplied at a strength of 275 mg and used as a NON-STEROID ANTI-INFLAMMATORY DRUG to treat period pain, migraine, pain after surgery, bone or muscle problems including sprains, strains, and lumbo-sacral pain.

Dose: 2 tablets immediately, then 1 tablet every 6-8 hours as needed to a maximum of 4 tablets a day after the first day; migraine 3 tablets immediately then 1-2 tablets as needed.
Availability: NHS and private prescription.
Side effects: rash, stomach intolerance, headache, tinnitus, vertigo, blood changes.
Caution: in pregnant women, nursing mothers, the elderly, and in patients with a history of gastro-intestinal lesions, or suffering from kidney or liver disease.
Not to be used for: patients under 16 years, or for patients suffering from peptic ulcer, ASPIRIN or anti-inflammatory induced allergy.
Not to be used with: anti-coagulants, hydantoins, sulphonylureas, LITHIUM, ß-BLOCKERS, METHOTREXATE, PROBENECID, FRUSEMIDE.
Contains: NAPROXEN sodium
Other preparations:

Synkavit
(Roche)

A white, scored tablet supplied at a strength of 10 mg and used as vitamin K to prevent bleeding.

Dose: adults 1-4 tablets a day, neonatal haemorrhage 1 tablet a day for 3-4 days before labour; children 1/2 -2 tablets a day.
Availability: NHS and private prescription.
Side effects: anaemia, jaundice.
Caution: in premature infants.
Not to be used for:
Not to be used with:
Contains: MENADIOL DIPHOSPHATE.
Other preparations:

Synogist
(Townendale)

A shampoo used as an anti-fungal, anti-bacterial treatment for seborrhoea of the scalp.

Dose: shampoo twice a week for 4 weeks, then once a week.
Availability: NHS, private prescription, over the counter.
Side effects:
Caution: keep out of the eyes.
Not to be used for:
Not to be used with:
Contains: SODIUM SULPHOSUCCINATED UNDECYLENIC MONOALKYLOLAMIDE.
Other preparations:

Synphase
(Syntex)

White tablets and yellow tablets used as an oestrogen, progestogen contraceptive.

Dose: 1 tablet a day for 21 days starting on day 5 of the period.
Availability: NHS and private prescription.
Side effects: enlarged breasts, bloating and fluid retention, cramps, leg pains, mood change, reduction in sexual desire, headaches, nausea, vaginal erosion, discharge, and bleeding, weight gain, skin changes.
Caution: in patients suffering from high blood pressure, diabetes, vascular disorders, asthma, depression, kidney disease, multiple sclerosis, womb diseases. Your doctor may advise you not to smoke, to have regular examinations. You should stop treatment at the first sign of serious symptoms such as severe headache or jaundice. Treatment should be stopped before surgery.
Not to be used for: pregnant women, or for patients suffering from sickle-cell anaemia, history of heart disease or thrombosis, liver disorders, some cancers, undiagnosed vaginal bleeding, some ear, skin, and kidney disorders.
Not to be used with: RIFAMPICIN, TETRACYCLINES, GRISEOFULVIN, barbiturates, PHENYTOIN, PRIMIDONE, CARBAMAZEPINE, ETHOSUXIMIDE, CHLORAL HYDRATE, DICHLORALPHENAZONE.
Contains: ETHINYLOESTRADIOL, NORETHISTERONE.
Other preparations:

Syntaris
(Syntex)

A spray supplied at a strength of 25 micrograms and used as a corticosteroid treatment for rhinitis, hay fever.

Dose: adults 2 sprays into each nostril 2-3 times a day at first reducing according to response; children over 5 years 1 spray into each nostril 3 times a day.
Availability: NHS and private prescription.
Side effects: temporary itching.
Caution: in pregnant women, and in patients suffering from ulcerated nose, trauma, or who have undergone nasal surgery, or who are being transferred from systemic steroids.
Not to be used for: children under 5 years or for patients suffering from untreated nose or eye infections.
Not to be used with:
Contains: FLUNISOLIDE.
Other preparations:

Syntopressin
(Sandoz)

A nasal spray used as a hormone treatment for diabetes insipidus (a condition causing excess thirst and urination).

Dose: adults 1-2 sprays into one or both nostrils 3-7 times a day; children as advised by the physician.
Availability: NHS and private prescription.
Side effects: nausea, stomach pain, desire to defaecate, blocked nose and ulceration.
Caution: in pregnant women and in patients suffering from asthma, epilepsy, or heart failure.
Not to be used for: patients suffering from vascular disease.
Not to be used with:
Contains: LYPRESSIN.
Other preparations:

Syraprim
(Wellcome)

A white, scored tablet supplied at strengths of 100 mg, 300 mg and used as an antibiotic treatment for respiratory and urinary infections.

Dose: adults respiratory infections 200 mg twice a day, urinary infections 300 mg once a day; children 6 months-6 years 50 mg twice a day, 6-12 years 100 mg twice a day.
Availability: NHS and private prescription.
Side effects: stomach disturbances, skin reactions, folate (vitamin) deficiency.
Caution: in patients suffering from kidney disease or folate (vitamin) deficiency. Your doctor may advise that patients on prolonged treatment should undergo regular blood tests.
Not to be used for: infants under 6 months, pregnant women, or for patients with severe kidney disease where the blood levels can not be regularly checked.
Not to be used with:
Contains: TRIMETHOPRIM.
Other preparations: Syraprim Injection.

Sytron
(Parke-Davis)

An elixir used as an iron supplement to treat iron-deficiency anaemia.

Dose: adults 1 5 ml teaspoonful 3 times a day at first increasing gradually to 2 teaspoonsful 3 times a day; children 0-1 year $\frac{1}{2}$ teaspoonful twice a day, 1-5 years $\frac{1}{2}$ teaspoonful 3 times a day, 6-12 years 1 teaspoonful 3 times a day.
Availability: NHS, private prescription, over the counter.
Side effects: nausea, diarrhoea.
Caution:
Not to be used for:
Not to be used with: TETRACYCLINES.
Contains: SODIUM IRON EDETATE.
Other preparations:

T Gel
(Neutrogena)

A shampoo used as an anti-psoriatic treatment for dandruff, seborrhoea, and psoriasis of the scalp.

Dose: shampoo 1-2 times a week.
Availability: NHS, private prescription, over the counter.
Side effects: irritation.
Caution:
Not to be used for: patients suffering from acute psoriasis.
Not to be used with:
Contains: COAL TAR EXTRACT.
Other preparations:

Tachyrol
(Duphar)

A white, scored tablet supplied at a strength of 0.2 mg and used as a source of vitamin D to treat rickets, osteomalacia, underactive para-thyroid gland, kidney osteodystrophy (bone problems due to kidney disease).

Dose: adults 1 a day at first adjusted as needed; children as advised by the physician.
Availability: NHS, private prescription, over the counter.
Side effects: raised blood or urine calcium levels.
Caution: in patients suffering from kidney disease. Blood calcium should be checked regularly.
Not to be used for:
Not to be used with: barbiturates, anti-convulsant drugs.
Contains: DIHYDROTACHYSTEROL.
Other preparations:

Tagamet
(S K B)

A green tablet supplied at strengths of 200 mg, 400 mg, 800 mg and used as an H_2 BLOCKER to treat duodenal and gastric ulcers, hiatus hernia, dyspepsia.

Dose: children over 1 year 25-30 mg per 1 kg body weight a day, adults 800 mg at night or 400 mg twice a day, maintenance 400 mg at night or 200 mg twice a day.
Availability: NHS and private prescription.
Side effects: diarrhoea, rash, tiredness, dizziness, liver changes,

breast swelling; rarely kidney, pancreas, bone marrow, joint, and muscle problems; headache.
Caution: in impaired kidney function. Ensure cancer has not been missed as a diagnosis. Monitor patients on long-term therapy.
Not to be used for:
Not to be used with: oral anticoagulants, PHENYTOIN, THEOPHYLLINE.
Contains: CIMETIDINE.
Other preparations: Tagamet syrup, injections, infusions. ALGITEC (S K B) in combination with alginic acid, DYSPAMET (Bridge).

---

talampicillin *see* Talpen

Talpen
(S K B)

A red tablet supplied at a strength of 250 mg and used as a penicillin treatment for infections.

Dose: adults 1 tablet 3 times a day; children under 2 years 3-7 mg per kg body weight 3 times a day, over 7 years ¹/₂ tablet 3 times a day.
Availability: NHS and private prescription.
Side effects: allergy, stomach disturbances.
Caution: in patients suffering from severe kidney or liver disease, or glandular fever.
Not to be used for:
Not to be used with:
Contains: TALAMPICILLIN hydrochloride.
Other preparations: Talpen Syrup.

Tambocor
(3M Riker)

A white, scored tablet supplied at a strength of 100 mg and used as an anti-arrhythmic treatment for abnormal heart rhythm.

Dose: 1 tablet twice a day at first for 3-5 days, then reduce the dose to the minimum necessary to keep symptoms under control.
Availability: NHS and private prescription.

Side effects: dizziness, disturbed vision..
Caution: in pregnant women and in patients suffering from kidney or liver problems, some heart muscle disorders. Your doctor may advise blood tests to check electrolytes and blood levels.
Not to be used for: children and for patients suffering from severe heart conduction block.
Not to be used with: DIGOXIN and some other heart drugs.
Contains: FLECAINIDE acetate.
Other preparations: Tambocor Injection.

Tamofen *see* Nolvadex-D
(Tillotts)

---

tamoxifen citrate *see* Nolvadex-D

Tampovagan
(Norgine)

A pessary used as an oestrogen treatment for atrophic or menopausal inflammation of the vagina.

Dose: 2 pessaries in the vagina at night.
Availability: NHS and private prescription.
Side effects: enlarged breasts, bloating and fluid retention, cramps, leg pains, mood change, reduction in sexual desire, headaches, nausea, vaginal erosion, discharge and bleeding, weight gain, skin changes.
Caution: in patients suffering from high blood pressure, diabetes, vascular disorders, asthma, depression, kidney disease, multiple sclerosis, womb diseases. Your doctor may advise you not to smoke, to have regular examinations. You should stop treatment at the first sign of serious symptoms such as severe headache or jaundice. Treatment should be stopped before surgery.
Not to be used for: children, pregnant women, or for patients suffering from sickle-cell anaemia, history of heart disease or thrombosis, liver disorders, some cancers, undiagnosed vaginal bleeding, some ear, skin, and kidney disorders.
Not to be used with: DIURETICS, anti-hypertensives, and drugs that

change liver enzymes.
Contains: STILBOESTEROL, LACTIC ACID.
Other preparations:

Tanderil
(Zyma)

An ointment used as a NON-STEROID ANTI-INFLAMMATORY DRUG to treat eye inflammation.

Dose: apply into the eye 2-5 times a day.
Availability: NHS and private prescription.
Side effects: swelling, redness, rarely blood changes
Caution: in patients suffering from glaucoma, weeping infections.
Not to be used for:
Not to be used with:
Contains: OXYPHENBUTAZONE.
Other preparations:

---

tannic acid *see* Phytex

---

tar *see* Gelcosal, Gelcotar, Polytar Liquid

Tarcortin
(Stafford-Miller)

A cream used as a steroid, anti-psoriatic treatment for eczema, psoriasis, other skin disorders.

Dose: apply to the affected area at least twice a day.
Availability: NHS and private prescription.
Side effects: fluid retention, suppression of adrenal glands, thinning of the skin may occur.
Caution: use for short periods of time only.
Not to be used for: patients suffering from acne or any other skin infections caused by tuberculosis, ringworm, viruses, or fungi, or con-

tinuously especially in pregnant women.
Not to be used with:
Contains: HYDROCORTISONE, COAL TAR EXTRACT.
Other preparations:

Tavegil
(Sandoz)

A white, scored tablet supplied at a strength of 1 mg and used as an antihistamine treatment for allergic rhinitis, dermatoses, urticaria, allergy to other drugs.

Dose: adults 1 tablet night and morning; children $1/2$ -1 tablet night and morning.
Availability: NHS, private prescription, over the counter.
Side effects: drowsiness, reduced reactions, rarely dizziness, dry mouth, palpitations, gastro-intestinal disturbances.
Caution:
Not to be used for:
Not to be used with: sedatives, MAOIS, alcohol.
Contains: CLEMASTINE.
Other preparations: Tavegil Elixir.

Tears Naturale
(Alcon)

Drops used to lubricate dry eyes.

Dose: 1-2 drops into the eye as needed.
Availability: NHS, private prescription, over the counter.
Side effects:
Caution:
Not to be used for: patients who wear soft contact lenses.
Not to be used with:
Contains: DEXTRAN, HYPROMELLOSE.
Other preparations:

Tedral *see* Theophylline
(Parke-Davis)

Teejel
(Napp Consumer)

A gel used as an antiseptic, analgesic treatment for mouth ulcers, stomatitis, gingivitis, glossitis, teething, uncomfortable dentures.

Dose: rub gently into the affected area every 3-4 hours.
Availability: NHS, private prescription, over the counter.
Side effects:
Caution:
Not to be used for: infants under 4 months.
Not to be used with:
Contains: CHOLINE SALICYLATE, CETALKONIUM CHLORIDE.
Other preparations:

Tegretol
(Geigy)

A white, scored tablet or a white, scored, oblong tablet according to strengths of 100 mg, 200 mg, 400 mg and used as an anti-convulsant, analgesic treatment for manic depression, epilepsy, neuralgia.

Dose: 400 mg a day in divided doses at first increasing gradually until symptoms are controlled and up to a maximum of 1.6 g a day. For epilepsy adults 100-200 mg 1-2 times a day at first increasing usually to 800 mg-1.2 g a day up to a maximum of 1.6 g; children up to 1 year 100-200 mg a day, 1-5 years 200-400 mg a day, 5-10 years 400-600 mg a day, 10-15 years 600 mg-1 g a day.
Availability: NHS and private prescription.
Side effects: stomach upset, double vision, dry mouth, drowsiness, dizziness, fluid retention, low blood sodium, blood changes, rash, acute kidney failure, jaundice.
Caution: in pregnant women and nursing mothers. Your doctor may advise that blood tests should be made regularly.
Not to be used for: nursing mothers or for patients suffering from heart conduction block.
Not to be used with: anti-coagulants taken by mouth, MAOIS, contraceptive pill, ERYTHROMYCIN, ISONIAZID, CIMETIDINE, DEXTROPROPOXYPHENE, DILTIAZEM, VERAPAMIL, VILOXAZINE, steroids, PHENYTOIN, LITHIUM.
Contains: CARBAMAZEPINE.
Other preparations: Tegretol Liquid.

---

temazepam *see also* Normison

A capsule supplied at strengths of 10 mg, 15 mg, 20 mg, 30 mg and used as a sleeping preparation to treat sleeplessness.

Dose: elderly 5-15 mg before going to bed; adults 10-30 mg before going to bed; in severe cases a maximum of 60 mg may be taken if needed.
Availability: NHS and private prescription.
Side effects: drowsiness, confusion, unsteadiness, low blood pressure, rash, changes in vision, changes in libido, retention of urine. Risk of addiction increases with dose and length of treatment. May impair judgement.
Caution: in the elderly, pregnant women, nursing mothers, in women during labour, and in patients suffering from lung disorders, kidney or liver disorders. Avoid long-term use and withdraw gradually.
Not to be used for: children, or for patients suffering from acute lung diseases, some chronic lung diseases, some obsessional and psychotic diseases.
Not to be used with: alcohol, anti-convulsants, other tranquillizers.
Contains:
Other preparations: Temazepam Elixir, Temazepam Planpak.

Temgesic
(Reckitt & Colman)

A white tablet supplied at a strength of 0.2 mg and used as a opiate to control pain.

Dose: 1-2 tablets under the tongue every 6-8 hours or as needed.
Availability: NHS and private prescription.
Side effects: drowsiness, nausea, sweating, dizziness.
Caution: in pregnant women, women in labour, and in patients suffering from breathing or liver problems, or patients addicted to or with a history of addiction to narcotics.
Not to be used for: children.
Not to be used with: MAOIS or sedatives.
Contains: BUPRENORPHINE hydrochloride.
Other preparations: Temgesic Injection.

Tenavoid
(Leo)

An orange, oval tablet used as a DIURETIC/sedative combination to treat premenstrual syndrome.

Dose: 1 tablet 3 times a day, starting 5-7 days before the beginning of the period.
Availability: NHS and private prescription.
Side effects: rash, sensitivity to light, blood changes, reduced powers of judgement and performance.
Caution: in patients suffering from diabetes, gout, weak liver. Potassium supplements may be needed.
Not to be used for: children or for patients suffereing from severe kidney weakness, acute intermittent porphyria (a rare blood disorder), alcoholism, history of epilepsy.
Not to be used with: LITHIUM, DIGITALIS, anti-hypertensives, alcohol, sedatives.
Contains: BENDROFLUAZIDE, MEPROBAMATE.
Other preparations:

T

Tenif
(Stuart)

A reddish-brown capsule used as a calcium blocker/ß-BLOCKER to treat high blood pressure, angina.

Dose: 1 capsule a day at first increasing to 2 capsules a day if needed; elderly a maximum oof 1 capsule a day.
Availability: NHS and private prescription.
Side effects: flushing, headache, dizziness, dry eyes, rash, fluid retention.
Caution: in patients suffereing from asthma or heart failure, kidney or liver disease, diabetes, or patients undergoing anaesthesia.
Not to be used for: children, pregnant women, nursing mothers, or for patients suffering from heart failure, block, or shock.
Not to be used with: CIMETIDINE, QUINIDINE, heart depressants.
Contains: ATENOLOL, NIFEDIPINE.
Other preparations: BETA-ADALAT (Bayer).

Tenoret 50
(Stuart)

A brown capsule used as a ß-BLOCKER/THIAZIDE DIURETIC to treat high blood pressure especially for the elderly.

Dose: 1 capsule a day.
Availability: NHS and private prescription.
Side effects: cold hands and feet, sleep disturbance, slow heart rate, tiredness, wheezing, heart failure, stomach upset.
Caution: in pregnant women, nursing mothers, and in patients suffering from diabetes, kidney or liver disorders, asthma. May need to be withdrawn before surgery. Withdraw gradually. Your doctor may advise additional treatment with diuretics or digitalis.
Not to be used for: children or patients suffering from heart block or failure.
Not to be used with: VERAPAMIL, CLONIDINE withdrawal, some anti-arrhythmic drugs and anaesthetics, RESERPINE, some anti-hypertensives, ergot alkaloids, CIMETIDINE, sedatives, SYMPATHOMIMETICS, INDOMETHACIN.
Contains: ATENOLOL, CHLORTHALIDONE.
Other preparations:

Tenoretic
(Stuart)

A brown tablet used as a ß-BLOCKER/THIAZIDE DIURETIC to treat high blood pressure.

Dose: 1 tablet a day.
Availability: NHS and private prescription.
Side effects: cold hands and feet, sleep disturbance, slow heart rate, tiredness, wheezing, heart failure, stomach upset.
Caution: in pregnant women, nursing mothers, and in patients suffering from diabetes, kidney or liver disorders, asthma. May need to be withdrawn before surgery. Withdraw gradually. Your doctor may advise additional treatment with diuretics or digitalis.
Not to be used for: children or for patients suffering from heart block or failure.
Not to be used with: VERAPAMIL, CLONIDINE withdrawal, some anti-arrhythmic drugs and anaesthetics, RESERPINE, some anti-hypertensives, ergot alkaloids, CIMETIDINE, sedatives, SYMPATHOMIMETICS, INDOMETHACIN.

Contains: ATENOLOL, CHLORTHALIDONE.
Other preparations:

Tenormin
(Stuart)

An orange capsule supplied at a strength of 100 mg and used as a ß-BLOCKER to treat angina, abnormal heart rhythm, high blood pressure.

Dose: 50-100 mg a day.
Availability: NHS and private prescription.
Side effects: cold hands and feet, sleep disturbance, slow heart rate, tiredness, wheezing, heart failure, stomach upset.
Caution: in pregnant women, nursing mothers, and in patients suffering from diabetes, kidney or liver disorders, asthma. May need to be withdrawn before surgery. Withdraw gradually. Your doctor may advise additional treatment with diuretics or digitalis.
Not to be used for: children or for patients suffering from heart block or failure.
Not to be used with: VERAPAMIL, CLONIDINE withdrawal, some anti-arrhythmic drugs and anaesthetics, RESERPINE, some anti-hyperten-sives, ergot alkaloids, CIMETIDINE, sedatives, SYMPATHOMIMETICS, IN-DOMETHACIN.
Contains: ATENOLOL.
Other preparations: Tenormin Injection, Tenormin Syrup, Tenormin LS. ANTIPRESSAN (Berk).

---

tenoxicam *see* **Mobiflex**

Tensium *see* **Valium**
(DDSA)

Tenuate Dospan
(Merrell Dow)

A white, oblong, scored tablet supplied at a strength of 75 mg and used as an appetite suppressant to treat obesity.

Dose: 1 tablet a day in the middle of the morning.
Availability: controlled drug.
Side effects: tolerance, addiction, mental disturbances, sleepless-ness, nervousness, agitation.
Caution: in patients suffering from high blood pressure, angina, abnormal heart rhythm, peptic ulcer, or women in the first three months of pregnancy. Do not use for prolonged periods.
Not to be used for: children, or for patients suffering from hardening of the arteries, overactive thyroid, severe high blood pressure, glau-coma, or with a history of alcoholism or drug addiction.
Not to be used with: MAOIS, SYMPATHOMIMETICS, METHYLDOPA, GUANETHID-INE, sedatives, other obesity drugs.
Contains: DIETHYLPROPION HYDROCHLORIDE.
Other preparations:

Teoptic
(Dispersa)

Drops used as a ß-BLOCKER to treat hypertension of the eye, open angle glaucoma, some secondary glaucomas.

Dose: 1 drop into the eye twice a day.
Availability: NHS and private prescription.
Side effects: burning, stinging, and painful sensations of the eye, blurred vision, redness, corneal inflammation.
Caution: in patients suffering from heart conduction block, heart failure, diabetes.
Not to be used for: children, pregnant women, or for patients suffering from heart failure, asthma, chronic obstructive lung disease, or for those who wear soft contact lenses.
Not to be used with: systemic ß-blockers.
Contains: CARTEOLOL HYDROCHLORIDE.
Other preparations:

terazosin *see* **Hytrin**

terbutaline *see* Bricanyl, Bricanyl Expectorant, Monovent

Tercoda
(Sinclair)

A syrup used as an opiate, expectorant, antussive, sputum softener to treat bronchitis.

Dose: 1-2 5 ml teaspoonsful 3 times a day.
Availability: private prescription and over the counter.
Side effects: constipation.
Caution: in patients suffering from asthma.
Not to be used for: children , or for patients suffering from liver disease.
Not to be used with: MAOIS.
Contains: CODEINE PHOSPHATE, TERPIN HYDRATE, CINEOLE, MENTHOL, PEP-PERMINT OIL, PUMILIO PINE OIL.
Other preparations:

terfenadine *see* Triludan

terodiline hydrochloride *see* Micturin

Terolin *see* Micturin
(KabiVitrum)

Teronac
(Sandoz)

A white, scored tablet supplied at a strength of 2 mg and used as an appetite suppressant to treat obesity.

Dose: 1 tablet a day after breakfast.
Availability: controlled drug.

Side effects: tolerance, addiction, mental disturbances, constipation, dry mouth, sweating, sleeplessness, urgent need to urinate and defaecate, impotence. Do not use for prolonged periods.
Caution: care in patients suffering from coronary heart disease, severe agitation, enlarged prostate.
Not to be used for: children, the elderly, pregnant women, nursing mothers, or for patients suffering from peptic ulcer, glaucoma, severe kidney, liver or heart disease, abnormal heart rhythms, severe high blood pressure, or with a history of mental illness alcoholism, or drug addiction.
Not to be used with: MAOIS, GUANETHIDINE, DEBRISOQUINE, thyroid drugs, SYMPATHOMIMETICS, psychostimulants, anti-diabetic drugs, alcohol.
Contains: MAZINDOL.
Other preparations:

---

terpin hydrate *see* **Copholco, Copholcoids, Tercoda**

Terpoin
(Hough, Hoseason)

An elixir used as an opiate treatment for dry cough.

Dose: 1 5 ml teaspoonful every 3 hours.
Availability: private prescription and over the counter.
Side effects: constipation.
Caution: in patients suffering from asthma.
Not to be used for: children under 5 years, or for patients suffering from liver disease.
Not to be used with: MAOIS.
Contains: CODEINE PHOSPHATE, CINEOLE, MENTHOL.
Other preparations:

Terra-Cortril
(Pfizer)

Drops used as an antibiotic, corticosteroid treatment for infections of the outer ear.

Dose: 2-4 drops into the ear 3 times a day.

Availability: NHS and private prescription.
Side effects: additional infection, rarely allergy.
Caution:
Not to be used for: children, pregnant women, or for patients suffering from perforated ear drum, or viral, fungal, tubercular, or acute weeping infections.
Not to be used with:
Contains: OXYTETRACYCLINE hydrochloride, HYDROCORTISONE acetate, POLYMYXIN B SULPHATE.
Other preparations:

Terra-Cortril Spray
(Pfizer)

A spray used as an antibiotic, steroid treatment for weeping and infected eczema, insect bites, weeping intertrigo.

Dose: apply to the affected area 2-4 times a day.
Availability: NHS and private prescription.
Side effects: fluid retention, suppression of adrenal glands, thinning of the skin may occur.
Caution: use for short periods of time only.
Not to be used for: children or for patients suffering from acne or any other skin infections caused by tuberculosis, ringworm, viruses, or fungi, or continuously especially in pregnant women.
Not to be used with:
Contains: OXYTETRACYCLINE hydrochloride.
Other preparations: Terra-Cortril Ointment, Terra-Cortril Nystatin.

Terramycin *see* Tetracycline
(Pfizer)

Tertroxin
(Glaxo)

A white, scored tablet supplied at a strength of 20 micrograms and used as a thyroid hormone to treat severe thyroid deficiency, to test for thyrotoxicosis.

Dose: adults10-20 micrograms a day at first, increasing every 7 days to 80-100 micrograms a day in 2-3 divided doses; children 5 micrograms a day at first.
Availability: NHS and private prescription.
Side effects: abnormal heart rhythm, chest pain,rapid heart rate, muscle cramp, headache, restlessness, flushing, excitability, sweating, diarrhoea, rapid weight loss.
Caution: in nursing mothers.
Not to be used for: patients suffering from cardiovascular problems or where effort causes anginal pain.
Not to be used with: anti-coagulants, TRICYCLICS, PHENYTOIN, CHOLES-TYRAMINE.
Contains: LYOTHYRONINE sodium.
Other preparations:

---

testosterone *see* Restandol

Tetmosol
(ICI)

A solution used as a scabicide to treat scabies.

Dose: dilute and apply to the body as directed.
Availability: NHS, private prescription, over the counter.
Side effects:
Caution: keep out of the eyes.
Not to be used for:
Not to be used with: alcohol.
Contains: MONOSULFIRAM.
Other preparations: Tetmosol Soap.

---

tetrabenazine *see* Nitoman

Tetrabid *see* Tetracycline
(Organon)

Tetrachel *see* **Tetracycline**
(Berk)

Tetracycline
(Lederle)

An orange capsule supplied at a strength of 250 mg and used as an antibiotic treatment for infections.

Dose: 1-2 tablets 4 times a day.
Availability: NHS and private prescription.
Side effects: stomach disturbances, allergy, additional infections.
Caution: in patients suffering from liver or kidney disease.
Not to be used for: children, nursing mothers, or women during the latter half of pregnancy.
Not to be used with: milk, antacids, mineral supplements, the contraceptive pill.
Contains: TETRACYCLINE HYDROCHLORIDE.
Other preparations: Tetracycline Tablets, Tetracycline Syrup, Tetracycline Injection, Tetracycline V. ACHROMYCIN (Lederle), BERKMYCEN (Berk), CHYMOCYCLAR (Rorer), DETECLO (Lederle), IMPERACIN (ICI), MINOCIN (Lederle), MYSTECLIN (Squibb), OXYMYCIN (DDSA), OXYTETRACYCLINE, TOPICYCLINE (Norwich Eaton).

---

tetracycline hydrochloride *see* **Achromycin, Tetracycline, Topicycline**

Tetralysal *see* **Tetracycline**
(Farmitalia CE)

Tetrex *see* **Tetracycline**
(Bristol-Myers)

---

thenyldiamine *see* **Hayphryn**

Theo-Dur *see* Theophylline
(Astra)

Theodrox
(3M Riker)

A white tablet used as a broncho-dilator to treat bronchial spasm brought on by asthma, chronic bronchitis.

Dose: 1 tablet 4 times a day including 1 tablet at night.
Availability: NHS, private prescription, over the counter.
Side effects: rapid heart rate, nausea, stomach upset, headache, sleeplessness, abnormal heart rhythms.
Caution: in pregnant women, nursing mothers, and in patients suffering from heart or liver disease, peptic ulcer.
Not to be used for: children.
Not to be used with: CIMETIDINE, ERYTHROMYCIN, CIPROFLOXACIN, INTERFERON.
Contains: AMINOPHYLLINE, ALUMINIUM HYDROXIDE GEL.
Other preparations:

Theophylline
(Pharmax)

A white, elongated, scored tablet supplied at a strength of 300 mg and used as a broncho-dilator to treat brochial spasm brought on by asthma, bronchitis, emphysema.

Dose: 1 tablet every 12 hours increasing by $\frac{1}{2}$ tablet if needed.
Availability: NHS and private prescription.
Side effects: rapid heart rate, nausea, stomach upset, headache, abnormal heart rhythms.
Caution: in pregnant women, nursing mothers, and in patients suffering from heart or liver disease, or peptic ulcer.
Not to be used for: children.
Not to be used with: CIMETIDINE, ERYTHROMYCIN, CIPROFLOXACIN, INTERFERON.
Contains: THEOPHYLLINE.
Other preparations: NUELIN SA (3M Riker), PRO-VENT (Wellcome), SABIDAL SR (Zyma), SLO-PHYLLIN (Lipha), TEDRAL (Parke-Davis), THEO-DUR (Astra), UNIPHYLLIN-CONTINUS (Napp).

theophylline *see* **Biophylline, Franol, Theophylline**

Thephorin
(Sinclair)

A white tablet supplied at a strength of 25 mg and used as an antihistamine to treat allergies.

Dose: 1-2 tablets 3 times a day before 4.00 in the afternoon.
Availability: NHS, private prescription, over the counter.
Side effects: dry mouth, stomach upset, rarely drowsiness.
Caution:
Not to be used for: children.
Not to be used with: sedatives, MAOIS, anti-cholinergics, alcohol.
Contains: PHENINDAMINE tartrate.
Other preparations:

Theraderm
(Westwood)

A gel used as an anti-bacterial, skin softener to treat acne.

Dose: wash and dry the affected area, then apply 1-2 times a day.
Availability: NHS, private prescription, over the counter.
Side effects: irritation, peeling.
Caution: keep out of the eyes, nose, mouth.
Not to be used for:
Not to be used with:
Contains: BENZOYL PEROXIDE.
Other preparations:

---

thiabendazole *see* **Mintezol**

---

thiamine *see* **Abidec, Allbee with C, Apisate, BC 500, BC 500 with Iron, Becosym, Benerva, Calcimax, Concavit, Fefol-Vit Spansule, Fesovit Spansule, Fesovit Z Spansule,**

Galfervit, Ketovite, Labiton, Lipflavonoid, Lipotriad, Metatone, Multivite, Octovit, Orovite, Orovite 7, Polyvite, Pregnavite Forte F, Surbex T, Tonivitan, Tonivitan B, Verdiviton, Villescon

---

thiethylperazine maleate *see* Torecan

---

thioridazine *see* Melleril

---

thurfyl salicylate *see* Transvasin,

Thymoxamine
(SNP)

Drops used as an alpha-blocker for pupil constriction.

Dose: 1 drop into the eye as needed.
Availability: NHS and private prescription.
Side effects: temporary irritation, redness, lid dropping.
Caution:
Not to be used for:
Not to be used with:
Contains: THYMOXAMINE hydrochloride.
Other preparations:

---

thymoxamine hydrochloride *see* Opilon, Thymoxamine

---

tiaprofenic acid *see* Surgam SA

Tiempe *see* **Monotrim**
(DDSA)

Tigason
(Roche)

A buff-coloured or a buff/orange capsule according to strengths of 10 mg, 25 mg and used as a vitamin A derivative to treat psoriasis, palmoplantar pustulosis, ichthyosis, Darier's disease (skin disorders).

Dose: 0.75 mg per kg body weight a day in divided doses at first up to a maximum of 75 mg a day according to response.
Availability: NHS (for hospital use only).
Side effects: dryness, erosion of mucous membranes, alopecia, liver poisoning, change in serum lipids, nausea, headache, sweating, anorexia.
Caution: children should only undergo short-term treatment. Women of child-bearing age should take contraceptive precautions for at least 2 years after treatment ceases.
Not to be used for: pregnant women or for patients suffering from liver or kidney disease.
Not to be used with: VITAMIN A, METHOTREXATE.
Contains: ETRETINATE.
Other preparations:

Tilade
(Fisons)

An aerosol supplied at a strength of 2 mg and used as a bronchial anti-inflammatory drug to treat blocked airway, bronchial asthma, asthmatic bronchitis, asthma.

Dose: 2 sprays twice a day up to a maximum of 2 sprays 4 times a day if needed.
Availability: NHS and private prescription.
Side effects: headache, nausea.
Caution: in pregnant women.
Not to be used for: children.
Not to be used with:
Contains: SODIUM NEDOCROMIL.
Other preparations:

Tildiem
(Lorex)

An off-white tablet supplied at a strength of 60 mg and used as a calcium antagonist to treat angina.

Dose: 60 mg 3 times a day increasing as need to up to 480 mg day in divided doses; elderly 60 mg twice a day at first.
Availability: NHS and private prescription.
Side effects: nausea, headache, rash, slow heart rate, ankle swelling, heart conduction block.
Caution: your doctor may advise that the heart rate be measured regularly especially in the elderly and in patients suffering from kidney or liver problems.
Not to be used for: children, pregnant women or for patients suffering from slow heart rate or heart block.
Not to be used with: ß-BLOCKERS, DIGITALIS.
Contains: DILTIAZEM hydrochloride.
Other preparations:

Timodine
(Lloyds)

A cream used as a steroid, disinfectant, anti-fungal treatment for skin disorders, nappy rash with thrush.

Dose: apply a small quantity to the affected area 3 times a day or when the nappy is changed.
Availability: NHS and private prescription.
Side effects: fluid retention, suppression of adrenal glands, thinning of the skin may occur.
Caution: use for short periods of time only.
Not to be used for: patients suffering from acne or any other skin infections caused by tuberculosis, ringworm, viruses, or fungi, or continuously especially in pregnant women.
Not to be used with:
Contains: NYSTATIN, HYDROCORTISONE, BENZALKONIUM CHLORIDE, DIMETHICONE.
Other preparations:

---

timolol *see* **Blocadren, Prestim, Timoptol**

Timoped
(Reckitt & Colman)

A cream used as an anti-fungal treatment for athlete's foot and similar skin infections.

Dose: rub gently into the affected area twice a day and allow to dry.
Availability: NHS, private prescription, over the counter.
Side effects:
Caution:
Not to be used for:
Not to be used with:
Contains: TOLNAFTATE, TRICLOSAN.
Other preparations:

Timoptol
(MSD)

Drops used as a ß-BLOCKER to treat hypertension of the eye, glaucomas.

Dose: 1 drop into the eye twice a day.
Availability: NHS and private prescription.
Side effects: eye irritation, systemic ß-blocker effects.
Caution: in pregnant women, nursing mothers. Treatment should be withdrawn gradually.
Not to be used for: children or patients suffering from asthma, heart conduction block, heart failure.
Not to be used with: VERAPAMIL, anti-hypertensives, ADRENALINE.
Contains: TIMOLOL maleate.
Other preparations:

Tinaderm-M
(Kirby-Warrick)

A cream used as an anti-fungal treatment for skin and nail infections
.

Dose: apply to the affected area 2-3 times a day.
Availability: NHS
Side effects:
Caution:
Not to be used for:
Not to be used with:
Contains: TOLNAFTATE, NYSTATIN.
Other preparations:

Tineafax
(Wellcome)

An ointment used as an anti-fungal treatment for athlete's foot and similar skin infections.

Dose: apply to the affected area twice a day at first then once a day.
Availability: NHS, private prescription, over the counter.
Side effects:
Caution:
Not to be used for:
Not to be used with:
Contains: ZINC UNDECENOATE, ZINC NAPHTHENATE.
Other preparations: Tineafax Powder.

---

tinidazole *see* Fasigyn

Tinset
(Janssen)

A white, scored tablet supplied at a strength of 30 mg and used as an antihistamine treatment for allergies including rhinitis, urticaria.

Dose: adults 1-2 tablets twice a day; children over 5 years half adult dose.
Availability: NHS and private prescription.
Side effects: drowsiness, reduced reactions.
Caution:
Not to be used for: children under 5 years.

Not to be used with: sedatives, MAOIS, alcohol.
Contains: OXATOMIDE.
Other preparations:

---

tioconazole *see* **Trosyl**

Tisept
(Seton-Prebbles)

A solution in a sachet used as a disinfectant for cleansing and disinfecting wounds and burns, changing dressings, obstetrics.

Dose: use neat as needed.
Availability: NHS, private prescription, over the counter.
Side effects:
Caution:
Not to be used for:
Not to be used with:
Contains: CHLORHEXIDINE GLUCONATE, CETRIMIDE.
Other preparations:

Titralac
(3M Riker)

A white tablet used as a calcium supplement.

Dose: to be adjusted for individuals.
Availability: NHS, private prescription, over the counter.
Side effects:
Caution:
Not to be used for:
Not to be used with: TETRACYCLINES.
Contains: CALCIUM CARBONATE, GLYCINE.
Other preparations:

Tobralex
(Alcon)

Drops used as an aminoglycoside, antibiotic treatment for eye infections.

Dose: 1-2 drops every 4 hours or up to 2 drops every hour in severe infections.
Availability: NHS and private prescription.
Side effects: temporary irritation.
Caution:
Not to be used for:
Not to be used with:
Contains: TOBRAMYCIN.
Other preparations:

---

tobramycin *see* Tobralex

---

tocainide *see* Tonocard

---

tocopheryl *see* Ephynal, Ketovite, Octovit

Tofranil
(Geigy)

A red-brown, triangular tablet or red-brown, round tablet according to strengths of 10 mg, 25 mg and used as an anti-depressant to treat depression, night-time bed wetting in children

Dose: adults 25 mg 3 times a day for 3 days, then increasing to 50 mg 3-4 times a day; elderly 10 mg at night at first increasing to 10-25 mg 3 times a day; children 6-7 years 25 mg, 8-11 years 50-75 mg before going to bed for 6-8 weeks then withdraw gradually.
Availability: NHS and private prescription.
Side effects: dry mouth, constipation, urine retention, blurred vision, palpitations, drowsiness, sleeplessness, dizziness, hands shaking,

low blood presure, weight change, skin reactions, jaundice or blood changes. Loss of sexual desire may occur.
Caution: in nursing mothers or in patients suffering from heart disease, thyroid disease, epilepsy, diabetes, some other psychiatric conditions. Your doctor may advise regular blood tests.
Not to be used for: children under 6 years, pregnant women, or for patients suffering from heart attacks, liver disease, heart block.
Not to be used with: alcohol, ANTI-CHOLINERGICS, ADRENALINE, MAOIS, barbiturates, other anti-depressants, anti-hypertensives.
Contains: IMIPRAMINE hydrochloride.
Other preparations: Tofranil Syrup.

Tolanase
(Upjohn)

A white, scored tablet supplied at strengths of 100 mg, 250 mg and used as an anti-diabetic treatment for diabetes

Dose: 100-250 mg a day in divided doses to a maximum of 1 g a day.
Availability: NHS and private prescription.
Side effects: allergy including skin rash.
Caution: in the elderly and in patients suffering from kidney failure.
Not to be used for: children, pregnant women, nursing mothers, during surgery, or for patients suffering from juvenile diabetes, liver or kidney disorders, stress, infections.
Not to be used with: ß-BLOCKERS, MAOIS, steroids, DIURETICS, alcohol, anti-coagulants, lipid-lowering agents, ASPIRIN, some antibiotics (RIFAMPICIN, sulphonamides, CHLORAMPHENICOL), GLUCAGON, CYCLOPHOSPHAMIDE.
Contains: TOLAZAMIDE.
Other preparations:

---

tolazamide *see* Tolanase

---

tolbutamide *see* Rastinon

Tolectin
(Cilag)

An ivory/blue capsule supplied at a strength of 400 mg and used as a NON-STEROID ANTI-INFLAMMATORY DRUG to treat rheumatoid arthritis, osteoarthritis, ankylosing spondylitis, other joint dsorders.

Dose: 1 capsule 3 times a day at first, then 2-4 capsules a day.
Availability: NHS and private prescription.
Side effects: stomach pain, fluid retention, rash.
Caution: in pregnant women, nursing mothers, and in patients suffering from kidney disease or a history of gastro-intestinal disease.
Not to be used for: children or patients suffering from peptic ulcer or allergy to ASPIRIN/non-steroid anti-inflammatory drugs.
Not to be used with:
Contains: TOLMETIN.
Other preparations:

Tolerzide
(Bristol-Myers)

A lilac tablet used as a ß-BLOCKER/THIAZIDE DIURETIC to treat high blood pressure.

Dose: 1 tablet a day.
Availability: NHS and private prescription.
Side effects: cold hands and feet, sleep disturbance, slow heart rate, tiredness, wheezing, heart failure, stomach upset.
Caution: in pregnant women, nursing mothers, and in patients suffering from diabetes, kidney or liver disorders, asthma. May need to be withdrawn before surgery. Withdraw gradually. Your doctor may advise additional treatment with diuretics or digitalis.
Not to be used for: children, patients suffering from heart block or failure.
Not to be used with: VERAPAMIL, CLONIDINE withdrawal, some anti-arrhythmic drugs and anaesthetics, RESERPINE, some anti-hypertensives, ergot alkaloids, CIMETIDINE, sedatives, SYMPATHOMIMETICS, INDOMETHACIN.
Contains: SOTALOL hydrochloride, HYDROCHLOROTHIAZIDE.
Other preparations:

tolmetin *see* **Tolectin**

---

tolnaftate *see* **Timoped, Tinaderm-M**

Tonivitan
(Medo)

A brown capsule used as a multivitamin treatment for vitamin deficiency.

Dose: 1-3 capsules 3 times a day.
Availability: private prescription and over the counter.
Side effects:
Caution:
Not to be used for:
Not to be used with:
Contains: VITAMIN A, THIAMINE, NICOTINIC ACID, ASCORBIC ACID, CALCIFEROL, DRIED YEAST.
Other preparations:

Tonivitan A & D
(Medo)

A syrup used as a vitamin A and D, and minerals tonic.

Dose: adults and children over 10 years 2 5 ml teaspoonsful 3 times a day; infants under 1 year $^1/_2$ teasspoonful 3 times a day, 1-10 years 1 teaspoonful 3 times a day.
Availability: private prescription and over the counter.
Side effects:
Caution:
Not to be used for:
Not to be used with:
Contains: VITAMIN A, CALCIFEROL, FERRIC AMMONIUM CITRATE, CALCIUM GLYCEROPHOSPHATE, MANGANESE GLYCEROPHOSPHATE, COPPER SULPHATE.
Other preparations:

Tonivitan B
(Medo)

A syrup used as a vitamin B and minerals tonic.

Dose: adults 1-2 5 ml teaspoonsful 3 times a day; children as advised by the physician.
Availability: over the counter and private prescription.
Side effects:
Caution:
Not to be used for:
Not to be used with: levodopa.
Contains: THIAMINE hydrochloride, RIBOFLAVINE, PYRIDOXINE hydrochloride, NICOTINAMIDE, CALCIUM GLYCEROPHOSPHATE, MANGANESE GLYCEROPHOSPHATE.
Other preparations:

Tonocard
(Astra)

A yellow tablet supplied at strengths of 400 mg, 600 mg and used as an anti-arrhythmic drug to treat abnormal heart rhythms.

Dose: 1.2 g a day in 2-3 divided doses.
Availability: NHS and private prescription.
Side effects: tremor, dizziness, stomach upset, white cell changes, SLE (a multisystem disorder).
Caution: in the elderly and pregnant women, and in patients suffering from severe liver or kidney disease or uncompensated heart failure.
Not to be used for: children or patients suffering from heart conduction block.
Not to be used with: other anti-arrhythmics.
Contains: TOCAINIDE hydrochloride.
Other preparations: Tonocard Injection.

Topal
(ICI)

A cream tablet used as an antacid to treat oesophagitis, heartburn, gastritis.

Dose: adults 1-3 tablets 3-4 times a day between meals and at

bedtime, children half adult dose.
Availability: NHS, private prescription, over the counter.
Side effects: occasionally constipation.
Caution:
Not to be used for: infants.
Not to be used with: TETRACYCLINE antibiotics.
Contains: ALUMINIUM HYDROXIDE, MAGNESIUM CARBONATE, ALGINIC ACID.
Other preparations:

Topiclens
(S & N)

A solution in a sachet used to wash out the eyes, wounds, or burns.

Dose: use as needed.
Availability: NHS, private prescription, over the counter.
Side effects:
Caution: throw away any remaining solution.
Not to be used for:
Not to be used with:
Contains: SODIUM CHLORIDE.
Other preparations:

Topicycline
(Norwich Eaton)

A solution used as an antibiotic treatment for acne.

Dose: apply freely to the affected area twice a day.
Availability: NHS and private prescription.
Side effects: stinging or burning sensations.
Caution: in pregnant women, nursing mothers, and in patients suffering from kidney disease. Keep out of the eyes, nose, mouth, etc.
Not to be used for: children.
Not to be used with:
Contains: TETRACYCLINE hydrochloride.
Other preparations:

Topilar
(Syntex)

A cream used as a steroid treatment for skin disorders, psoriasis.

Dose: apply to the affected area twice a day.
Availability: NHS and private prescription.
Side effects: fluid retention, suppression of adrenal glands, thinning of the skin may occur.
Caution: use for short periods of time only.
Not to be used for: patients suffering from acne or any other skin infections caused by tuberculosis, ringworm, viruses, or fungi, or continuously especially in pregnant women.
Not to be used with:
Contains: FLUCLOROLONE acetonide.
Other preparations: Topilar Ointment.

Torbetol
(Torbet Laboratories)

A lotion used as an anti-bacterial treatment for acne.

Dose: apply to the affected area 3 times a day.
Availability: NHS, private prescription, over the counter.
Side effects:
Caution:
Not to be used for:
Not to be used with:
Contains: CETRIMIDE, BENZALKONIUM CHLORIDE, HEXACHLOROPHANE.
Other preparations:

Torecan
(Sandoz)

A white tablet supplied at a strength of 6.33 mg and used as an anti-emetic treatment for nausea, vomiting, vertigo.

Dose: 1 tablet 2-3 times a day.
Availability: NHS and private prescription.
Side effects: brain disturbances, anticholinergic symptoms, heart changes, allergies, rarely extrapyramidal symptoms (shaking and

rigidity).
Caution: in pregnant women and in patients suffering from liver disease, cardiovascular disease, bone marrow depression.
Not to be used for: severely depressed or unconscious patients.
Not to be used with: sedatives, alcohol, analgesics, anti-hypertensives, anti-depressants, anti-convulsants, anti-diabetics.
Contains: THIETHYLPERAZINE MALEATE.
Other preparations: Torecan Suppositories, Torecan Injection,

---

tramazoline *see* **Dexa-Rhinaspray**

Trancopal
(Winthrop)

A yellow tablet supplied at a strength of 200 mg and used as a tranquillizer in the short-term treatment of sleeplessness.

Dose: elderly 1 tablet at night; adults 2 tablets at night.
Availability: NHS and private prescription.
Side effects: nausea, dry mouth, headache, dizziness, lethargy, rash, jaundice
Caution: in pregnant women and in patients suffering from kidney or liver disease. Patients should be warned of reduced judgement and abilities.
Not to be used for: children.
Not to be used with: MAOIS, alcohol, sedatives.
Contains: CHLORMEZANONE.
Other preparations:

Trancoprin
(Winthrop)

A white, scored tablet used as an analgesic, muscle relaxant to treat muscle spasm, headache, period pain.

Dose: adults 1-2 tablets 3 times a day to a maximum of 8 tablets a day; elderly half normal adult dose.
Availability: private prescription only.

Side effects: drowsiness, constipation, flushes, dry mouth.
Caution: pregnant women and in patients suffering from kidney or liver disease or allergy to anti-inflammatory drugs.
Not to be used for: children or for patients suffering from peptic ulcer or haemophilia.
Not to be used with: anti-coagulants, anti-diabetics, hydantoins, sedatives, uric acid lowering drugs.
Contains: ASPIRIN, CHLORMEZANONE.
Other preparations:

Trandate
(Duncan, Flockhart)

An orange tablet supplied at strengths of 50 mg, 100 mg, 200 mg, 400 mg and used as an alpha- and ß-BLOCKER to treat angina with high blood pressure, high blood pressure of pregnancy.

Dose: 100-200 mg twice a day with food at first increasing as needed every 14 days to a maximum of 2.4 g a day in 3-4 divided doses; elderly 50 mg twice a day at first.
Availability: NHS and private prescription.
Side effects: cold hands and feet, sleep disturbance, slow heart rate, tiredness, wheezing, heart failure, stomach upset.
Caution: in pregnant women, nursing mothers, and in patients suffering from diabetes, kidney or liver disorders, asthma. May need to be withdrawn before surgery. Withdraw gradually. Your doctor may advise additional treatment with diuretics or digitalis.
Not to be used for: children or for patients suffering from heart block or failure.
Not to be used with: VERAPAMIL, CLONIDINE withdrawal, some anti-arrhythmic drugs and anaesthetics, RESERPINE, some anti-hypertensives, ergot alkaloids, CIMETIDINE, sedatives, SYMPATHOMIMETICS, INDOMETHACIN.
Contains: LABETALOL hydrochloride.
Other preparations: Trandate Injection, LABROCOL (Lagap).

---

tranexamic acid *see* Cyclokapron

Transiderm-Nitro
(Ciba)

Patches supplied at strengths of 5 mg, 10 mg and used as a NITRATE for the prevention of angina.

Dose: apply a patch to a hairless part of the chest every 24 hours on a differnt pleace each time.
Availability: NHS and private prescription.
Side effects: headache, rash, dizziness.
Caution: the treatement should be reduced gradually and replaced with decreasing doses of an oral nitrate.
Not to be used for: children
Not to be used with:
Contains: GLYCERYL TRINITRATE.
Other preparations:

Transvasin
(Lloyds)

A cream used as an analgesic rub for the relief of rheumatic and muscular pain.

Dose: massage into the affected area at least twice a day.
Availability: NHS, private prescription , over the counter.
Side effects:
Caution:
Not to be used for:
Not to be used with:
Contains: THURFYL SALICYLATE, ETHYL NICOTINATE, N-HEXYL NICOTINATE, BENZOCAINE.
Other preparations:

Tranxene
(Boehringer Ingelheim)

A pink/grey capsule or a maroon/ grey capsule according to strengths of 15 mg, 7.5 mg and used as a sedative to treat anxiety and depression.

Dose: elderly 7.5 mg a day; adults over 16 years 7.5-22.5 mg a day.

Availability: private prescription only.

Side effects: drowsiness, confusion, unsteadiness, low blood pressure, rash, changes in vision, changes in libido, retention of urine. Risk of addiction increases with dose and length of treatment. May impair judgement.

Caution: in the elderly, pregnant women, nursing mothers, in women during labour, and in patients suffering from lung disorders, kidney or liver disorders. Avoid long-term use and withdraw gradually.

Not to be used for: children under 16 years, or for patients suffering from acute lung diseases, some chronic lung diseases, some obsessional and psychotic diseases.

Not to be used with: alcohol, other tranquillizers, anti-convulsants.

Contains: CLORAZEPATE potassium.

Other preparations:

---

tranylcypromine sulphate *see* Parnate, Parstelin

Trasicor
(Ciba)

A white tablet, a beige tablet, or an orange tablet according to strengths of 20 mg, 40 mg, 80 mg, 160 mg and used as a ß-BLOCKER to treat angina, abnormal heart rhythm, high blood pressure.

Dose: adults 20-40 mg 2-3 times a day at first; children 1 mg per kg of bodyweight a day. For angina 40-160 mg 3 times a day to a maximum of 480 mg a day. For high blood pressure 80 mg twice a day at first increasing to 480 mg a day.

Availability: NHS and private prescription.

Side effects: cold hands and feet, sleep disturbance, slow heart rate, tiredness, wheezing, heart failure, stomach upset.

Caution: in pregnant women, nursing mothers, and in patients suffering from diabetes, kidney or liver disorders, asthma. May need to be withdrawn before surgery. Withdraw gradually. Your doctor may advise additional treatment with diuretics or digitalis.

Not to be used for: patients suffering from heart block or failure.

Not to be used with: VERAPAMIL, CLONIDINE withdrawal, some anti-arrhythmic drugs and anaesthetics, RESERPINE, some anti-hyperten

sives, ergot alkaloids, CIMETIDINE, sedatives, SYMPATHOMIMETICS, IN-
DOMETHACIN.
Contains: OXPRENOLOL hydrochloride.
Other preparations:

Trasidrex
(Ciba)

A red, coated tablet used as a ß-BLOCKER/thiazide to treat high blood
pressure.

Dose: 1 tablet every morning at first, increasing to 2 or more tablets
a day if needed.
Availability: NHS and private prescription.
Side effects: cold hands and feet, sleep disturbance, slow heart rate,
tiredness, wheezing, heart failure, stomach upset.
Caution: in pregnant women, nursing mothers, and in patients
suffering from diabetes, kidney or liver disorders, asthma. May need
to be withdrawn before surgery. Withdraw gradually. Your doctor may
advise additional treatment with diuretics or digitalis.
Not to be used for: children, or for patients suffering from heart block
or failure.
Not to be used with: VERAPAMIL, CLONIDINE withdrawal, some anti-
arrhythmic drugs and anaesthetics, RESERPINE, some anti-hypertensives, ergot alkaloids, CIMETIDINE, sedatives, SYMPATHOMIMETICS, IN-
DOMETHACIN.
Contains: OXPRENOLOL hydrochloride, PENTHIAZIDE.
Other preparations:

Travasept 100
(Baxter)

A solution used as an aminoglycocide antibiotic, anti-bacterial preparation for disinfecting wounds and burns.

Dose: use neat as needed.
Availability: NHS, private prescription, over the counter.
Side effects:
Caution:
Not to be used for:
Not to be used with:

Contains: CHLORHEXIDINE ACETATE, CETRIMIDE.
Other preparations:

Travogyn
(Schering)

A white, almond-shaped vaginal tablet supplied at a strength of 300 mg and used as an anti-fungal treatment for thrush or other infections of the vagina.

Dose: 2 tablets inserted together into the vagina as a single dose.
Availability: NHS and private prescription.
Side effects: irritation and burning.
Caution:
Not to be used for: children.
Not to be used with:
Contains: ISOCONAZOLE nitrate.
Other preparations: Travogyn Cream.

Traxam
(Lederle)

A clear gel used as a topical non-steroid anti-inflamatory rub to treat soft tissue injury such as strains, sprains, contusions.

Dose: massage gently into the affected area 2-4 times a day for up to 14 days up to a maximum of 25 g a day.
Availability: NHS and private prescription.
Side effects: mild local redness, dermatitis, itch.
Caution: in pregnant women, nursing mothers, and in patients suffering from asthma. Use only on unbroken skin and keep out of the eyes, nose, mouth etc. It should not be used with covering dressings.
Not to be used for: children or for patients suffering from allergy to ASPIRIN/anti-inflammatory drugs.
Not to be used with:
Contains: FELBINAC.
Other preparations:

---

trazodone *see* **Molipaxin**

Tremonil
(Sandoz)

A white, scored tablet supplied at a strength of 5 mg and used as an ANTI-CHOLINERGIC treatment for Parkinson's disease and senile tremor.

Dose: adults ¹/₂ tablet 3 times a day at first increasing gradually to 3-12 tablets a day in divided doses; elderly usually 3-6 tablets a day.
Availability: NHS and private prescription.
Side effects: anti-cholinergic effects, confusion at high doses.
Caution: in patients with marked disease of the autonomic nervous system. Dose should be reduced slowly.
Not to be used for: children or for patients suffering from enlarged prostate, glaucoma, abnormal heart rhythm, intestinal slowness, tardive dyskinesia (a movement disorder), myasthenia gravis (a muscle disorder).
Not to be used with: phenothiazines, antihistamines, anti-depressants, analgesics, alcohol.
Contains: METHIXENE hydrochloride.
Other preparations:

Trental
(Hoechst)

A pink, oblong tablet supplied at a strength of 400 mg and used as a blood cell altering drug to treat peripheral vascular problems.

Dose: 1 tablet 2-3 times a day.
Availability: NHS and private prescription.
Side effects: stomach disturbances, vertigo, flushes.
Caution: in patients suffering from low blood pressure, severe heart artery disease, kidney disease.
Not to be used for: children.
Not to be used with: anti-hypertensives.
Contains: OXPENTIFYLLINE.
Other preparations:

tretinoin *see* Retin-A

Tri-Adcortyl
(Squibb)

A cream used as an anti-fungal, anti-bacterial, steroid treatment for skin disorders where there is also inflammation, infection, or thrush.

Dose: apply to the affected area 2-4 times a day.
Availability: NHS and private prescription.
Side effects: fluid retention, suppression of adrenal glands, thinning of the skin may occur.
Caution: use for short periods of time only
Not to be used for: patients suffering from acne or any other skin infections caused by tuberculosis, ringworm, viruses, or fungi, or continuously especially in pregnant women.
Not to be used with:
Contains: TRIAMCINOLONE acetonide, NYSTATIN, NEOMYCIN, GRAMICIDIN.
Other preparations: Tri-Adcortyl Ointment.

Tri-Adcortyl Otic
(Squibb)

An ointment with an aural applicator used as an antibiotic, anti-fungal, corticosteroid treatment for inflammation of the external ear.

Dose: apply the ointment into the ear 2-4 times a day.
Availability: NHS and private prescription.
Side effects: additional infection.
Caution: in infants, pregnant women, and in patients suffering from perforated ear drum — avoid using over extended periods.
Not to be used for: patients suffering from tubercular or viral wounds.
Not to be used with:
Contains: TRIAMCINOLONE acetonide, NEOMYCIN sulphate, GRAMICIDIN, NYSTATIN.
Other preparations:

Tri-Cicatrin
(Calmic)

An ointment used as a steroid, anti-bacterial, anti-fungal treatment for skin disorders where there is also inflammation, infection, or thrush.

Dose: apply a small quantity to the affected area 1-3 times a day.
Availability: NHS and private prescription.
Side effects: fluid retention, suppression of adrenal glands, thinning of the skin may occur.
Caution: use for short periods of time only.
Not to be used for: patients suffering from acne or any other skin infections caused by tuberculosis, ringworm, viruses, or fungi, or continuously especially in pregnant women.
Not to be used with:
Contains: HYDROCORTISONE, NEOMYCIN, ZINC BACITRACIN, NYSTATIN.
Other preparations:

---

tri-potassium dicitrato bismuthate *see* De-Nol

---

triamcinolone acetonide *see* Adcortyl, Adcortyl in Orabase, Audicort, Aurecort, Ledercort, Ledercort Cream, Nystadermal, Tri-Adcortyl, Tri-Adcortyl Otic,

---

Triamco *see* Dyazide
(Norton)

---

triamterene *see* Dyazide, Dytac, Dytide, Frusene, Kalspare

---

triazolam *see also* Halcion

A tablet supplied at strengths of 0.125 mg, 1.25 mg and used as a sleeping tablet to treat sleeplessness.

Dose: elderly 0.125 mg before going to bed; adults 0.125-0.25 mg before going to bed.
Availability: NHS and private prescription.
Side effects: drowsiness, confusion, unsteadiness, low blood pressure, rash, changes in vision, changes in libido, retention of urine.

Risk of addiction increases with dose and length of treatment. May impair judgement.

Caution: in the elderly, pregnant women, nursing mothers, in women during labour, and in patients suffering from lung disorders, kidney or liver disorders. Avoid long-term use and withdraw gradually.

Not to be used for: children, or for patients suffering from acute lung diseases, some chronic lung diseases, some obsessional and psychotic diseases.

Not to be used with: alcohol, other tranquillizers, anti-convulsants.

Contains:

Other preparations:

Tribiotic
(3M Riker)

An aerosol used as an aminoglycoside antibiotic, anti-bacterial preparation to prevent and treat infection in surgery.

Dose: adequate.
Availability: NHS and private prescription.
Side effects: ear and kidney damage, sensitization.
Caution: in patients with large areas of affected skin.
Not to be used for: treating burns.
Not to be used with:
Contains: NEOMYCIN sulphate, BACITRACIN zinc, POLYMYXIN B SULPHATE.
Other preparations:

---

triclosan *see* **Aquasept, Manusept, Ster-Zac Bath Concentrate, Timoped, Triclosept**

Triclosept
(Hough, Hoseason)

A cream used as a disinfectant for disinfecting the hands and skin.

Dose: rub vigorously into the affected area until the cream has been absorbed.
Availability: NHS, private prescription, over the counter.

Side effects:
Caution:
Not to be used for:
Not to be used with:
Contains: TRICLOSAN.
Other preparations:

tricyclic anti-depressant

a drug used to treat depression but which may cause sedation and dryness of the mouth. Example AMITRYPTILINE *see* Tryptizol.

Tridesilon
(Lagap)

A cream used as a steroid treatment for skin disorders, psoriasis, eczema.

Dose: massage gently into the affected area 2-3 times a day.
Availability: NHS and private prescription.
Side effects: fluid retention, suppression of adrenal glands, thinning of the skin may occur.
Caution: use for short periods of time only.
Not to be used for: patients suffering from acne or any other skin infections caused by tuberculosis, ringworm, viruses, or fungi, or continuously especially in pregnant women.
Not to be used with:
Contains: DESONIDE.
Other preparations:

trifluoperazine *see* Parstelin, Stelazine

trifluperidol *see* Triperidol

Trilisate
(Napp)

An orange, oblong, scored tablet supplied at a strength of 500 mg and used as a salicylate to treat rheumatoid arthritis, osteoarthritis.

Dose: 2-3 tablets twice a day.
Availability: NHS and private prescription.
Side effects: stomach upsets, allergy, asthma.
Caution: in pregnant women, the elderly, or in patients with a history of allergy to aspirin, asthma, impaired kidney or liver function, indigestion.
Not to be used for: children, nursing mothers, or patients suffering from haemophilia, or ulcers.
Not to be used with: anti-coagulants (blood-thinning drugs), some anti-diabetic drugs, anti-inflammatory agents, METHOTREXATE, SPIRONOLACTONE, steroids, some antacids, some uric acid-lowering drugs.
Contains: CHOLINE MAGNESIUM TRISALICYLATE.
Other preparations:

---

trilostane *see* Modrenal

Triludan
(Merrell Dow)

A white, scored tablet supplied at a strength of 60 mg and used as an antihistamine treatment for allergies including hay fever and rhinitis.

Dose: adults 1 tablet twice a day or 2 tablets once a day; children 6-12 years ½ tablet twice a day.
Availability: NHS, private prescription, over the counter.
Side effects: rash, sweating, headache, mild stomach disturbances.
Caution:
Not to be used for: children under 6 years.
Not to be used with:
Contains: TERFENADINE.
Other preparations: Triludan Forte, Triludan Suspension.

---

trimeprazine *see* Vallergan

trimethoprim *see* Monotrim, Polytrim, Septrin, Syraprim, Trimopan

---

trimipramine maleate *see* Surmontil

Trimogal *see* Monotrim
(Lagap)

Trimopan
(Berk)

A white, scored tablet supplied at strengths of 100 mg, 200 mg and used as an antibiotic treatment for infections.

Dose: adults 200 mg twice a day; children use suspension.
Availability: NHS and private prescription.
Side effects: stomach disturbances, skin reactions, folate (vitamin) deficiency.
Caution: in the elderly, nursing mothers, and in patients suffering from kidney disease or folate deficiency. Your doctor may advise that patients undergoing prolonged treatment should have regular blood tests.
Not to be used for: infants under 4 months, pregnant women, or for patients suffering from severe kidney disease where blood tests cannot be carried out regularly.
Not to be used with: FOLATE INHIBITORS, anti-coagulants, anti-convulsants, anti-diabetics.
Contains: TRIMETHOPRIM.
Other preparations: Trimopan Suspension.

Trimovate
(Glaxo)

A cream used as an antibiotic, anti-fungal, steroid treatment in skin disorders in moist or covered places where there is also thrush or infection.

Dose: apply to the affected area 1-4 times a day.
Availability: NHS and private prescription.
Side effects: fluid retention, suppression of adrenal glands, thinning of the skin may occur.
Caution: use for short periods of time only.
Not to be used for: patients suffering from acne or any other skin infections caused by tuberculosis, ringworm, viruses, or fungi, or continuously especially in pregnant women.
Not to be used with:
Contains: CLOBETASONE BUTYRATE, NYSTATIN, CALCIUM OXYTETRACYCLINE.
Other preparations: Trimovate Ointment.

Trinordiol
(Wyeth)

Brown, white, and ochre tablets used as an oestrogen, progestogen contraceptive.

Dose: 1 tablet a day for 21 days starting on day 1 of the period.
Availability: NHS and private prescription.
Side effects: enlarged breasts, bloating and fluid retention, cramps, leg pains, mood change, reduction in sexual desire, headaches, nausea, vaginal erosion, discharge, and bleeding, weight gain, skin changes.
Caution: in patients suffering from high blood pressure, diabetes, vascular disorders, asthma, depression, kidney disease, multiple sclerosis, womb diseases. Your doctor may advise you not to smoke, to have regular examinations. You should stop treatment at the first sign of serious symptoms such as severe headache or jaundice. Treatment should be stopped before surgery.
Not to be used for: pregnant women, or for patients suffering from sickle-cell anaemia, history of heart disease or thrombosis, liver disorders, some cancers, undiagnosed vaginal bleeding, some ear, skin, and kidney disorders.
Not to be used with: RIFAMPICIN, TETRACYCLINES, GRISEOFULVIN, barbiturates, PHENYTOIN, PRIMIDONE, CARBAMAZEPINE, ETHOSUXIMIDE, CHLORAL HYDRATE, DICHLORALPHENAZONE.
Contains: ETHINYLOESTRADIOL, LEVONORGESTREL.
Other preparations:

Trinovum
(Cilag)

White tablets, pale peach tablets, and peach-coloured tablets used as an oestrogen, progestogen contraceptive.

Dose: 1 tablet a day for 21 days starting on day 1 of the period.
Availability: NHS and private prescription.
Side effects: enlarged breasts, bloating and fluid retention, cramps, leg pains, mood change, reduction in sexual desire, headaches, nausea, vaginal erosion, discharge, and bleeding, weight gain, skin changes.
Caution: in patients suffering from high blood pressure, diabetes, vascular disorders, asthma, depression, kidney disease, multiple sclerosis, womb diseases. Your doctor may advise you not to smoke, to have regular examinations. You should stop treatment at the first sign of serious symptoms such as severe headache or jaundice. Treatment should be stopped before surgery.
Not to be used for: pregnant women, or for patients suffering from sickle-cell anaemia, history of heart disease or thrombosis, liver disorders, some cancers, undiagnosed vaginal bleeding, some ear, skin, and kidney disorders.
Not to be used with: RIFAMPICIN, TETRACYCLINES, GRISEOFULVIN, barbiturates, PHENYTOIN, PRIMIDONE, CARBAMAZEPINE, ETHOSUXIMIDE, CHLORAL HYDRATE, DICHLORALPHENAZONE.
Contains: ETHINYLOESTRADIOL, LEVONORGESTREL.
Other preparations:

Triperidol
(Lagap)

A tablet supplied at strengths of 0.5 mg, 1 mg and used as a sedative to treat manic agitation.

Dose: up to 10 mg a day.
Availability: NHS and private prescription.
Side effects: muscle spasms, restlessness, hands shaking, dry mouth, urine retention, palpitations, low blood pressure, weight gain, changes in libido, low body temperature, breast swelling, menstrual changes, jaundice, blood and skin changes, drowsiness, rarely fits.
Caution: in pregnant women, nursing mothers and in patients suffering from severe liver disease, pyramidal or extrapyramidal

symptoms (tremor and rigidity).
Not to be used for: patients suffering from severe clinical depression.
Not to be used with: alcohol, tranquillizers, pain killers, anti-hypertensives, anti-depressants, anti-convulsants, anti-diabetic drugs, LEVODOPA.
Contains: TRIFLUPERIDOL.
Other preparations:

---

triprolidine hydrochloride *see* **Actidil, Actifed Compound, Pro-Actidil, Sudafed Plus**

Triptafen
(A & H)

A pink tablet used as an anti-depressant to treat depression with anxiety.

Dose: 1 tablet 3 times a day with 1 tablet at bed time if needed.
Availability: NHS and private prescription.
Side effects: dry mouth, constipation, urine retention, blurred vision, palpitations, drowsiness, sleeplessness, dizziness, hands shaking, low blood presure, weight change, skin reactions, jaundice or blood changes. Loss of sexual desire may occur.
Caution: in nursing mothers and in patients suffering from Parkinson's disease.
Not to be used for: children or for patients suffering from bone marrow depression.
Not to be used with: alcohol, ANTI-CHOLINERGICS, ADRENALINE, MAOIS, barbiturates, other anti-depressants, anti-hypertensives.
Contains: AMITRYPTILINE hydrochloride, PERPHENAZINE.
Other preparations: Triptafen-M.

Trisequens
(Novo-Nordisk)

Twelve blue tablets, 10 white tablets, and 6 red tablets used as a oestrogen, progestogen treatment for menopausal symptoms.

Dose: 1 tablet a day starting on the fifth day of the period if present, beginning with the blue tablets and continuing in sequence without a break.
Availability: NHS and private prescription.
Side effects: enlarged breasts, bloating and fluid retention, cramps, leg pains, mood change, reduction in sexual desire, headaches, nausea, vaginal erosion, discharge, and bleeding, weight gain, skin changes.
Caution: in patients suffering from high blood pressure, diabetes, vascular disorders, asthma, depression, kidney disease, multiple sclerosis, womb diseases. Your doctor may advise you not to smoke, to have regular examinations. You should stop treatment at the first sign of serious symptoms such as severe headache or jaundice. Treatment should be stopped before surgery.
Not to be used for: children, pregnant women, or for patients suffering from sickle-cell anaemia, history of heart disease or thrombosis, liver disorders, some cancers, undiagnosed vaginal bleeding, some ear, skin, and kidney disorders.
Not to be used with: DIURETICS, anti-hypertensives, and drugs that change liver enzymes, RIFAMPICIN, TETRACYCLINES, GRISEOFULVIN, barbiturates, phenytoin, PRIMIDONE, CARBAMAZEPINE, ETHOSUXIMIDE, CHLORAL HYDRATE, DICHLORALPHENAZONE.
Contains: OESTRADIOL, OESTRIOL, NORETHISTERONE acetate.
Other preparations:

T

Tropicamide
(SNP)

Drops used as an ANTI-CHOLINERGIC, short-acting pupil dilator.

Dose: 2 drops with 5 minutes between each drop, then 1-2 drops 30 minutes later if needed.
Availability: NHS and private prescription.
Side effects: temporary smarting.
Caution: care in infants.
Not to be used for: for patients suffering from narrow angle glaucoma.
Not to be used with:
Contains: TROPICAMIDE.
Other preparations:

---

tropicamide *see* **Mydriacyl, Tropicamide**

Tropium *see* **Librium**
(DDSA)

Trosyl
(Pfizer)

A solution used as an anti-fungal treatment for infections of the nails.

Dose: apply to the affected areas every 12 hours for 6-12 months.
Availability: NHS and private prescription.
Side effects: mild irritation.
Caution:
Not to be used for: pregnant women.
Not to be used with:
Contains: TIOCONAZOLE.
Other preparations:

---

trypsin *see* **Chymoral Forte**

Tryptizol
(Morson)

A blue tablet, yellow tablet, or brown tablet according to strengths of 10 mg, 25 mg, 50 mg and used as an anti-depressant to treat depression, bed wetting in children.

Dose: adults 75 mg a day in divided doses, increasing if needed to 150 mg a day; children 6-10 years 10-20 mg a day; 11-16 years 25-50 mg a day.
Availability: NHS and private prescription.
Side effects: dry mouth, constipation, urine retention, blurred vision, palpitations, drowsiness, sleeplessness, dizziness, hands shaking, low blood presure, weight change, skin reactions, jaundice or blood changes. Loss of sexual desire may occur.
Caution: in nursing mothers or in patients suffering from heart

disease, thyroid disease, epilepsy, diabetes, some other psychiatric conditions. Your doctor may advise regular blood tests.

Not to be used for: children under 6 years, pregnant women, or for patients suffering from heart attacks, liver disease, heart block.

Not to be used with: alcohol, ANTI-CHOLINERGICS, ADRENALINE, MAOIS, barbiturates, other anti-depressants, anti-hypertensives.

Contains: AMITRIPTYLINE hydrochloride.

Other preparations: Tryptizol Capsules, Tryptizol Syrup, Tryptizol Injection.

---

tryptophan *see* **Optimax, Pacitron**

Tuinal
(Eli LIlly)

An orange/blue capsule used as a barbiturate to treat sleeplessness in patients with barbiturate habit.

Dose: 1-2 tablets before going to bed

Availability: controlled drug.

Side effects: drowsiness, hangover, dizziness, allergies, headache, confusion, excitement.

Caution: in patients suffering from kidney or lung disease. Dependence (addiction) may develop.

Not to be used for: children, young adults, pregnant women, nursing mothers, the elderly, patients with a history of drug or alcohol abuse, or suffering from porphyria (a rare blood disorder), or in the management of pain.

Not to be used with: anti-coagulants (blood-thinning drugs), alcohol, other tranquillizers, steroids, the contraceptive pill, GRISEOFULVIN, RIFAMPICIN, PHENYTOIN, METRONIDAZOLE, CHLORAMPHENICOL.

Contains: QUINALBARBITONE sodium, AMYLOBARBITONE sodium.

Other preparations:

Tylex
(Cilag)

A red/white capsule used as an analgesic to relieve severe pain.

Dose: 1-2 tablets every 4 hours to a maximum of 6 tablets in 24 hours.
Availability: NHS and private prescription.
Side effects: tolerance, addiction, constipation, dizziness, sedation, nausea, dry mouth, blurred vision.
Caution: in the elderly, women in labour, and in patients suffering from underactive thyroid, or kidney or liver disease.
Not to be used for: children, pregnant women, nursing mothers, or for patients suffering from respiratory depression or blocked airways.
Not to be used with: MAOIS, sedatives.
Contains: PARACETAMOL, CODEINE PHOSPHATE.
Other preparations:

tyrothricin *see* **Tyrozets**

Tyrozets
(MSD)

A pink lozenge used as an antibiotic and local anaesthetic to treat mild mouth and throat disorders.

Dose: allow 1 lozenge to dissolve in the mouth every 3 hours to a maximum of 8 lozenges in 24 hours.
Availability: NHS, private prescription, over the counter.
Side effects: additional infection, blackening or soreness of mouth and tongue.
Caution:
Not to be used for:
Not to be used with:
Contains: TYROTHRICIN, BENZOCAINE.
Other preparations:

Ubretid Tablets
(Rorer)

A white, scored tablet supplied at a strength of 5 mg and used as an ANTI-CHOLINESTERASE to treat myasthenia gravis (a muscle disorder), post-operative bladder problems.

Dose: adults myasthenia gravis 1 tablet a day ¹/₂ hour before breakfast at first adjusting every 3-4 days up to 4 tablets a day; children up to 2 tablets a day. Otherwise 1 tablet a day or alternate days.
Availability: NHS and private prescription.
Side effects: nausea, vomiting, colic, diarrhoea, salivation.
Caution: in patients suffering from bronchial asthma, heart disease, peptic ulcer, epilepsy, Parkinson's disease.
Not to be used for: pregnant women, or for patients suffering from bowel or urinary blockage, or with weak circulation or in shock after surgery.
Not to be used with: muscle relaxants, HALOTHANE and CYCLOPROPANE, anaesthetics.
Contains: DISTIGMINE bromide.
Other preparations: Ubretid Injection.

Ultradil
(Schering)

A cream used as a steroid treatment for skin disorders, eczema.

Dose: apply to the affected area 3 times a day at first, then reduce as soon as possible.
Availability: NHS and private prescription.
Side effects: fluid retention, suppression of adrenal glands, thinning of the skin may occur.
Caution: use for short periods of time only.
Not to be used for: patients suffering from acne or any other skin infections caused by tuberculosis, ringworm, viruses, or fungi, or continuously especially in pregnant women.
Not to be used with:
Contains: FLUOCORTOLONE PIVALATE, FLUOCORTOLONE HEXANOATE.
Other preparations: Ultradil Ointment.

Ultralanum Plain Cream
(Schering)

A cream used as a steroid treatment for skin disorders.

Dose: apply to the affected area 2-3 times a day at first reducing to once a day as soon as possible.

Availability: NHS and private prescription.
Side effects: fluid retention, suppression of adrenal glands, thinning of the skin may occur.
Caution: use for short periods of time only.
Not to be used for: patients suffering from acne or any other skin infections caused by tuberculosis, ringworm, viruses, or fungi, or continuously especially in pregnant women.
Not to be used with:
Contains: FLUOCORTOLONE PIVALATE, FLUOCORTOLONE HEXANOATE.
Other preparations: Ultralanum Plain Ointment.

Ultraproct
(Schering)

A suppository supplied at a strength of 1 mg and used as a steroid, local anaesthetic, antihistamine treatment for haemorrhoids, anal fissure, proctitis, anal itch.

Dose: 1-3 times a day after passing motions.
Availability: NHS and private prescription.
Side effects: systemic corticosteroid effects.
Caution: do not use for prolonged periods; care in pregnant women.
Not to be used for: children.
Not to be used with:
Contains: FLUOCORTOLONE PIVALATE, FLUOCORTOLONE HEXANOATE, CINCHOCAINE HYDROCHLORIDE,
Other preparations: Ultraproct ointment

---

undecenoic acid *see* Audicort

Uniflu & Gregovite C
(Unigreg)

A red, oblong tablet and a yellow tablet used as an analgesic, opiate, antussive, xanthine, and antihistamine treatment for cold and flu symptoms.

Dose: 1 each of the tablets every 4 hours up to a maximum of 6 of each tablets in 24 hours.

Availability: private prescription and over the counter.

Side effects: constipation, drowsiness, reduced reactions, anxiety, hands shaking, irregular or rapid heart rate, dry mouth, excitement, rarely skin eruptions.

Caution: in patients suffering from asthma, kidney disease, diabetes.

Not to be used for: children, or for patients suffering from liver disease, heart or thyroid isorders.

Not to be used with: MAOIS, alcohol, sedatives, TRICYCLICS.

Contains: PARACETAMOL, CODEINE PHOSPHATE, CAFFEINE, DIPHENHYDRAMINE HYDROCHLORIDE, PHENYLEPHRINE HYDROCHLORIDE; ASCORBIC ACID.

Other preparations:

Unigest *see* Asilone
(Unigreg)

Unimycin *see* Tetracycline
(Unigreg)

Uniphyllin Continus *see* Theophylline
(Napp)

Uniroid
(Unigreg)

A suppository used as an antibiotic, steroid, local anaesthetic treatment for haemorrhoids, anal fissure, inflammation, anal itch.

Dose: 1 3 times a day after passing motions.

Availability: NHS and private prescription.

Side effects: systemic corticosteroid effects.

Caution: in pregnant women — do not use for prolonged periods.

Not to be used for: children or for patients suffering from tuberculous, fungal, and viral infections.

Not to be used with:

Contains: NEOMYCIN sulphate, POLYMYXIN B SULPHATE, HYDROCORTISONE, CINCHOCAINE HYDROCHLORIDE.
Other preparations: Uniroid ointment.

Unisept
(Seton-Prebbles)

A solution used as a disinfectant and general antiseptic.

Dose: use neat as needed.
Availability: NHS, private prescription, over the counter.
Side effects:
Caution:
Not to be used for:
Not to be used with:
Contains: CHLORHEXIDINE gluconate.
Other preparations:

Unisomnia *see* Mogadon
(Unigreg)

Univer *see* Cordilox
(Rorer)

---

urea hydrogen peroxide *see* Exterol

---

urea *see* Alphaderm, Calmurid HC, Psoradrate, Sential

Uriben *see* Negram
(RP Drugs)

Urisal
(Sterling Research Laboratories)

Orange-flavoured granules in sachets of 4 g used as an alkalizing agent to relieve the pain of cystitis.

Dose: the contents of 1 sachet dissolved in water 3 times a day for 3 days.
Availability: NHS, private prescription, over the counter.
Side effects:
Caution:
Not to be used for: children, pregnant women, or for patients suffering from heart disease, high blood pressure, or with a history of kidney disease.
Not to be used with:
Contains: SODIUM CITRATE.
Other preparations:

Urispas
(Syntex)

A white tablet supplied at a strength of 100 mg and used as an anti-spasmodic treatment for incontinence, abnormally frequent or urgent urination, bed wetting, painful urination.

Dose: 2 tablets 3 times a day.
Availability: NHS and private prescription.
Side effects: headache, nausea, tiredness, diarrhoea, blurred vision, dry mouth.
Caution: in patients suffering from glaucoma.
Not to be used for: children or for patients suffering from obstruction of the urinary or gastro-intestinal tracts.
Not to be used with:
Contains: FLAVOXATE HYDROCHLORIDE.
Other preparations:

Uromide
(Consolidated)

A yellow, capsule-shaped tablet supplied at a strength of 500 mg and

U

used as a sulphonamide/anaesthetic to treat urinary infections.

Dose: adults 2 tablets 3 times a day; children $^1/_2$ -1 tablet 3 times a day.
Availability: NHS and private prescription.
Side effects: anaemia, stomach disturbances, inflammation of the tongue, rash, low white blood cell count if prolonged treatment is given.
Caution: in patients suffering from kidney or liver disease. Your doctor may advise that patients on prolonged treatment should undergo regular blood tests.
Not to be used for: new-born infants or women during the late stages of pregnancy.
Not to be used with: FOLATE ANTAGONISTS (such as TRIMETHOPRIM), anti-diabetics taken by mouth.
Contains: SULPHACARBAMIDE, PHENAZOPYRIDINE HYDROCHLORIDE.
Other preparations:

---

ursodeoxycholic acid *see* Destolit

Ursofalk *see* Destolit
(Thames)

Uticillin
(S K B)

A white, oval tablet supplied at a strength of 500 mg and used as a penicillin to treat infections of the urinary tract.

Dose: adults 1-2 tablets 3 times a day; children 2-10 years 30-60 mg per kg body weight a day in 3 divided doses.
Availability: NHS and private prescription.
Side effects: allergy, stomach disturbances.
Caution: in patients with severe kidney disease.
Not to be used for: infants under 2 years.
Not to be used with:
Contains: CARFECILLIN sodium.
Other preparations:

Utovlan
(Syntex)

A white, scored tablet supplied at a strength of 5 mg and used as a progestogen for postponing menstruation, and to treat premenstrual syndrome, abnormal uterine bleeding, breast cancer, uterine and menstrual disorders.

Dose: normally 1 tablet 3 times a day for 10 days.
Availability: NHS and private prescription.
Side effects: liver disturbances, masculinization.
Caution: in patients suffering from migraine, epilepsy, diabetes.
Not to be used for: children or patients suffering from certain types of breast cancer, liver disease, abnormal vaginal bleeding, a history of thromboembolic disorders.
Not to be used with:
Contains: NORETHISTERONE.
Other preparations:

V-Cil-K
(Eli Lilly)

A white, scored tablet supplied at strengths of 125 mg, 250 mg and used as a penicillin to treat infections.

Dose: adults 125-250 mg every 4-6 hours; children under 1 year 62.5mg every 6 hours, 1-5 years 125 mg every 6 hours, over 5 years 125-250 mg every 6 hours.
Availability: NHS and private prescription.
Side effects: allergy, stomach disturbances.
Caution: in patients suffering from kidney disease.
Not to be used for:
Not to be used with:
Contains: PENICILLIN V POTASSIUM.
Other preparations: V-Cil-K Capsules, V-Cil-K Syrup, V-Cil-K Paediatric Syrup.

Valium
(Roche)

A white tablet, yellow tablet, or blue tablet according to strengths of 2 mg, 5 mg, 10 mg and used as a sedative to treat anxiety, acute alcohol withdrawal, and for the short-term treatment of sleeplessness where sedation during the day is not a difficulty, fear and sleepwalking at night in children, muscle spasm.

Dose: elderly 3-15 mg a day; adults 6-30 mg a day; children 1-5 mg a day.
Availability: NHS (when prescribed as a generic) and private prescription.
Side effects: drowsiness, reduced reactions, .
Caution: in pregnant women, nursing mothers, and in patients suffering from chronic lung weakness, kidney or liver disease. Avoid long-term treament and withdraw gradually.
Not to be used for: patients with acute lung weakness.
Not to be used with: alcohol, sedatives, anti-convulsants.
Contains: DIAZEPAM.
Other preparations: Valium Syrup, Valium Suppositories, Valium Injection. ALUPRAM (Steinhard), SOLIS (Galen), STESOLID (CP Pharmaceuticals), TENSIUM (DDSA)

Vallergan
(M & B)

A blue tablet supplied at a strength of 10 mg and used as an antihistamine treatment for itch, allergy.

Dose: adults 1 tablet 3-4 times a day; children over 2 years $^1/_4$ -$^1/_2$ tablet 3-4 times a day.
Availability: NHS and private prescription.
Side effects: drowsiness, reduced reactions, rash, elation, depression, convulsions on high doses, extrapyramidal reactions (shaking and rigidity), stomach disturbances.
Caution:
Not to be used for: infants under 2 years.
Not to be used with: sedatives, MAOIS, SYMPATHOMIMETICS, alcohol.
Contains: TRIMEPRAZINE tartrate.
Other preparations: Vallergan Syrup, Vallergan Forte Syrup.

Valoid
(Calmic)

A white, scored tablet supplied at a strength of 50 mg and used as an antihistamine treatment for vomiting, nausea, vertigo, labyrinthine disorders.

Dose: adults and children over 10 years 1 tablet 3 times a day; children 1-10 years $^1/_2$ tablet 3 times a day.
Availability: NHS and private prescription.
Side effects: drowsiness, reduced reactions, rarely skin eruptions.
Caution: in patients suffering from liver or kidney disease.
Not to be used for: infants under 1 year.
Not to be used with: alcohol, sedatives, some anti-depressants (MAOIS).
Contains: CYCLIZINE hydrochloride.
Other preparations: Valoid Injection.

Variclene
(Dermal)

A gel used as an antiseptic treatment for skin ulcers.

Dose: apply to the affected area and cover; repeat no later than 7 days after.
Availability: NHS and private prescription.
Side effects:
Caution:
Not to be used for:
Not to be used with:
Contains: BRILLIANT GREEN, LACTIC ACID.
Other preparations:

V

Vascardin
(Nicholas)

A white, scored tablet supplied at a strength of 10 mg, 30 mg and used as a NITRATE treatment for angina, and as an additional treatment for congestive heart failure.

Dose: 10-30 mg 4 times a day increasing according to response. For angina 5-10 mg under the tongue for an acute attack and 30-120 mg in divided doses or as required.

Availability: NHS and private prescription.
Side effects: headache, flushes.
Caution:
Not to be used for: children.
Not to be used with:
Contains: ISOSORBIDE DINITRATE.
Other preparations:

Vasocon-A
(Iolab)

Drops used as an antihistamine, sympathomimetic treatment for allergic conjunctivitis and other eye inflammations.

Dose: adults 1-2 drops into the eye every 3-4 hours; children over 2 years as advised by the physician.
Availability: NHS and private prescription.
Side effects: temporary smarting, headache, sleeplessness, rapid heart rate, drowsiness, congestion.
Caution: in patients suffering from diabetes, coronary disease, high blood pressure, overactive thyroid gland.
Not to be used for: infants under 2 years, patients suffering from glaucoma, or for those who wear soft contact lenses.
Not to be used with:
Contains: ANTAZOLINE phosphate, NAPHOZOLINE hydrochloride.
Other preparations:

Velosef
(Squibb)

A blue/orange capsule or a blue capsule according to strengths of 250 mg, 500 mg and used as a cephalosporin antibiotic to treat infections, and for the prevention of infections in surgery.

Dose: adults 1-2 g a day in 2-4 divided doses up to a maximum of 4 g a day; children 25-50 mg per kg body weight a day in 2-4 divided doses.
Availability: NHS and private prescription.
Side effects: allergy, stomach disturbances thrush, blood changes, change in liver, rise in urea level, positive Coomb's test.

Caution: in patients suffering from kidney disease or who are sensitive to penicillin.
Not to be used for:
Not to be used with: loop DIURETICS, aminoglycoside antibiotics.
Contains: CEPHRADINE.
Other preparations: Velosef Syrup, Velosef Injection.

Ventide
(A & H)

An aerosol supplied at a strength of 100 micrograms and used as a broncho-dilator to treat asthma.

Dose: adults 2 sprays 3-4 times a day; children 1-2 sprays 2-4 times a day.
Availability: NHS and private prescription.
Side effects: hand shaking, nervous tension, headache, hoarseness, thrush, dilation of the blood vessels.
Caution: in pregnant women, and in patients suffering from overactive thyroid gland, heart muscle disease, abnormal heart rhythms, angina, high blood pressure, tuberculosis of the lungs, or in those transferring from systemic steroids.
Not to be used for:
Not to be used with: SYMPATHOMIMETICS.
Contains: SALBUTAMOL, BECLOMETHASONE diproprionate.
Other preparations: Ventide Rotacaps, Ventide Paediatric Rotacaps.

V

Ventodisks
(A & H)

A pale-blue disc or a dark-blue disc according to strengths of 200 micrograms, 400 micrograms. and used as a broncho-dilator to treat bronchial spasm brought on by bronchial asthma, bronchitis, emphysema.

Dose: adults 200-400 micrograms as a single dose or 400 micrograms 3-4 times a day; children 200 micrograms or 200 micrograms 3-4 times a day.
Availability: NHS and private prescription.

Side effects: hand shaking, nervous tension, headache, dilation of the blood vessels.
Caution: in pregnant women and in patients suffering from high blood pressure, abnormal heart rhythms, angina, overactive thyroid gland, heart muscle disease.
Not to be used for:
Not to be used with: SYMPATHOMIMETICS.
Contains: SALBUTAMOL sulphate.
Other preparations:

Ventolin
(A & H)

A pink tablet supplied at strengths of 2 mg, 4 mg and used as a broncho-dilator to treat premature labour, bronchial spasm brought on by bronchial asthma, chronic bronchitis, emphysema

Dose: adults 2-4 mg 3-4 times a day; children 2-6 years 1-2 mg 3-4 times a day, 6-12 years 2 mg 3-4 times a day.
Availability: NHS and private prescription.
Side effects: rapid heart rate, anxiety, rise in blood sugar level, shaking of the hands, nervous tension, dilation of the blood vessels, headache.
Caution: in patients suffering from thyrotoxicosis or cardiovascular disease. Heart rate of mother and foetus should be monitored carefully when used for treatment of premature labour.
Not to be used for: children under 2 years, or for patients suffering from antepartum haemorrhage, toxaemia of pregnancy, cord compression, threatened abortion, or conditions where prolonging the pregnancy may be dangerous.
Not to be used with: ß-BLOCKERS, other ß-agonists, SYMPATHOMIMETICS.
Contains: SALBUTAMOL sulphate.
Other preparations: Ventolin Infusion, Ventolin Inhaler, Ventolin Spandets, Ventolin Rotacaps, Ventolin Injection, Ventolin Infusion, Ventolin Respirator, Ventolin Nebules. VOLMAX (Duncan, Flockhart), AEROLIN AUTO (3M Riker).

Veractil
(M & B)

A white, scored tablet supplied at a strength of 25 mg and used as a sedative to treat schizophrenia, and manic depression especially where sedation is needed.

Dose: 1 tablet at night increasing gradually as advised.
Availability: NHS and private prescription.
Side effects: muscle spasms, restlessness, hands shaking, dry mouth, urine retention, palpitations, low blood pressure, weight gain, changes in libido, low body temperature, breast swelling, menstrual changes, jaundice, blood and skin changes, drowsiness, rarely fits.
Caution: in pregnant women, nursing mothers, and in patients suffering from epilepsy, liver disease, cardiovascular disease, Parkinson's disease.
Not to be used for: children, the elderly, patients in unconscious states, or patients suffering from bone marrow depression
Not to be used with: alcohol, tranquillizers, pain killers, anti-hypertensives, anti-depressants, anti-convulsants, anti-diabetic drugs, LEVODOPA.
Contains: METHOTRIMEPRAZINE.
Other preparations:

Veracur
(Typharm)

V

A gel used as a skin softener to treat warts.

Dose: apply to the wart twice a day and cover, rubbing down with a pumice stone between treatments.
Availability: NHS, private prescription, over the counter.
Side effects:
Caution: do not apply to healthy skin.
Not to be used for: warts on the face or anal and genital areas.
Not to be used with:
Contains: FORMALDEHYDE.
Other preparations:

---

verapamil *see* **Cordilox, Cordilox 160, Glauline, Securon, Securon SR**

Verdiviton
(Squibb)

A liquid used as a vitamin B complex for maintaining vitamin B complex levels.

Dose: 3 5 ml teaspoonsful 3 times a day before food.
Availability: private prescription and over the counter.
Side effects:
Caution:
Not to be used for: children or for patients suffering from hepatitis, alcoholism.
Not to be used with: levodopa.
Contains: GLYCEROPHOSPHATES OF CALCIUM, SODIUM, POTASSIUM, AND MANGANESE, CYANOCOBALAMIN, D-PANTHENOL, NICOTINAMIDE, PYRIDOXINE, RIBOFLAVINE, THIAMINE, alcohol.
Other preparations:

Vermox
(Janssen)

A suspension used as a vermicide to treat worms.

Dose: adults and children over 2 years 1 5 ml teaspoonful morning and evening for 3 days or 1 5 ml teaspoonful repeated after 2-3 weeks according to the type of infestation.
Availability: NHS and private prescription.
Side effects: stomach upset.
Caution:
Not to be used for: children under 2 years or pregnant women.
Not to be used with:
Contains: MEBENDAZOLE.
Other preparations: Vermox Tablets.

Verrugon
(Pickles)

An ointment with corn rings and plasters used as a skin softener to treat warts.

Dose: protect healthy skin, apply the ointment to the wart, and cover

with a plaster, rubbing down with a pumice stone between treatments.
Availability: NHS, private prescription, over the counter.
Side effects:
Caution: do not apply to healthy skin.
Not to be used for: warts on the face or anal and genital areas.
Not to be used with:
Contains: SALICYLIC ACID.
Other preparations:

Vertigon Spansule *see* Stemetil
(S K B)

Verucasep
(Galen)

A gel used as a virucidal, anhidrotic treatment for viral warts.

Dose: apply twice a day, paring down any hard skin around the wart.
Availability: NHS, private prescription, over the counter.
Side effects: stains the skin.
Caution: do not apply to healthy skin.
Not to be used for: warts on the face or anal and genital areas.
Not to be used with:
Contains: GLUTARALDEHYDE.
Other preparations:

V

Vibramycin
(Pfizer)

A green capsule supplied at a strength of 100 mg and used as a tetracycline treatment for pneumonia, respiratory, stomach, soft tissue, eye, and urinary infections.

Dose: adults 2 capsules with food or drink on the first day then 1 capsule a day; children 4 mg per kg body weight with food or drink on the first day then 2 mg per kg body weight a day.
Availability: NHS and private prescription.
Side effects: stomach disturbances, allergy, additional infections,

discoloured teeth, other tooth changes, reduced rate of growth of one of the lower leg bones.

Caution: in patients suffering from liver disease.

Not to be used for: children under 8 years, nursing mothers, women in the last half of pregnancy, or even for pregnant women at all unless no other treatment is possible.

Not to be used with: antacids, mineral supplements.

Contains: DOXYCYCLINE hydrochloride.

Other preparations: NORDOX (Panpharma).

Vibramycin 50
(Pfizer)

A green/cream capsule supplied at a strength of 50 mg and used as an antibiotic treatment for acne.

Dose: 1 capsule a day with food or drink for 6-12 weeks.

Availability: NHS and private prescription.

Side effects: stomach disturbances, allergies.

Caution: in patients suffering from liver disease.

Not to be used for: nursing mothers or women in the last half of pregnancy.

Not to be used with: antacids, mineral supplements.

Contains: DOXYCYCLINE hydrochloride.

Other preparations:

V

Vibrocil
(Zyma)

A spray, drops, or gel used as an antihistamine, antibiotic, SYMPATHOMIMETIC treatment for rhinitis, hay fever, sinusitis.

Dose: adults 3 sprays, 3-4 drops, or a little gel into each nostril 3-4 times a day; children under 6 years 1-2 drops or a little gel into each nostril 3-4 times a day, 6-12 years 3-4 drops or a little gel into each nostril 3-4 times a day.

Availability: NHS and private prescription.

Side effects:

Caution: in patients suffering from cardiovascular disease, high blood pressure overactive thyroid gland. Do not use for extended

periods.
Not to be used for:
Not to be used with: MAOIS.
Contains: DIMETHINDENE maleate, PHENYLEPHRINE, NEOMYCIN sulphate.
Other preparations:

Videne Powder
(3M Riker)

A powder used as an antiseptic treatment for infections in wounds and burns.

Dose: dust the affected area lightly with the powder.
Availability: NHS, private prescription, over the counter.
Side effects:
Caution:
Not to be used for:
Not to be used with:
Contains: POVIDONE-IODINE.
Other preparations: Videne Solution, Videne Tincture, Videne Surgical Scrub.

---

viderabine *see* Vira-A

Vidopen
(Berk)

A pink/red capsule supplied at a strength of 250 mg, 500 mg and used as a penicillin to treat respiratory, eye, nose, and throat, soft tissue, and urinary infections.

Dose: adults and children over 20 kg body weight 250 mg-1 g 4 times a day; children under 20 kg body weight 200 mg per kg a day in divided doses.
Availability: NHS and private prescription.
Side effects: allergy, stomach disturbances.
Caution: in patients suffering from kidney disease or glandular fever.
Not to be used for:

Not to be used with:
Contains: AMPICILLIN trihydrate.
Other preparations: Vidopen Syrup.

Villescon
(Boehringer Ingelheim)

An orange tablet used as a tonic.

Dose: adults 1 tablet after breakfast and 1 tablet before 4 pm each day for 1-2 weeks; children 5-8 years use liquid; 8-12 years 1 tablet a day.
Availability: private prescription only.
Side effects: rapid heart rate, nausea, colic, sleeplessness.
Caution:
Not to be used for: children under 5 years or for patients suffering from thyrotoxicosis, epilepsy.
Not to be used with: MAOIS, LEVODOPA.
Contains: PROLINTANE hydrochloride, THIAMINE mononitrate, RIBOFLAVINE, PYRIDOXINE hydrochloride, NICOTINAMIDE, ASCORBIC ACID.
Other preparations: Villescon Liquid.

V **viloxazine hydrochloride** *see* **Vivalan**

Vioform-Hydrocortisone
(Zyma)

A cream used as a steroid, anti-bacterial, anti-fungal treatment for skin disorders, infected skin in the anal and genital areas.

Dose: apply to the affected area 1-3 times a day.
Availability: NHS and private prescription.
Side effects: fluid retention, suppression of adrenal glands, thinning of the skin may occur.
Caution: use for short periods of time only.
Not to be used for: patients suffering from acne or any other skin infections caused by tuberculosis, ringworm, viruses, or fungi, or continuously especially in pregnant women.
Not to be used with:

Contains: CLIOQUINOL, HYDROCORTISONE.
Other preparations: Vioform-Hydrocortisone Ointment.

Vira-A
(Parke-Davis)

An ointment used as an anti-viral treatment for herpes keratoconjunctivitis.

Dose: insert 1 cm length of ointment in to the corner of the eye 5 times a day until it is healed and then twice a day for another 7 days.
Availability: NHS and private prescription.
Side effects: irritation, corneal inflammation, pain, fear of light, punctal occlusion.
Caution:
Not to be used for: children.
Not to be used with:
Contains: VIDARABINE.
Other preparations:

Virudox
(Bioglan)

A transparent, colourless solution used as an anti-viral treatment for herpes, shingles.

Dose: apply 4 times a day for 4 days within 2-3 days of the appearance of the rash.
Availability: NHS and private prescription.
Side effects: local stinging, taste change.
Caution: keep away from eyes, mucous membranes, and clothing.
Not to be used for: children, pregnant women, nursing mothers.
Not to be used with:
Contains: IDOXURIDINE, DIMETHYL SULPHOXIDE.
Other preparations:

V

Visclair
(Sinclair)

A yellow tablet supplied at a strength of 100 mg and used as a mucus softener to treat bronchitis, phlegm.

Dose: adults 2 tablets 3-4 times a day for 6 weeks then 2 tablets twice a day; children over 5 years 1 tablet 3 times a day.

Availability: private prescription and over the counter.

Side effects: stomach upset.

Caution:

Not to be used for: children under 5 years.

Not to be used with:

Contains: METHYLCYSTEINE HYDROCHLORIDE.

Other preparations:

Viskaldix
(Sandoz)

A white, scored tablet used as a ß-BLOCKER to treat high blood pressure.

Dose: 1 tablet in the morning at first, then increase to 2-3 tablets a day after 2-3 weeks.

Availability: NHS and private prescription.

Side effects: cold hands and feet, sleep disturbance, slow heart rate, tiredness, wheezing, heart failure, stomach upset.

Caution: in pregnant women, nursing mothers, and in patients suffering from diabetes, kidney or liver disorders, asthma. May need to be withdrawn before surgery. Withdraw gradually. Your doctor may advise additional treatment with DIURETICS or digitalis.

Not to be used for: children or for patients suffering from heart block or failure.

Not to be used with: VERAPAMIL, CLONIDINE withdrawal, some anti-arrhythmic drugs and anaesthetics, RESERPINE, some anti-hypertensives, ergot alkaloids, CIMETIDINE, sedatives, SYMPATHOMIMETICS, INDOMETHACIN.

Contains: PINDOLOL, CLOPAMIDE.

Other preparations:

Visken
(Sandoz)

A white, scored tablet supplied at stregths of 5 mg, 15 mg and used as a ß-BLOCKER to treat angina, high blood pressure.

Dose: 2.5-5 mg up to 3 times a day. High blood pressure 10-15 mg a day at first increasing if needed at weekly intervals to 45 mg a day.
Availability: NHS and private prescription.
Side effects: cold hands and feet, sleep disturbance, slow heart rate, tiredness, wheezing, heart failure, stomach upset.
Caution: in pregnant women, nursing mothers, and in patients suffering from diabetes, kidney or liver disorders, asthma. May need to be withdrawn before surgery. Withdraw gradually. Your doctor may advise additional treatment with DIURETICS or DIGITALIS.
Not to be used for: children or for patients suffering from heart block or failure.
Not to be used with: VERAPAMIL, CLONIDINE withdrawal, some anti-arrhythmic drugs and anaesthetics, RESERPINE, some anti-hypertensives, ergot alkaloids, CIMETIDINE, sedatives, SYMPATHOMIMETICS, IN-DOMETHACIN.
Contains: PINDOLOL.
Other preparations:

Vista-Methasone
(Daniel)

Drops used as a corticosteroid treatment for inflammation of the nasal passages or eyes where there is no infection present, infected inflammation of the ear.

V

Dose: 2-3 drops into each nostril twice a day, 2-3 drops into the ear every 3-4 hours, or 1-2 drops into the eye every 2 hours at first then as needed.
Availability: NHS and private prescription.
Side effects: additional infection, rise in eye pressure, thinning of the cornea, fungal infection, cataract.
Caution: in infants and pregnant women — avoid using over extended periods.
Not to be used for: patients suffering from viral, fungal, or tubercular infections of the nose, perforated ear drum.
Not to be used with:
Contains: BETAMETHASONE sodium phosphate.
Other preparations: Vista-Methasone N.

Vita-E
(Bioglan)

An ointment used as an anti-oxidant to treat wounds, bed sores, burns, skin ulcers.

Dose: apply to the affected area as needed.
Availability: NHS, private prescription, over the counter.
Side effects:
Caution:
Not to be used for: patients suffering from overactive thyroid gland.
Not to be used with: fish liver oils, DIGITALIS, INSULIN.
Contains: D-ALPHA-TOCOPHERYL ACETATE.
Other preparations:

---

vitamin A *see* **Concavit, Ketovite, Halycitrol, Multivite, Octovit, Orovite 7, Polyvite, Ro-A-Vit, Tonivitan, Tonivitan A & D**

---

vitamin C (ascorbic acid) *see* **Abidec, Allbee with C, BC 500, BC 500 with Iron, Concavit, Dalivit Drops, Fefol-Vit Spansule, Ferrograd C, Fesovit Spansule, Fesovit 2 Spansule, Galfervit, Givitol, Irofol C, Lipoflavonoid, Multivite, Octovit, Optimax, Oralcer, Orovite, Orovite 7, Polyvite, Pregnavite Forte F, Redoxon, Surbex T, Tonivitan, Uniflu & Gregovite C, Villescon.**

---

vitamin D *see* **Halycitrol, Ketovite**

---

vitamin E *see* **Concavit**

Vivalan
(ICI)

A yellow tablet supplied at a strength of 50 mg and used as an antidedpressant to treat depression, especially in patients for whom sedation is not required.

Dose: adults usually 6 tablets a day in divided doses up to a maximum of 8 tablets a day; elderly 2 tablets a day at first.
Availability: NHS and private prescription.
Side effects: nausea, headache, impaired reactions, anti-cholinergic effects, jaundice, convulsions.
Caution: in pregnant women and in patients with suicidal tendencies, or suffering from heart disease including congestive heart failure, heart block, epilepsy.
Not to be used for: children, nursing mothers, or patients suffering from mania, severe liver disease, history of peptic ulcer, recent heart attack.
Not to be used with: MAOIS, alpha blockers, CLONIDINE, PHENYTOIN, LEVODOPA, sedatives.
Contains: VILOXAZINE hydrochloride.
Other preparations:

Volital
(LAB)

A white, scored tablet supplied at a strength of 20 mg and used as a brain stimulant to treat movement disorders in children.

Dose: children 6-12 years $1/2$ -1 tablet twice a day in the morning and afternoon.
Availability: NHS and private prescription.
Side effects: dizziness, sweating, palpitations, headache.
Caution:
Not to be used for: children under 6 years or for adults.
Not to be used with: MAOIS.
Contains: PEMOLINE.
Other preparations:

Volmax *see* Ventolin
(Duncan, Flockhart)

Voltarol
(Geigy)

A yellow tablet or brown tablet according to strengths of 25 mg, 50 mg and used as a NON-STEROID ANTI-INFLAMMATORY DRUG to treat bone or muscular problems, rheumatoid arthritis, osteoarthritis, ankylosing spondylitis, acute gout, chronic juvenile arthritis.

Dose: adults 75-150 mg a day in 2-3 divided doses; children 1-3 mg per kg body weight a day in divided doses.
Availability: NHS and private prescription.
Side effects: passing stomach pain, nausea, headache, rash, fluid retention, rarely blood changes, stomach bleeding, abnormal liver or kidney function.
Caution: in pregnant women, nursing mothers, the elderly, or patients suffering from kidney, liver, or heart weakness, recent proctitis, blood abnormalities, history of gastro-intestinal lesions. Your doctor may advise regular check-ups.
Not to be used for: patients suffering from asthma, peptic ulcer, or allergy to aspirin/non-steroid anti-inflammatory drugs.
Not to be used with: SALICYLATES, METHOTREXATE, LITHIUM, DIGOXIN, DIURETICS.
Contains: DICLOFENAC sodium.
Other preparations: Voltarol Retard, Voltarol Suppositories. RHUMAL-GAN (Lagap).

W

warfarin *see* Marevan

Warticon
(Cph)

A solution with applicators used as a cell softener and remover to treat warts on the penis.

Dose: apply twice a day for 3 days and repeat after 7 days if needed.
Availability: NHS and private prescription.
Side effects: irritation.
Caution:
Not to be used for: children.
Not to be used with:

Contains: PODOPHYLLOTOXIN.
Other preparations:

Waxsol
(Norgine)

Drops used as a wax softener to remove ear wax.

Dose: fill the ear with the solution for 2 nights before they are to be syringed.
Availability: NHS, private prescription,over the counter.
Side effects: temporary irritation.
Caution:
Not to be used for: patients suffering from inflammation of the ear or perforated ear drum.
Not to be used with:
Contains: sodium DOCUSATE.
Other preparations:

Welldorm
(SNP)

A purple, oval tablet supplied at a strength of 650 mg and used as a sedative-hypnotic to treat sleeplessness or to sedate children when elixir is used.

Dose: 2-3 tablets before going to bed.
Availability: NHS and private prescription.
Side effects: nausea, vomiting, headache, rash, rarely blood changes.
Caution: in nursing mothers.
Not to be used for: patients suffering from acute intermittent porphyria (a rare blood disorder), severe kidney, liver, or heart disease, gastric inflammation.
Not to be used with: alcohol, sedatives, anti-coagulants
Contains: DICHLORALPHENAZONE.
Other preparations:

X

---

xamoterol *see* **Corwin**

Xanax
(Upjohn)

A white, oval, scored tablet or a pink, oval, scored tablet according to strengths of 0.25 mg, 0.5 mg and used as a sedative for the short-term treatment of anxiety and depression.

Dose: elderly 0.25 mg 2-3 times a day; adults 0.25-0.5 mg 3 times a day to a maximum of 3 mg a day.
Availability: private prescription only.
Side effects: drowsiness, confusion, unsteadiness, low blood pressure, rash, changes in vision, changes in libido, retention of urine. Risk of addiction increases with dose and length of treatment. May impair judgement.
Caution: in the elderly, pregnant women, nursing mothers, in women during labour, and in patients suffering from lung disorders, kidney or liver disorders. Avoid long-term use and withdraw gradually.
Not to be used for: children, or for patients suffering from acute lung diseases, some chronic lung diseases, some obsessional and psychotic diseases.
Not to be used with: alcohol, other tranquillizers, anti-convulsants.
Contains: ALPRAZOLAM.
Other preparations:

---

xipamide *see* Diurexan

---

xylometazoline hydrochloride *see* Otrivine, Otrivine-Antistin (Ciba), Otrivine-Antistin (Zyma)

Xyloproct
(Astra)

A suppository used as a local anaesthetic and steroid treatment for haemorrhoids, anal itch, anal fissure and fistula.

Dose: 1 at night and after passing motions.
Availability: NHS and private prescription.
Side effects: systemic corticosteroid effects.

Caution: do not use for prolonged periods; care in pregnant women.
Not to be used for: patients suffering from tuberculous, fungal, or viral infections
Not to be used with:
Contains: LIGNOCAINE, ALUMINIUM ACETATE, ZINC OXIDE, HYDROCORTISONE acetate.
Other preparations: Xyloproct ointment.

Yomesan
(Bayer)

A yellow tablet supplied at a strength of 500 mg

and used to treat tapeworm.
Dose: as advised by the physician.
Availability: NHS, private prescription, over the counter.
Side effects: stomach upset, lightheadedness, itch.
Caution:
Not to be used for:
Not to be used with: alcohol.
Contains: NICLOSAMIDE.
Other preparations:

Yutopar
(Duphar)

A buff, scored tablet supplied at a strength of 10 mg and used as a ß-agonist to treat premature labour, foetal asphyxiation in labour.

Dose: 1 tablet about 30 minutes before ending intravenous treatment, 1 tablet every 2 hours for 24 hours, and then 1-2 tablets every 4-6 hours.
Availability: NHS and private prescription.
Side effects: rapid heart rate, anxiety, rise in blood sugar level.
Caution: in patients suffering from diabetes, cardiovascular disease, or maternal thyrotoxicosis. The heart rate of mother and foetus should be checked carefully.
Not to be used for: children or for patients suffering from antepartum bleeding, toxaemia of pregnancy, cord compression, threatened abortion, or where prolonging the pregnancy might be dangerous.

Y

Not to be used with: MAOIS, ß-BLOCKERS, other ß-agonists.
Contains: RITODRINE hydrochloride.
Other preparations: Yutopar Injection.

Z Span Spansule
(S K B)

A blue/clear capsule used as a zinc supplement for the prevention and treatment of zinc deficiency.

Dose: adults and children over 1 year 1 capsule 1-3 times a day.
Availability: NHS, private prescription, over the counter.
Side effects: stomach upset.
Caution: in patients suffering from kidney failure.
Not to be used for: infants under 1 year.
Not to be used with: TETRACYCLINES.
Contains: ZINC SULPHATE MONOHYDRATE.
Other preparations:

Zaditen
(Sandoz)

A white, scored tablet supplied at a strength of 1 mg and used as an antihistamine preparation for the prevention of bronchial asthma, and the treatment of allergic rhinitis, conjunctivitis.

Dose: adults 1-2 tablets twice a day with food; children over 2 years 1 tablet twice a day with food.
Availability: NHS and private prescription.
Side effects: drowsiness, reduced reactions, dizziness, dry mouth.
Caution:
Not to be used for: children under 2 years.
Not to be used with: alcohol, sedatives, anti-diabetics taken by mouth.
Contains: KETOTIFEN.
Other preparations: Zaditen Capsules, Zaditen Elixir.

Z

Zadstat *see* Flagyl
(Lederle)

Zantac
(Glaxo)

A white tablet supplied at strengths of 150 mg, 300 mg and used as an H_2 blocker to treat duodenal and gastric ulcers, oesophagitis, dyspepsia, reduction of gastric acid.

Dose: children over 8 years up to 150 mg twice a day, adults 150 mg twice a day or 300 mg at bedtime for 28 days, 150 mg at bedtime thereafter.
Availability: NHS and private prescription.
Side effects: headache, dizziness, occasionally hepatitis, low platelet counts, low white blood cell counts, allergy, confusion, breast symptoms.
Caution: exclude malignant disease. Care in pregnant women, nursing mothers, and in patients suffering from impaired kidney function.
Not to be used for:
Not to be used with:
Contains: RANITIDINE.
Other preparations: Zantac dispensible, Zantac syrup, Zantac injection.

Zarontin
(Parke-Davis)

An orange capsule supplied at a strength of 250 mg and used as an anti-convulsant to treat epilepsy.

Dose: adults and children over 6 years 2 tablets a day increasing as needed by 1 tablet a day every 4-7 days up to 8 tablets a day; children under 6 years 1 tablet a day at first increasing according to response.
Availability: NHS and private prescription.
Side effects: stomach and brain disturbances, rash, blood changes, SLE (a multisystem disorder).
Caution: in pregnant women, nursing mothers, and in patients suffering from kidney or liver disease. Dose should be decreased gradually.
Not to be used for:
Not to be used with:
Contains: ETHOSUXIMIDE.
Other preparations: Zarontin Syrup.

Z

Zestril
(ICI)

A white, pink, or red tablet according to strengths of 2.5 mg, 5 mg, 10 mg, 20 mg and used as an ACE INHIBITOR to treat congestive heart failure in addition to DIURETICS and DIGITALIS, high blood pressure.

Dose: 2.5 mg once a day at first increasing over 2-4 weeks to 5-20 mg once a day.
Availability: NHS and private prescription.
Side effects: low blood pressure, kidney failure, rash, dizziness,diarrhoea, cough, tiredness, palpitations, chest pain, weakness.
Caution: in nursing mothers and in patients suffering from kidney disease.
Not to be used for: children, pregnant women, or for patients suffering from some heart diseases.
Not to be used with: DIURETICS, potassium supplements, INDOMETHACIN.
Contains: LISINOPRIL.
Other preparations:

---

zidovudine *see* Retrovir

Zinamide
(MSD)

A white, scored tablet supplied at a strength of 500 mg and used as an anti-tubercular drug in the additional treatment for tuberculosis.

Dose: 20-35 mg per kg body weight to a maximum of 3 g a day in divided doses.
Availability: NHS and private prescription.
Side effects: hepatitis.
Caution: in patients with a history of gout or diabetes. Your doctor may advise that liver function and blood should be checked regularly.
Not to be used for: children or for patients suffering from liver disease.
Not to be used with:
Contains: PYRAZINAMIDE.
Other preparations:

Z

zinc bacitracin *see* **hydroderm**

---

zinc naphthenate *see* **Tineafax**

---

zinc oxide *see* **Anugesic-HC, Anusol HC, Mutilind, Xyloproct**

---

zinc sulphate monohydrate *see* **Fefol Z Spansule, Fesovit Z Spansule, Octovit, Solvazinc, Z Span Spansule**

---

zinc undecenoate *see* **Tineafax**

Zinnat
(Glaxo)

A white tablet supplied at strengths of 125 mg, 250 mg and used as a cephalosporin antibiotic to treat respiratory, ear, nose, and throat, skin, soft tissue, and urinary infections.

Dose: adults usually 250 mg twice a day, urinary infections 125 mg twice a day, gonorrhoea 1 g as one dose; children over 5 years usually 125 mg twice a day.
Availability: NHS and private prescription.
Side effects: stomach disturbances, allergy, colitis, blood changes, thrush, change in liver chemistry, positive Coomb's test.
Caution: in pregnant women, nursing mothers, and in patients who are sensitive to penicillin.
Not to be used for:
Not to be used with:
Contains: CEFUROXIME AXETIL.
Other preparations:

Z

Zirtek
(A & H)

A white, oblong, scored tablet supplied at a strength of 10 mg and used as an antihistamine treatment for rhinitis, allergy.

Dose: 1 tablet a day in the morning.
Availability: NHS and private prescription
Side effects: drowsiness, dizziness, headache, agitation, stomach disturbances, dry mouth.
Caution: in pregnant women and in patients suffering from kidney disease.
Not to be used for: children, nursing mothers.
Not to be used with: sedatives, alcohol.
Contains: CETIRIZINE DIHYDROCHLORIDE.
Other preparations:

Zocor
(MSD)

A peach-coloured, oval tablet or a tan, oval tablet according to strengths of 10 mg, 20 mg and used as a lipid-lowering agent to treat raised cholesterol.

Dose: 10-40 mg taken at night.
Availability: NHS and private prescription.
Side effects: headache, indigestion, diarrhoea, tiredness, rash, constipation, wind nausea.
Caution: in patients suffering from liver disease. Your doctor may advise liver and eye checks.
Not to be used for: pregnant women, nursing mothers, or for patients suffering from liver disease.
Not to be used with: DIGOXIN, some anti-coagulants.
Contains: SIMVASTATIN.
Other preparations:

Z Zovirax
(Wellcome)

A blue, shield-shaped tablet supplied at strengths of 200 mg, 400 mg, 800 mg and used as an anti-viral treatment for genital herpes, other skin herpes, shingles.

Dose: adults shingles1 800 mg tablet 5 times a day every 4 hours for 7 days; other herpes infections 200 mg 5 times a day for 5 days; reduced doses for prevention or in children.
Availability: NHS and private prescription.
Side effects: irritation (local use).
Caution: in patients suffering from kidney damage; drink plenty of fluids.
Not to be used for:
Not to be used with: PROBENECID.
Contains: ACYCLOVIR.
Other preparations: Zovirax Suspension, Zovirax Cream, Zovirax Infusion.

Zovirax Ointment
(Wellcome)

An ointment used as an anti-viral treatment for herpes simplex infection of the cornea.

Dose: insert 1 cm length of ointment into the corner of the eye 5 times a day every 4 hours for at least 3 days after healing.
Availability: NHS and private prescription.
Side effects: mild smarting, superficial punctate inflammation of the cornea.
Caution:
Not to be used for:
Not to be used with:
Contains: ACYCLOVIR.
Other preparations:

zuclopenthixol *see* Clopixol

Zyloric
(Calmic)

A white tablet supplied at a strength of 100 mg, 300 mg and used as an enzyme blocker to treat gout, and for the prevention of uric acid and calcium oxalate stones.

Dose: 100-300 mg a day at first, then 200-600 mg a day.
Availability: NHS and private prescription.
Side effects: skin reactions, nausea, acute gout.
Caution: in pregnant women, the elderly, and in patients suffering from kidney or liver disease. Be sure to drink plenty of fluids.
Not to be used for: children or for patients suffering from acute gout.
Not to be used with: anti-coagulants, CHLORPROPAMIDE, MERCAPTO-PURINE, AZATHIOPRINE.
Contains: allopurinol.
Other preparations: ALORAL (Lagap), ALULINE (Steinhard), CAPLENAL (Berk), COSURIC (DDSA), HAMARIN (Nicholas).

Z

For each of the medicines described in detail in this book, there is a paragraph headed 'Not to be used with'. This paragraph includes other medicines, groups of medicines, substances such as alcohol, or even foods which should not be taken at the same time as the drug described. This is because the medicine may interact with one or more of the substances mentioned in an unpleasant, harmful, or potentially dangerous way. On the other hand, for an individual patient, there may be no serious interaction at all.

The purpose of the chart set out below is to depict, using a simple and familiar technique, whether or not major 'families' of medicines have been found to interact with one another in any way. It does not attempt to show the degree of interaction. To work out whether or not a medicine you have been prescribed is likely to interact with any other substance, just pick out the family to which it belongs in the vertical column, and trace it horizontally across the chart. Where a '●' occurs, trace down the chart and you will find the name of the substance with which it may interact.

For detailed information concerning interactions, you should, of course, refer to the 'Not to be used with' paragraph for the particular medicine you have been prescribed.

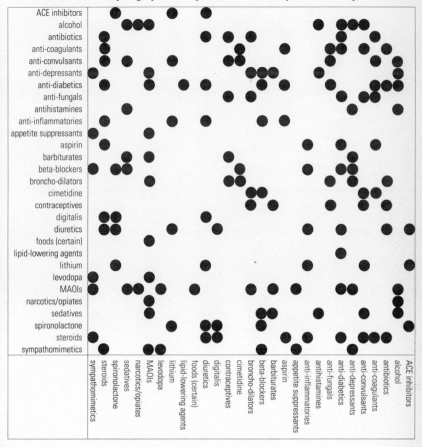